Second Edition

Handbook of Clinical Psychopharmacology

Edited by

Joe P. Tupin, M.D.
Richard I. Shader, M.D.
David S. Harnett, M.D.

Jason Aronson Inc., Northvale, New Jersey, London

Copyright © 1988 by Jason Aronson Inc.

10 9 8 7 6 5 4 3 2 1

All rights reserved. Printed in the United States of America. No part of this book may be used or reproduced in any manner whatsoever without written permission from *Jason Aronson Inc.* except in the case of brief quotations in reviews for inclusion in a magazine, newspaper, or broadcast.

The publisher gratefully acknowledges the following permissions from:

C.V. Mosby Company to use charts in chapter 17.
British Journal of Psychiatry to use figure in chapter 14.
American Psychiatric Association to use table in chapter 6.
American Journal of Psychiatry to use table in chapter 8.
Journal of Clinical Psychiatry to use table in chapter 10.
Journal of Clinical Psychopharmacology to use table in chapter 3.

Library of Congress Cataloging-in-Publication Data

Handbook of clinical psychopharmacology.
    Second ed. of: Clinical handbook of psychopharmacology
edited by Alberto DiMascio and Richard I. Shader. [1970]
    Includes bibliographies and index.

    1. Psychopharmacology—Handbooks, manuals, etc.
I. Tupin, Joe P., 1934–   . II. Shader, Richard I.,
1935–   . III. Harnett, David S. IV. Clinical handbook of psychopharmacology. [DNLM: 1. Psychopharmacology.
2. Psychotropic Drugs. QV 77 H2356]
RM315.H343 1988   616.89'18   7   87-33442
ISBN 0-87668-997-7

Manufactured in the United States of America.

Contents

Foreword — vii
Preface — ix

1 Psychosis
Joseph R. Magliozzi, M.D.,
and *Charles B. Schaffer*, M.D. — 1

2 Depressive Disorders
Alan F. Schatzberg, M.D. — 49

3 Stress, Fear, and Anxiety
Richard I. Shader, M.D. — 73

4 Mania
David L. Dunner, M.D. — 97

5	**Violence**	
	Joe P. Tupin, M.D.	111
6	**Substance Abuse**	
	Domenic A. Ciraulo, M.D., and *Ann Marie Ciraulo*, R.N.	121
7	**Memory Disturbance and Cognitive Impairment in the Elderly**	
	Patricia I. Rosebush, M.D. and *Carl Salzman*, M.D.	159
8	**Child Psychiatry Problems**	
	Barbara J. Coffey, M.D.	211
9	**Eating Disorders**	
	Harrison G. Pope, Jr., M.D., and *James I. Hudson*, M.D.	245
10	**Treatment-Resistant Problems**	
	David N. Osser, M.D.	269
11	**Atypical Depression**	
	Ronald W. Pies, M.D.	329

Contents

12 Attention Deficit Disorder, Residual Type (ADD, RT) or Adult Hyperactivity

Paul H. Wender, M.D.   **357**

13 Drug Combinations and Interactions

Charles B. Schaffer, M.D., *Patrick T. Donlon*, M.D., and *Linda C. Schaffer*, M.D.   **375**

14 Psychotherapy and Psychopharmacology

David S. Harnett, M.D.   **401**

15 Rational Use of Serum Drug Concentration Monitoring

H. Friedman, M.D., and *David J. Greenblatt*, M.D.   **425**

16 Liability Issues and Malpractice Prevention

Thomas G. Gutheil, M.D.   **439**

17 Glossary of Pharmacological Terms

Joseph R. Magliozzi, M.D., and *Joe P. Tupin*, M.D.   **455**

Index   **467**

Foreword

This volume, the second edition of the *Handbook of Clinical Psychopharmacology*, is dedicated to the memory and contributions of Alberto DiMascio, Ph.D. (1928-1978). Published in the tenth year after his death, this edition deals with his concerns about clinical psychopharmacology. Al wanted to be sure that clinicians in the field were kept up-to-date on new developments and changing practices in clinical care. The first edition grew out of a statewide lecture series for mental health professionals in public sector hospitals and outpatient programs that he and I developed.

Al became a professor of psychiatry (psychopharmacology) at Tufts University School of Medicine. Unfortunately, his untimely death occurred the year before I, too, moved to Tufts. To honor his memory and his commitment to teaching, the American College of Neuropsychopharmacology in 1980 established the Alberto DiMascio Memorial Lecture series to be given annually at Tufts. To complement this lecture series, the Department of Psychiatry at Tufts in 1983 initiated a two-day course, called the Psychopharmacology Update. For this annual conference, topics are chosen that represent either the cutting-edge issues in clinical care or the thorny problems that benefit from regular re-examination and review. We have included in this edition selected topics from the Update plus invited contributions to provide balance and scope. Typical of the latter is the chapter in this edition by Magliozzi and Schaffer on antipsychotic drugs; typical of the former is the Pope and Hudson chapter on eating disorders. Prior to 1970, when the first edition of the *Handbook of Clinical Psychopharmacology* was published, eating disorders were poorly understood, psychopharmacological treatment was at best nonspecific, and most seriously ill patients were hospitalized to keep them alive through forced feeding. The *Handbook* is not intended as a textbook. Rather, we have selected as topics those areas about which trainees have asked the most questions over the last several years, or for which we receive numbers of patient referrals to our clinical programs at the New England Medical Center Hospitals.

Dr. Joe P. Tupin has been a friend and colleague for more than twenty-five years. He and I shared many joyful hours with Al DiMascio from the mid-1960s until Al's tragic death in 1978. It seemed appropriate to turn to Joe to take the lead in editing this edition. We were also assisted by Dr. David S. Harnett, who is course director for our Annual Update. We share the view that the material in this edition is timely, of clinical relevance, and written with attention to our major audience—those of you who are concerned with patient care and want to keep up-to-date with our slowly growing but consistently more effective array of treatment approaches to problems of mind, brain, and behavior.

We would also like to acknowledge the invaluable and untiring assistance of Dr. Vivian P. Halfin, Kathleen Fabiano, and Susan White.

Richard I. Shader, M.D.

Professor and Chairman,
Department of Psychiatry
Tufts University School of Medicine
and Psychiatrist-in-Chief,
New England Medical Center

Preface

There have been significant advances in the field of psychopharmacology since the first edition of this handbook nearly twenty years ago. Most clinicians cannot keep up with all of these. However, the diligent clinician can maintain a good knowledge-base in this field by reading scientific journals, attending scientific and research meetings, and turning to reference books. This volume is designed to provide basic background and facilitate the continued development of clinical skills for the student and experienced professional. It is organized around typical clinical problems, not theoretical, biochemical, or pharmacological structures. New medications have been introduced since 1970. Of primary importance was the introduction of lithium, a drug useful both for the initial control of manic symptoms and for prevention of manic and depressive episodes. Of equal interest has been the application of psychopharmacological agents to a variety of unexpected conditions. Antidepressants are now used for phobias and panic attacks. Lithium has application in the treatment of violence. Other examples abound.

In this edition, contributors explain basic pharmacological concepts and terminology. Concepts of elimination half-life, absorption rates, and volume of distribution have direct clinical application and must be understood; increased sophistication is required in the choice and administration of psychopharmacological agents. The difference among various benzodiazepines is typified by the differences in absorption rates, peak blood values, elimination of half-life times, and similar pharmacological characteristics. These play a role in determining the selection of the drug for the patient. A short-acting drug may be best for patients potentially sensitive to oversedation, for example, the elderly. Conversely, some individuals may require long-term management with a benzodiazepine, and can avoid the peaks and valleys of pharmacological effect of a longer-acting medication monitored to achieve the desired effect without oversedation. By bringing pharmacological concepts back into the consultation room, patients and professionals will benefit.

The chapters are authored by acknowledged experts in the field of psychopharmacology, and many chapters grew out of work by staff at Tufts University and the University of California, Davis. All of the contributors are active researchers, clinicians, and teachers, whose work emphasizes the importance of psychopharmacology in the education of mental health professionals.

The orientation of the book will be useful to the busy practitioner who may need to "brush up" on the pharmacological management of a particular complex problem. The structure of the book offers direct access to specific clinical issues. Most practitioners realize that use of medications alone, without appropriate integration into psychotherapeutic, educational, or behavioral techniques is not a complete management approach. These other dimensions are not dealt with in detail here, but this in no way reflects their lack of importance.

The editors realize the complex legal, ethical, and clinical challenges to the modern practitioner who is faced with liability challenges relating to involuntary treatment. These must be balanced on the other side with patient and family interests, as well as ethical and practical considerations relating to utilization of scarce resources.

A chapter on legal concerns is therefore included. The field of psychopharmacology is not determined by clinical considerations alone. Such a book could not have been exhaustive because it seemed prudent to maintain readability rather than to maintain an encyclopedic approach. We trust that clinicians will find it helpful and relevant to their practice and that it will give them a good basis for understanding and applying future developments.

Joe P. Tupin, M.D.
Richard Shader, M.D.
David S. Harnett, M.D.

1

Psychosis

Joseph R. Magliozzi, M.D.
Charles B. Schaffer, M.D.

The discovery in the early 1950s that derivatives of *Rauwolfia serpentina* and phenothiazine were effective in the tranquilization of patients with certain agitated and psychotic conditions led not only to major changes in the treatment of mental illness but to equally revolutionary changes in the conceptualization of mental disorders. It is not an exaggeration to say that the burgeoning use of these agents in the 1950s and 1960s was a principal factor in the movement away from institutionalization of the mentally ill. Recognition that symptoms of the major psychoses and other mental illnesses could, at least in part, be ameliorated by these agents, has reduced the need for long-term custodial treatment, saved millions of dollars, and provided relief for those suffering disabling mental symptoms.

Despite these advances, schizophrenia, the disorder for which the antipsychotics are indicated, remains elusive and confounding of any parsimonious etiological hypothesis and treatment strategy. The modern concept is that schizophrenia is not a discrete illness at all but rather a heterogeneous collection of mental disorders characterized by psychotic thinking, abnormal perceptions, marked constricted emotional expression, and markedly impaired social and occupational functioning. Moreover, it has recently been recognized that not all schizophrenics are helped by these agents and that, in those who are helped, antipsychotics may be helpful, but only for a limited number of manifestations of the illness.

It has, in fact, become useful to regard these agents as nonspecific for the schizophrenic symptom constellation and, as the name implies, specific to the processes of psychosis no matter what the setting of these processes. The symptoms most likely to yield to antipsychotic therapy are agitation, fury, mania, hallucinations, delusions, catatonia, and accelerated and disorganized thinking processes.

In addition to these therapeutic limitations, antipsychotic drugs are recognized to have serious adverse effects. The development of treatment strategies for these complications has been one of the most challenging enterprises of modern psychiatry and neurology and has led to the development of basic insights into brain and central nervous system functions.

In summary, a specific, curative chemotherapeutic regimen for schizophrenia remains to be developed. In the meantime, the dopamine-blocking class of agents must be regarded as the mainstay of treatment of acute psychoses and an important tool in the long-term management of the chronically mentally ill.

INDICATIONS FOR ANTIPSYCHOTIC MEDICATION

Schizophrenia

Antipsychotic medications are currently the most often used drugs for treating schizophrenia in both acute and maintenance phases. Of the five classes of antipsychotic drugs available in the United States, the phenothiazines, butyrophenones, thioxanthenes, dibenzoxapines, and dihydroindoles have been documented to possess efficacy in treatment of manifestations of acute schizophrenia and in preventing relapse. More relevant to the clinician is the high-potency/low-potency distinction that affords some basis upon which to choose among this often bewildering array of medications. In recent years, it has become generally accepted in all but a few situations that the so-called low-potency agents represented by chlorpromazine and thioridazine are being replaced by higher-potency agents such as haloperidol.

The low-potency agents may be useful when sedative and anxiolytic properties are desired. As will be discussed more extensively in the section on extrapyramidal effects, thioridazine causes fewer extrapyramidal motor symptoms than any antipsychotic medication currently available in the United States. This may prompt the clinician to occasionally use a low-potency agent. Since 1975, however, so-called high-potency agents have been the mainstay of acute and maintenance treatment of the schizophrenic patient.

Haloperidol is the best studied of these agents. It is available in tablet, concentrate, and short- and long-acting parenteral forms, and is well absorbed with an oral bioavailability of 60–80% (1). It has moderate sedative properties, low anticholinergic properties, and moderate alpha-1 and alpha-2 blocking effects (2). It has become the drug of choice for treatment of schizophrenia, especially maintenance treatment, and is relatively well tolerated. There is, however, a high incidence of extrapyramidal effects with this medication (2).

The thioxanthene derivative, thiothixene, is comparable to haloperidol. It is slightly less potent in clinical situations but paradoxically has a very much higher affinity for the dopamine$_2$ (DA-2) receptor. It has similar sedative properties as haloperidol, a very low alpha-1 and alpha-2 adrenergic and anticholinergic binding activity and a very high incidence of extrapyramidal side effects.

Fluphenazine is also a commonly used high-potency agent. It has a very high affinity for the DA-2 receptor in human caudate nucleus (2) and it is low in anticholinergic, sedative, and hypotensive effects. It is available in oral concentrate, tablet, short- and long-acting parenteral formulations, the latter of which has proved most useful in the maintenance phase of treatment and in treatment with noncompliant individuals. Fluphenazine has a very high incidence of extrapyramidal motor reactions, including akathisia, and for this reason is poorly tolerated. It is almost devoid of sedative effects and is consequently useful in individuals for whom, for occupational reasons, sedation may not be a desirable effect.

Molindone (Moban), an indole derivative, is also considered a high-potency drug. It has a profile similar to fluphenazine with low incidences of sedative, anticholinergic, and hypotensive actions.

Other than the general statement that high-potency agents are now preferred over lower-potency agents, there is no consistent paradigm that has been successful in matching a given neuroleptic with a given patient. Most authors recommend that a neuroleptic agent be chosen on the basis of prior drug response or family history of drug response (although there may be a few patients who do not fit this pattern). Other empirical guidelines for the selection of a neuroleptic agent are discussed in a later section.

Dosage and Administration

A fairly wide range of therapeutic doses for antipsychotic medication exists in current practice. There may be, however, a wide overlap between doses associated with clinical response and doses associated with side effects, especially extrapyramidal effects. Doses of 2–100 mg daily of haloperidol, or the equivalent, have been utilized in the nongeriatric age group. Geriatric age group doses below 2 mg/day are observed to be somewhat more efficacious. The initial promise of megadose strategies has not been fulfilled, although there may be a very rare patient who requires the 100–120 mg/day of haloperidol or the equivalent for improvement. As is discussed later, there may be up to a 100-fold variation in plasma concentration of these agents (3). This may explain some of the variability in dosages required for symptom control. Table 1–1 gives a rough conversion guide between the various antipsychotic medications in general use in the United States along with affinities for the DA-2 receptor.

Time Course and Response

The response time of these agents has been relatively well characterized. In the first few days to a number of weeks, excessive activity and grossly disorganized or combative motor behavior is the first constellation of symptoms noted to subside. Subsequently, the perceptual features of delusions and hallucinations and thought disorder are reduced. Finally, improvement in socialization and personal hygiene occurs. The most rapid changes occur within the first 3 weeks, and there is very little change noted after 2–3 weeks of treatment. A lack of any response or a very slow response after 6–8 weeks of treatment should prompt a reassessment of the compliance factor.

If compliance is assured, then the strategy of increasing the dose to the equivalent of 60–80 mg/day of haloperidol gradually for 6–8 weeks is indicated followed by a change in neuroleptic. In some cases, a trial of reducing the dose to approximately half of the unsuccessful

TABLE 1-1 Relative Potencies and Affinities for the DA-2 Receptor of Antipsychotic Medication Currently in Use in the United States

Drug	Trade Name	Milligram Potency Relative to Chlorpromazine (=100)		Affinity for DA-2 Receptor[a2]
		Hollister, 1973[4]	Davis[5]	
Phenothiazines				
Aliphatic				
Chlorpromazine	Thorazine	100	100	5.3
Triflupromazine	Vesprin	25	28	36
Piperidine				
Thioridazine	Mellaril	100	100	3.8
Mesoridazine	Serentil	50	51	5.3
Piperacetazine	Quide	10	14	—
Piperazine				
Carphenazine	Proketazine	25	28	—
Acetophenazine	Tindal	20	19	—
Prochlorperazine	Compazine	15	15	14
Perphenazine	Trilafon	10	10	71
Butaperazine	Repoise	10	13	—
Trifluoperazine	Stelazine	5	5	38
Fluphenazine	Prolixin	2	2	125
Thioxanes				
Chlorprothixene	Taractan	100	—	13
Thiothixene	Navane	4	3	222[b]
Butyrophenones				
Haloperidol	Haldol	2	2	25
Indoles				
Molindone	Moban	10[6]	10	0.83
Dibenzoxazpines				
Loxapine	Loxitane	10[6]	—	1.4

[a] 10^{-7} x/Kp; where Kp = equilibrium dissociation constant in molarity
[b] CIS isomer

dose may be indicated prior to changing to a new drug. In the future, it is expected that monitoring of plasma levels will be useful in assessing drug efficacy and/or failure following an adequate trial period (4).

Limitations of Chemotherapy for Schizophrenia

It is clear that antipsychotic medications make the difference between the prognosis of years of immersion in a psychotic experience and only intermittent manifestations of psychotic symptoms. This effect could potentially allow an individual to be productive and socially active; however, this potential has not been fulfilled. It has recently become apparent that the symptoms of social withdrawal, blunted and inappropriate affect, apathy, and inhibition of volition, which nineteenth-century authors such as Eugin Blueler claimed to be the hallmarks of schizophrenia, are not responsive to neuroleptics and may become quite predominant when the more active, positive symptoms—hallucinations, delusions, agitation, and thought disorders—are ameliorated by antipsychotic medications (7,8). Moreover, it has become apparent that individuals presenting with predominantly negative symptoms are not improved much by administration of antipsychotic medications (9–12).

So far, the management of negative symptoms of social withdrawal, blunted affect, and impaired social functioning remains elusive; however, alprazolam has been shown to be efficacious in open study, and blind trials are currently underway (13). Lack of response to neuroleptic agents is relatively common, with approximately 9% of all schizophrenic patients showing a poor response to neuroleptics even at therapeutically adequate doses (14). It is important to attempt to identify these individuals, as treatment with antipsychotic medication contributes nothing to their outcome, and these individuals may be at very high risk for developing dyskinesias.

Combination Drug Therapy

While the practice of polypharmacy early in the antipsychotic drug era was widely experimented with and even advocated by some authors, experience over the past three decades has shown that use of multiple antipsychotic agents confers no clear advantage and is to be discouraged. The practice, however, of using drugs with two entirely different activities, such as an antipsychotic plus an antidepressant or an antipsychotic plus lithium or even an antipsychotic plus a benzodiazepine or sedative antihistaminic drug, may be justified. For example, if sedation is desired in an acutely psychotic patient, the combination of a high-potency antipsychotic plus an antihistaminic sedative medication, such as diphenhydramine, is indicated. Combinations such as lithium plus a neuroleptic for mania, and an antidepressant plus a neuroleptic for psychotic depression, also have a rational pharmacological basis and are often useful.

ORGANIC BRAIN SYNDROMES

Primary Dementias

As noted in the preceding sections, the most clinically relevant classification of the antipsychotic agents is the high-potency/low-potency classification. In the literature there is a division of opinion as to whether the low-potency or high-potency agents are most useful in the psychotic and agitated components of senile and presenile dementias (15). Because of the high risk of cardiovascular problems in the elderly population, we advocate, where possible, the use of high-potency antipsychotic agents, such as haloperidol in the elderly or cardiovascular risk-prone patient. In the younger patient, in whom cardiovascular or other risk factors can be excluded, the low-potency, more sedative agents, such as thioridazine, mesoridazine, or chlorpromazine, are indicated. These agents are especially useful in the management of the highly explosive and combative behavior seen in young, brain-damaged persons. Treatment with antipsychotic agents in these individuals should be limited to obtaining control with carbamazepine, beta blockers, or lithium recommended for long-term treatment.

For the psychotic manifestations of Alzheimer's disease, Pick's disease, and other dementias, haloperidol or thiothixene with or without a sedating agent (such as diazepam or chloral hydrate) appears to be the best initial approach. Dosage schedules for this combination are exemplified by the following schedule: haloperidol

(Haldol) 0.5–3 mg t.i.d. for 48–72 hours with or without a sedative such as diazepam or lorazepam just before bedtime (16). Because of the possibility of a very long half-life in the elderly population and resultant accumulation of drug levels, it has been recommended that, after 48–72 hours of this regimen, the drug dose be cut by one-half to two-thirds, resulting in a total daily dose of 0.5–3 mg/day. This can usually be given as a single daily dose. This author recommends that the dose be given at approximately 4–6 P.M. daily, or at dinnertime if the patient shows an exacerbation of his or her disturbed behavior in the early evening hours (sundown). Occasionally patients will require splitting the dose with one-third of the total daily dose to be given in the morning and two-thirds either at dinner or at bedtime.

If sedation is desired, a benzodiazepine, such as lorazepam, should be chosen. An alternative to the use of a benzodiazepine is an antihistaminic compound, such as diphenhydramine, which then can be administered in the later hours of the day to achieve sedation. Advantages of the antihistaminic compounds are simultaneous protection against extrapyramidal tract effects and a general low incidence of confusion, dyscontrol, and anticholinergic reactions in this class of drug. Disadvantages include a tendency to weight-gain and the rapid development of tolerance to sedation. Advantages to the benzodiazepine compounds include an anxiolytic effect and a sedative effect. Disadvantages include the development of tolerance and the possibility of increasing confusion and out-of-control behavior.

Substance-Induced Organic Mental Disorders

Alcohol. Antipsychotic agents generally have no place in the treatment of either uncomplicated alcohol intoxication or alcohol idiosyncratic intoxication. Their use in alcohol withdrawal and alcohol-withdrawal delirium was initially advocated but has been largely replaced by the benzodiazepines. The use of low doses of neuroleptics in the treatment of alcoholic hallucinosis is somewhat more controversial but has occasional advocates. Antipsychotic medications are generally of no value in the treatment of alcoholic amnestic disorder unless the disorder is accompanied by severe behavioral regression in which case a trial of low-dose antipsychotic agents may be helpful. Similarly, antipsychotics are of no value in the treatment of dementia associated with alcoholism except to ameliorate uncontrollable behavior.

Barbiturates and opioids. Antipsychotic medications are generally accepted to have no value in the treatment of barbiturate- or opioid-intoxication or withdrawal.

Psychostimulants. In the case of the psychostimulants cocaine and the amphetamines, antipsychotic medications are indicated in states of prominent paranoid, delusional, or hallucinatory activity. Every attempt should be made, however, to treat these states non-pharmacologically. They generally resolve within a few days, and pharmacological intervention should be limited. However, since these agents are thought to exert their effects via dopaminergic mechanisms and since their states of intoxication closely resemble functional psychoses, antipsychotic agents may be rapidly and dramatically effective in these conditions.

In withdrawing these agents, the lethargic, withdrawn, and occasionally profoundly depressed state may be exacerbated by the use of antipsychotic agents. Moreover, the patient may be at very high risk for the occurrence of extrapyramidal effects during this phase. For this reason, the lowest possible dosage for the shortest length of time with the maximal possible period of observation should be employed. Careful attention to differential diagnosis must be emphasized as states of sympathomimetic intoxication frequently coexist with functional psychoses, such as schizophrenia, affective disorders, and personality disorders.

Phencyclidine (PCP) or similarly acting drug. States of intoxication, delirium, and mixed organic mental disorder due to this class of drugs should generally not be treated with antipsychotic agents. It is estimated, however, that a fair number of these states are inadvertently treated with antipsychotic agents because they so closely resemble the functional psychotic states. In treating these conditions, it must be remembered that the use of the low-potency antipsychotic agents is much more hazardous than treatment with the high-potency antipsychotic agents. For this reason, the high-potency antipsychotic agents, such as haloperidol, should be used in situations of diagnostic uncertainty. Since psychotic states from these drugs may persist for a considerable period of time, a somewhat longer course of treatment with antipsychotic agents may be required. Possible complications of antipsychotic treatment of a PCP-induced psychotic or delirious state include hypertension or hypotension and possibly an increased risk of malignant neuroleptic syndrome.

Once the diagnosis is established, which usually can be accomplished by detection of PCP in the urine, the patient should be switched to a safer drug such as benzodiazepine. Even under such circumstances, benzodiazepine may not "hold" a severe PCP-induced psychosis or delirium, and antipsychotic agents may be required. In these circumstances, the clinician must weigh the considerable risks of an undermedicated PCP-induced psychosis, including suicide, violence to others, or self-mutilation against the risks of the antipsychotic medications. Under these conditions, frequent monitoring of all vital signs is indicated.

A PCP-induced state is often indistinguishable from acute schizophrenia or mania. However, certain physical signs, such as anesthesia, horizontal and occasionally vertical nystagmus, hypertension, and finding of the drug on toxicology screen may help to differentiate these conditions.

Hallucinogen-Induced Organic Mental Disorders

Hallucinogens, such as LSD, psilocybin and mescaline generally produce hallucinoses and delusional states of a relatively short duration. Generally, nonpharmacological approaches are recommended.

Cannabis. Antipsychotic agents have no role in the treatment of cannabis-induced intoxication of delusional disorder.

Caffeine. Antipsychotics generally have no role in management of intoxication from caffeine.

Other or unspecified substances. As a general rule, in the undiagnosed case, antipsychotic agents are most effective in treatment of hallucinosis or delusional states. They have intermediate efficacy in the treatment of agitated but nonpsychotic states, including affective disorders, and very low efficacy in the treatment of dementias, amnestic disorders, and personality disorders, and in fact, may exacerbate signs of delirium. Another rule is that the low-potency agents should be avoided in the undiagnosed case. When antipsychotic agents are used to manage an acute toxic syndrome, close observation and frequent monitoring of vital signs is essential. Perhaps the most important caveat is that diagnostic efforts should begin immediately and specific treatments initiated as soon as possible.

Other Nonsubstance Abuse Organic Mental Disorders

As previously mentioned, antipsychotic agents are most useful for disturbances characterized by hallucinosis, delusional syndrome, combativeness, and affective features, especially when these features are present with a clear sensorium. As clouding of these sensoriums occurs and features of delirium appear, the antipsychotic medications become less useful and may actually exacerbate the delirium and impede diagnostic efforts.

Antipsychotic agents should be used with great caution when the risk of seizures is expected to be high. This includes conditions in which epileptoid states are part of the differential diagnosis or in cases of trauma or increased intercranial pressure. Also, patients in delirium or epileptoid states frequently manifest very exaggerated extrapyramidal symptoms which may lead to the development of neuroleptic malignant syndrome and attendant complications. Furthermore, the neuroleptic malignant syndrome itself may present as a psychotoform encephalopathy or delirium and, of course, in this state any further dopamine blockade could be fatal.

ANTIPSYCHOTICS IN BORDERLINE AND OTHER PERSONALITY DISORDERS

Although not considered a principal diagnostic feature of the borderline personality disorder, psychotic episodes of a brief but intense nature are considered by many clinicians as being a highly characteristic feature of this disorder (17). These psychotic episodes are characterized by the following five types of psychotic phenomena:

1. affective with frequent depression and feelings of worthlessness,
2. dissociative phenomena with depersonalization and derealization,

3. visual and auditory perceptual distortion,
4. paranoid ideation,
5. self-boundary confusion.

Similarly, borderline individuals have been noted to have an increased vulnerability to the substance-induced organic disorders mentioned earlier. Although the practice is somewhat controversial, some clinicians have employed antipsychotic agents in the management of the above phenomena in the context of borderline personality disorder. Some caveats are in order: as mentioned in the section on organic brain syndromes, states in which visual and auditory perceptual distortions and paranoid ideation predominate are the most likely to respond to antipsychotic agents. The conditions in which affective states predominate are generally of intermediate responsivity, with excitement and maniacal states being more responsive than depressive states. Dissociative states may show either no response or a negative response to antipsychotic medications. The anxiety and the self-boundary confusion of the borderline patient is often of a free-floating type and is generally nonresponsive to antipsychotic agents. The depersonalization, derealization, anxiety, and self-boundary confusion symptoms may actually be intensified by the uncomfortable feelings of restlessness and akathisia generated by antipsychotic medications.

Low doses of high-potency antipsychotic agents are generally recommended for these individuals and should only be used when the highly responsive symptoms of paranoia and perceptual disturbances occur in a particularly threatening or disabling way. The use of antidepressants, lithium, or benzodiazepines in the control of the depressive, excited, and highly anxious manifestations of the borderline state has been recommended by some clinicians.

Mania

Stabilization with lithium is the primary goal in treating the most acutely manic patients. Antipsychotics may frequently be necessary to initially suppress the severe manic symptoms until the lithium takes effect, which may be several days to 2 weeks. In studies comparing the efficacy of an antipsychotic versus lithium, antipsychotics are superior to lithium in rapid control of manic symptoms (18). In addition to suppressing psychotic symptoms in acute manics, the antipsychotics are also effective in decreasing other clinically related symptoms, including sleep disturbances, increased motor activity, irritability, intrusiveness, lability, aggressive behavior, and pressured speech. When these severe symptoms are under control with antipsychotics, the patient is more manageable and cooperative, and lithium therapy can be initiated. The antipsychotics can gradually be tapered off after 1-2 weeks when a therapeutic serum level of lithium has been maintained.

Most clinicians prefer to treat acute symptoms with haloperidol because larger doses can be given parenterally and in frequent intervals without the fear of dangerous cardiovascular side effects. Acutely manic patients treated with the potent antipsychotics often experience acute extrapyramidal side effects (EPS). These can usually be managed with antiparkinsonian agents. Some manic patients may take several weeks to respond to lithium, and antipsychotic medication should be continued in these patients for longer periods of time.

For those manic patients who cannot tolerate lithium or do not respond to this agent, continued therapy with antipsychotics, although less desirable, is necessary. Unfortunately, these patients may require long-term maintenance therapy with antipsychotics if manic episodes are frequent and severe.

In preliminary research studies, newer antimanic agents such as carbamazepine, valproic acid, and clonazepam have shown some promise in the treatment of acute mania and may eventually replace antipsychotics as a second-line treatment (19). Electroconvulsive therapy (ECT) should be considered when pharmacotherapy is not successful.

Psychotic Depression

Antipsychotics are often used in combination with antidepressants in the treatment of patients who suffer from major depressive episodes with psychotic features. In most studies, the efficacy of this combined therapy is usually greater (50-75%) when compared to the effectiveness of antidepressants or antipsychotics alone (usually under 50%) (20). Electroconvulsive therapy is still the superior treatment for this disorder with a success rate of 75-90%. When the combined therapy is used, antipsychotic therapy can be started alone or simultaneously with antidepressant therapy. When the two families of medications are used simultaneously, care should be taken to avoid additive adverse affects. For example, one should avoid combining antidepressants and antipsychotics that have significant anticholinergic properties. Some medications have fixed dosages, but we prefer the use of antipsychotics and antidepressants separately. This allows greater flexibility in adjusting one or both agents for target symptoms and for controlling adverse affects.

Once the patient has been stabilized on the combined therapy, it is not known how long both agents should be maintained simultaneously. Additional controlled studies are needed to determine if antipsychotics are required along with antidepressant agents after the acute episode.

Catatonia

Until recently, the term catatonia has been synonymous with schizophrenia. In the past decade there has been a rekindling of interest in this clinical entity as a result of research in clinical phenomenology, neuroendocrinology, and psychopharmacology. This research has resulted in a reconceptualization of the meaning of catatonia.

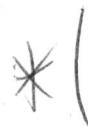

Three important factors have necessitated a different approach in the evaluation and treatment of the catatonic patient. First, rather than a subtype of schizophrenia, catatonia should be considered a nonspecific syndrome (constellation of signs and symptoms) which can be associated with a wide variety of both medical and psychiatric disorders (21). Indeed, most patients presenting with catatonic features are more likely to be suffering from a major affective disorder than schizophrenia (22). Second, catatonia is not rare. On the contrary, there is a great likelihood of encountering the syndrome. This makes it imperative that clinicians of all primary-care specialties be aware of the differential diagnosis and special management problems associated with catatonic patients. Third, catatonia can be a life-threatening condition, either as a result of undiagnosed medical problems or complications of the catatonic state itself. This risk is another argument for an aggressive diagnostic workup and thorough familiarity with the likely causes and complications of the catatonic syndrome.

There are no pathognomonic signs or symptoms of catatonia. Most experts in this field suggest that the diagnosis be made by the presence of one or more of the following signs: mutism, posturing, rigidity, stereotypic motor activity, automatic obedience, negativism, waxy flexibility, catalepsy, or stupor (23). Other signs often associated with catatonia include grimacing, echolalia, echopraxia, excitement, or retardation.

No double-blind control studies address the treatment of catatonia. Once medical disorders have been ruled out, most clinicians use antipsychotic medications to bring the patient out of the catatonic state by decreasing the severe symptoms noted above. Aggressive parenteral use of potent neuroleptics is indicated during the first 24 hours, which usually results in reduction of the most extreme catatonic symptoms. During this period, the patient must be reevaluated on a frequent basis, since these same antipsychotic medications can cause a catatonic condition. Deterioration or lack of improvement with the use of antipsychotics would suggest either a drug reaction or failure to diagnose an underlying medical disorder.

Electroconvulsive therapy has been used in catatonic states when pharmacotherapy is not successful or when quick results are mandatory and an affective disorder is suspected. Antidepressant therapy or lithium may be used for catatonic patients suffering from affective disorders. These drugs are usually not effective during the acute states of catatonia and are difficult to administer orally to the catatonic patient. Most clinicians start these medications when the catatonic patient has been stabilized with antipsychotic drugs.

Chronic Pain

Although antipsychotics are not drugs of first choice in the treatment of chronic pain states, some pain patients report beneficial results with these agents. There are some reports indicating that phenothiazine can serve as adjunctive therapy to antidepressant medication (24). A few studies have claimed success with the use of antipsychotics alone in patients with chronic pain (25).

Headache syndromes may also respond to antipsychotic therapy. In one double-blind study, low-dose fluphenazine was found to be effective in the treatment of chronic tension headaches (26). In another trial, chlorpromazine was found to be useful in some patients with chronic cluster headaches which had been unresponsive to more conventional therapy (27). Although phenothiazine antipsychotics were once thought to have the ability to potentiate narcotic-induced analgesia, recent reports fail to confirm this property.

Gilles de la Tourette's Syndrome

Gilles de la Tourette's syndrome is characterized by involuntary movements of functionally related skeletal muscles and vocalizations. The movements or tics are usually rapid, unexpectedly repetitive, and of a brief duration and changing intensity. The tics are also multiple and usually involve the head but can frequently involve other parts of the body. Vocal tics are frequently present and can be characterized by sounds, words, or less commonly, coprolalia. All symptoms can be voluntarily suppressed for short periods. The disorder usually starts before age 10 and can have a fluctuating chronic course. There is a continuum of presentation of symptoms from those that are minor and hardly noticeable to those that are grotesque and socially disabling. Most experts feel that Tourette's syndrome is a primary neurological movement disorder caused by a defect in neurotransmitter function in the basal ganglia (28).

Many different families of medicines have been tried in the treatment of Tourette's syndrome. Thus far, the neuroleptics, especially haloperidol, have proved to be the most successful agents in ameliorating the symptoms of Tourette's syndrome (29). Haloperidol causes symptom improvement in 60–90% of patients with Tourette's syndrome. Currently, it is the drug treatment of choice for this disorder. The range of doses used to treat the Tourette's patient is usually lower than those employed in psychiatric disorders. Some authors recommend starting as low as 0.25 mg/day (in children) with an upper limit of 10–15 mg/day. A common dose range of 1–5 mg/day is employed in the average Tourette's patient.

Other dopamine antagonists reported to be effective in this disorder are pimozide, penfluridol, and most of the members of the phenothiazine antipsychotics (29). Several other major families of medications have been tried in the treatment of this disorder, but the results thus far have been inconclusive.

The initiation of treatment with haloperidol for Tourette's patients should not be done in a cavalier fashion. Most Tourette's patients experience significant side effects to this medication, even at very low doses. The types of side effects are similar to those seen in other populations in which haloperidol is used for its antipsychotic affect. These include the full range of extrapyramidal symptoms, including sedation.

The decision to treat a Tourette's patient is based on several factors including the severity of the symptoms, the patient's tolerance to the symptoms, the patient's age, and the patient's sensitivity to side effects of haloperidol. Since the course of Tourette's symptoms waxes and wanes, maintenance therapy with haloperidol necessitates constant reevaluation of dosage and presence of adverse affects. As in the case with other psychiatric patient populations, Tourette's patients who require long-term maintenance administration of antipsychotics are probably at risk to develop tardive dyskinesia.

Postpartum Psychosis

There are three major psychiatric disorders that can occur following delivery: major affective disorders (either manic or depressive episodes), schizophrenic disorders, and organic mental disorders. Any one of these three disorders can cause an illness of psychotic proportions. However, these major psychiatric disorders are actually not unique to the postpartum psychosis per se. Any postpartum psychotic syndrome that does not qualify for the above three categories is grouped under the heading "atypical psychosis" in DSM-III. Some recent studies suggest that the most common cause of postpartum psychosis is affective disorder, especially manic-depressive disorders (30).

Since there is no major psychiatric disorder unique to the postpartum period, the somatic treatments for affective disorders, schizophrenic disorders, and selected organic mental disorders are the same as would be utilized for non-postpartum patients. Major depressive episodes following delivery are usually treated with antidepressant medication with the addition of antipsychotic agents if the depression has psychotic features. Electroconvulsive therapy should also be considered when medication is not successful. Lithium carbonate is the treatment of choice for manic episodes in the postpartum patient, but antipsychotic medication is often needed to reduce the acute symptoms until the onset of the effect of lithium. Psychotic symptoms of postpartum patients should also be treated with antipsychotic medication.

Acutely Psychotic Medical-Surgical Patients

Occasionally, patients suffering from life-threatening medical disorders require treatment for acute psychotic symptoms. In this situation, intravenous (I.V.) haloperidol has been used with considerable success. Although this route of administration of haloperidol has not been approved by the U.S. Food and Drug Administration (FDA), preliminary studies indicate that it can be quite effective and safe when used with caution.

Two recent studies have shown that I.V. haloperidol can be used in a wide variety of medical emergencies. Cassem and Sos administered haloperidol intravenously to acutely agitated or psychotic patients after cardiac surgery or myocardial infarction (31). Ten of these patients received I.V. haloperidol in doses ranging from 2 to 135 mg within 24 hours. This treatment was safe and effective for most of the patients.

In a second study, Dudley and associates treated 20 patients with life-threatening illnesses who required immediate control of psychotic symptoms (32). The patients' primary psychiatric diagnoses included schizophrenia, organic brain syndrome, and mania. The medical diagnoses included gastrointestinal bleeding, severe burns, or trauma. The dose of I.V. haloperidol ranged from 2.5 to 25 mg over a 2-minute period. The authors reported that agitation of psychosis was successfully controlled in every patient permitting medical treatment.

ADVERSE EFFECTS OF ANTIPSYCHOTICS

Extrapyramidal Reactions

The effects of antipsychotic medication on the extrapyramidal motor system can be classified into two general types: those resulting from acute administration of neuroleptics and those following or upon withdrawal from antipsychotic medication.

Following acute administration of neuroleptics, five general extrapyramidal motor syndromes have been identified. The first is a syndrome of hypokinesis, tremor, and rigidity, which is similar to naturally occurring Parkinson's disease. The second is a condition of restlessness and inability to sit still, known as akathisia. The third is an acute spasmodic condition of the tongue and neck resembling spastic torticollis. The fourth is a high-amplitude facial tremor simulating the motion of the snout of a rabbit and known as the rabbit syndrome. The fifth is a neurological catastrophe manifested by extreme muscular rigidity, dystonia, hyperthermia, and delirium and is known as the neuroleptic malignant syndrome (NMS). All five of these syndromes result from the blockade of central post-synaptic dopamine receptors by neuroleptic agents, although other mechanisms may be important in the production of the acute dystonias, akathisia, and NMS.

These effects are reversible by three basic strategies. The first is the addition to a neuroleptic of an anticholinergic medication. Blockage of dopamine at the striatal sites results in a heightened activity of cholinergic cells, which is thought to underlie the hypokinetic state. Blockade of acetylcholine at these sites overcomes this heightened activity and restores the system to normal. Agents commonly used for this purpose are benzotropine, trihexiphenidyl, and procyclidine. They are most effective against the symptoms of hypokinetic rigidity and acute dystonia, somewhat less effective for the symptom of akathisia, and essentially ineffective in NMS. Appropriate dosages and frequencies of administration are shown in Table 1-2.

The second strategy for overcoming dopaminergic blockage is to reduce the dose of dopamine blocker itself or to change to an agent with a low propensity for this effect, such as thioridazine. This strategy has the advantage of being the most economical both clinically and monetarily. It is useful in all of the general types of extrapyramidal conditions. Its chief drawback is that it can be associated with a recurrence of psychotic symptoms. For the latter reason, it is most often used during the maintenance phase of treatment when dosages may be more safely reduced without risk of exacerbating psychotic symptoms. Consequently, a very common scenario is for the clinician to utilize antiparkinson drugs in combination with a higher dosage of neuroleptic drugs during the early phases of treatment, then to reduce neuroleptic dosage and reduce or discontinue antiparkinson drug dosage during the maintenance phases of treatment. Recently, however, it has come to be recognized that while discontinuation of antiparkinson agents is a desirable goal, it may not easily be achieved in practice, since extrapyramidal effects recur frequently when antiparkinson drugs are discontinued (33).

The last strategy for dealing with disorders caused by dopamine blockage is to administer a dopamine agonist. For practical pur-

TABLE 1-2 Drugs Used in the Treatment of Neuroleptic-Induced Extrapyramidal Disorders

Drug	Trade Name	Indication	Daily Dose Range	Comments
Anticholinergic Agent				
Benztropine Maleate	Cogentin	Acute Dystonia, Parkinsonism, Akinesia, Akathisia	2–8 mg	1–2 mg i.m. for acute dystonic reactions. Potential for abuse
Trihexyphenidyl	Artane	Acute Dystonia, Parkinsonism, Akinesia, Akathisia	1–15 mg	Not available in parenteral formulation. Potential for abuse
Procyclidine	Kemadrin	Acute Dystonia, Parkinsonism, Akinesia, Akathisia	7.5–20 mg	Not available in parenteral formulation.
Dopamine Agonists				
Amantadine	Symmetrel	Parkinsonism, Akinesia, Akathisia	100–300 mg	Not available in parenteral formulation.
Bromocriptine	Parlodel	Neuroleptic Malignant Syndrome	15–80 mg	Not available in parenteral formulation. Give only if patient can swallow. Do not administer via nasogastric tube.

Benzodiazapines			
Diazepam	Valium	Akathisia	2–20 mg	Poorly absorbed intramuscularly. Oral administration usually suffices. Potential for abuse
Lorazepam	Ativan	Akathisia Early Neuroleptic Malignant Syndrome	0.5–6 mg	Available parenterally. Well absorbed intramuscularly. Some success in NMS if treatment started early in course. Potential for abuse.
Miscellaneous Agents			
Diphenhydramine (antihistamine/anticholinergic)	Benadryl	Acute Dystonia Torticollis Akathisia	50–200 mg	Administer 25–50 mg. I.V. or i.m. for acute dystonia or torticollis May repeat × 1
Dantrolene Sodium (muscle relaxant)	Dantrium	Neuroleptic Malignant Syndrome	1–12 mg/kg I.V. in four divided doses	Use if patient cannot swallow, switching to bromocriptine as soon as patient can swallow.

poses, the dopamine agonists most commonly utilized in the United States are amantadine and bromocriptine. Amantadine hydrochloride is an agent that increases the availability of intrasynaptic dopamine by blockage of presynaptic autoreceptors. It is moderately useful for pseudoparkinsonian symptoms, akathisia, and chronic symptoms. Its use is somewhat limited by a dosage ceiling of 300 mg/day. Severe withdrawal effects including the development of neuroleptic malignant syndrome have been reported in association with amantadine withdrawal (34). Its chief advantage is that it does not characteristically produce anticholinergic effects such as dry mouth, urinary retention, confusion, and memory loss that the anticholinergic agents produce. This is particularly important in the elderly or demented patient.

Bromocriptine is a direct dopamine agonist. It stimulates postsynaptic dopamine receptors and directly overcomes the effects of antipsychotic agents. Bromocriptine has been found to be the most valuable in the treatment of NMS (35). Its value in the other conditions mentioned above has not been thoroughly investigated. Further information on dosage and administration is given in Table 1–2, and a full discussion of NMS follows.

While the use of antiparkinsonian agents and amantadine or dosage reduction are generally effective in the alleviation of extrapyramidal symptoms, there are occasional situations in which these strategies are inadequate. This occurs most often in the treatment of acute dystonic reactions, such as the spastic torticollis and also the peculiar and quite uncomfortable effect of akathisia. In the former situation, administration of I.V. or intravascular diphenhydramine may be particularly valuable. In the latter situation, use of diphenhydramine or amantadine or a benzodiazepine may be necessary to ameliorate akathisia.

Akathisia is probably the most common of all extrapyramidal side effects and it is certainly the most frequently overlooked (36). It has been postulated as the major cause of medication noncompliance, apparent failure to respond to medication, impulsivity and violence, and even suicide attempts. While most texts describe akathisia as being accompanied by visible signs of motor restlessness, such as rhythmic movements of the lower extremities, tapping of the feet, or pacing about, akathisia need not manifest these features and may be manifested only by complaints of anxiety, hostility, and other apparently functional symptoms. A high index of suspicion, perseverance in trying different regimens, a high degree of compassion, and sound therapeutic alliance are indispensable for the management of this all-too-common and very uncomfortable effect of neuroleptics.

The Neuroleptic Malignant Syndrome

In the past four to five years, a catastrophic neurological syndrome has been identified which, because of its partial resemblance to the malignant hyperthermia induced by volatile anesthetics, has been termed the neuroleptic malignant syndrome (NMS). Its incidence has been reported in the range of 0.5–1% of those receiving neuroleptics. Mortality has been calculated as 14% of those receiving oral and 37% of those receiving parenteral neuroleptics. It is manifested by the following cardinal features: hyperthermia, muscular rigidity, autonomic instability, and encephalopathy. The last is manifested by signs ranging from delirium to stupor and coma. Temperature may be as high as 42° C. Associated findings include leukocytosis, elevation of serum creatine phosphokinase (CPK), and transaminases, myoglobinuria, and occasionally slowing of the electroencephalogram (EEG). As mentioned earlier, mortality may be high, up to 20%, and even in nonlethal outcomes, irreversible dementia and dyskinesias have been noted.

This syndrome has been thought to be secondary to an almost total blockade of central dopamine pathways and dysregulation of central adrenergic and hypothalamic mechanisms. Whether or not skeletal muscle abnormalities involving the sarcoplasmic reticulum predispose to the condition is not known at this time and is the subject of active investigation.

The treatment of this syndrome is generally threefold. The first component consists of aggressive life-support measures, including I.V. hydration, vital signs and laboratory monitoring, and intubation and mechanical ventilation if necessary. Ice baths may be used to reduce fever; antipyretics are contraindicated. Use of dantrolene I.V. at a dosage of 0.25 mg/kg body weight, q.i.d., to 3 mg/kg, q.i.d., will usually provide enough skeletal muscle relaxation to permit oral medication with bromocriptine, which has recently been found to be the most efficacious agent in the management of neuroleptic malignant syndrome (37). Patients who are able to swallow should be treated with 5–20 mg q.i.d., p.o. When a positive response has been noted, the medication should be continued for at least 10 days and the dosage reduced incrementally to prevent recurrence of the initial symptoms. Bromocriptine produces consistent and often dramatic results and may also reduce the risk of irreversible neurological sequelae of this condition.

Risk factors for the neuroleptic malignant syndrome are just beginning to be identified. In general, the high potency neuroleptic agents, such as haloperidol are thought to be of greater risk than the lower potency agents, although reactions have occurred with chlorpromazine and thioridazine. The syndrome does not appear to be dose-related and has been observed following a single dose of these medications. It is more commonly seen with serial use, although patients may tolerate a medication for months before developing the syndrome. Perhaps other concomitant factors such as transient fever or dehydration are necessary to initiate the syndrome or perhaps the syndrome can only occur in certain individuals that have central or peripheral factors making them more vulnerable.

The prolonged use of long-acting neuroleptic medications may be a risk factor for the development of NMS. Individuals who are mentally retarded or who have organic brain syndromes may develop NMS if treated for long periods with neuroleptics. Withdrawal from dopamine agonists, such as amantadine, L-dopa, and bromocriptine has also been associated with NMS, especially in patients receiving these medications for idiopathic parkinsonism. A summary of treatment strategies for neuroleptic malignant syndrome is shown in Table 1–2.

Tardive Dyskinesia

The other main side effect of neuroleptics on the extrapyramidal motor system arises not from the blockage of dopamine receptor sites, but from the emergence of a supersensitivity to dopamine. As a general principle in neuronal systems, when input to a neuron is reduced over time, the target cell develops an increased responsivity to the stimulus. This has been shown in experimental and accidental mechanical neuronal injury and, in this circumstance, is known as denervation supersensitivity. One can think of a cell whose postsynaptic dopamine receptors are blocked by a neuroleptic agent as being chemically denervated. This chemically denervated cell would then develop hypersensitivity to a neurotransmitter, in this case, dopamine, whose receptors are blocked. These are the events that are believed to lead to the development of tardive dyskinesia, a complication of long-term treatment with neuroleptics.

The dyskinesias are characterized by low amplitude movements that commonly involve the oral and facial musculature and produce a rhythmic movement of the tongue, lips, and cheeks. These movements may simulate puckering of the mouth or chewing gum, and also may result in rhythmic protrusion of the tongue. Often, especially in the early stages, these movements are not noted while the patient is resting comfortably but may be brought out by asking him or her to perform a voluntary movement, such as touching the thumb to each of the other fingers of the hand rapidly. The dyskinetic movements, however, may not be initially manifested in the oral region but may be manifested by tapping movements of the fingers.

The course of such movements is quite varied, but it has become clear that many such cases are progressive and even irreversible. Progression, when it occurs, does so from the oral areas to the more distal structures, such as the hands, fingers, feet, and toes. It finally progresses to the axial musculature to produce a full-blown chorea reminiscent of the advanced stages of Huntington's chorea or Wilson's disease. Movements may be secondarily exacerbated by anxiety. Alternately, a state of heightened anxiety and possibly even increased psychosis may accompany the progression and spread of the dyskinesia.

Risk factors. An overall prevalence of tardive dyskinesia of 20–40% in patients chronically treated with neuroleptics has been estimated (38). Of considerable recent interest has been the attempt to identify risk factors that predispose toward the development of this condition. Although the results have, in fact, often been complications, the most consistently identified risk factors are age and use of high-potency neuroleptics. The following risk factors have been inconsistently identified: female gender, history of organicity, total lifetime neuroleptic dose, and exposure to prophylactic antiparkinsonian medication (39,40).

Interventions. The clinician should periodically perform a systematic assessment of the patient in order to detect the earliest possible manifestations of tardive dyskinesia. If symptoms are observed, the first and least disrupting step is to taper off any antiparkinsonian medication. This usually leads to a remission of dyskinetic symptoms, especially if they were initially minimal. The next step is to lower the patient's dose of antipsychotic medication to the minimum amount necessary to prevent relapse. In the process of doing so, intensification of the dyskinetic movements is to be expected. If the dyskinetic movements become intolerable or if psychotic symptoms should reappear, then the neuroleptic dose should be increased to the minimum amount required to suppress the most intolerable of the dyskinetic or psychotic symptoms. After a few weeks, dosage tapering should commence again, even more gradually. The clinician may at this point wish to undertake a thorough diagnostic reassessment of the patient with the goal of making a diagnosis, such as bipolar disorder, in which maintenance treatment with lithium carries a much lower risk of tardive dyskinesia. If this cannot be done and if the dyskinesia is severe, changing to a roughly equivalent dose of a low-potency neuroleptic may be useful.

Frequently, dyskinetic movements are first discovered during a dosage reduction or tapering of neuroleptics. Such dyskinesias have been called withdrawal dyskinesias, and there is some evidence that they may be mechanistically and prognostically distinct from dyskinesias that appear on a constant neuroleptic dose. Specifically, withdrawal dyskinesias are thought to have a somewhat better prognosis than the emergent dyskinesias. No consistent, distinguishing features have been discovered so far that would indicate a preference in treatment.

Pharmacological treatment of tardive dyskinesia has been extremely disappointing. Almost every type of psychotherapeutic agent has been attempted, including benzodiazepines, beta blockers, lithium, antidepressants, and cholinomimetics. Benzodiazepines may have a nonspecific effect based upon their sedative and anxiolytic effects. In our experience, tardive dyskinesia can be exacerbated by anxiety and is occasionally accompanied by considerable free-floating anxiety. Any success noted with the beta blockers may also be due to this effect. Assessment is very complicated as the dyskinesias themselves have quite a variable course. The most promising pharmacological interventions to date appear to be the depleting agents reserpine and tetrabenazine (41).

Prevention. Preventing tardive dyskinesia centers around the principle of keeping neuroleptic doses and levels as low as possible. It is clear that the main risk factors are dose and exposure over time. It is generally accepted that long-term drug-free periods are of value in preventing tardive dyskinesia, but whether briefer drug holidays are of any benefit is more controversial. The issue of whether long-term prophylactic antiparkinson medication contributes to tardive dyskinesia is also somewhat controversial, but most clinicians advocate reduction and elimination of prophylactic antiparkinsonian medications if at all possible. There is no evidence that use of any one antipsychotic medication offers an advantage over another given at the same equivalent dosage. However, there is some evidence that certain properties, such as the ability to block both pre- and postsynaptic dopamine receptors, as found in the very high-potency agents, may contribute to tardive dyskinesia. Furthermore, certain neuroleptics with atypical features, such as clozapine, thioridazine, and sulpiride are currently being looked at as being possibly safer than the other available neuroleptics in this regard.

Cardiovascular effects. The effects of antipsychotics on the cardiovascular system can be divided into three major areas: autonomic, electrocardiographic (EKG) changes, and direct action on the heart.

Autonomic effects. Antipsychotic medications can cause postural hypotension and reflex tachycardia as a result of peripheral alpha-adrenergic blockage and possibly an additional central action. These adverse effects are more frequently seen with chlorpromazine (CPZ), thioridazine, and mesoridazine. The postural hypotensive effect caused by CPZ is possibly enhanced by direct vasodilation effect on the peripheral blood vessels. This adverse effect can be quite severe and can result in dangerous falls. Some patients develop a tolerance to this effect after a few days or weeks of therapy. In other patients, the symptom persists and requires a decrease in dosage or a change to another family of antipsychotics. The risk of postural hypotension is increased with parenteral administration. In more severe cases, more acute treatment is necessary. Epinephrine should be avoided as a pressor agent because it has a beta-adrenergic activity and could lower the blood pressure even further with potentially fatal results. Geriatric patients are especially sensitive to postural hypotension, and falls in this age group often result in hip fractures.

Electrocardiographic (EKG) Changes. The most common EKG changes seen with antipsychotic medications include prolonged

QT interval, depression of the ST segment, blunting or inversion of the T wave, increased length of the PR interval and increase in U wave amplitude. EKG changes are most frequently associated with the use of thioridazine and, less commonly, CPZ. Usually these EKG changes do not effect cardiac functions and are reversible when the agent is discontinued. The most troublesome effect of thioridazine is its tendency to prolong ventricular repolarization which increases the chances of developing a reentry arrhythmia. CPZ has been reported to have an antiarrhythmic effect which could be a quinidine-type property or a local anesthetic effect.

There have been rare cases of sudden death reported in association with the use of antipsychotic agents. The role of the antipsychotic agent as a primary cause of sudden death remains controversial. It is postulated that antipsychotics may cause sudden death from fatal arrhythmia or a severe, acute episode of postural hypotension. Thioridazine and CPZ have been most frequently mentioned in association with reported cases of sudden death. Thioridazine seems to be incriminated at a greater frequency than other agents. Until further definitive research is done in this area, clinicians should avoid using CPZ or thioridazine in patients with known heart disease, pre-existing postural hypotension or arrhythmias.

Direct Effect on the Heart. Phenothiazines, especially CPZ, are felt to possess a negative iontropic (direct depressant action) effect on the heart. It is unclear whether this effect is clinically significant. For this reason caution should be used when using phenothiazines on patients with a known history of heart failure.

Sedation

Drowsiness or excessive sedation is a common adverse effect associated with use of thioridazine or CPZ. This side effect is often dose-related and commonly diminishes over the first several days-to-weeks of administration of these two agents. In agitated patients, the sedative effect can be helpful in controlling behavioral problems. However, many patients find drowsiness undesirable and uncomfortable, especially those who require alertness to function. Oversedation can also be experienced by patients given more potent antipsychotics, such as piperazine, phenothiazines, or haloperidol, when large oral doses or parenteral administration are required. Although somnolence is frequently seen in oversedated patients, this hypnotic effect is different from that seen with most central nervous system depression because the patient is easily arousable in this state.

Dermatological Side Effects

Skin reactions to the antipsychotic agents are not uncommon. There are three major types. The first is a hypersensitivity reaction that can take several common forms including urticarial, maculopapular, petechial, or edematous. These eruptions usually occur between the first and eighth week after initiation of treatment and resolve after discontinuation of the offending agent. In rare cases, exfoliate dermatitis can occur, and this reaction can be life-threatening and require vigorous treatment including epinephrine, steroids, and supportive measures. About 5% of patients taking CPZ develop a skin rash. Usually a cross sensitivity is rare, and the patient can be switched to another family of antipsychotic drugs. The rashes usually occur on the face, neck, upper chest, and extremities.

Photosensitivity is the second major class of skin reactions to antipsychotic agents, especially to CPZ. This reaction resembles a severe sunburn. It is a result of the drug combining with proteins in the malpighian layer of the skin, producing free radicals, which are thought to cause severe sunburn even from mild exposure to direct sunlight. Less commonly, phenothiazines other than CPZ can also cause this effect. If this photosensitivity reaction does occur, exposure to the sun should be avoided for up to 4-6 weeks after discontinuation of the drug to allow for elimination of the drug stored in the epidermis. Commercial sunscreens containing benzophenone lotion are available, and their application to the exposed area may prevent this problem.

A third dermatological reaction to antipsychotics is a form of hyperpigmentation, which was seen usually in schizophrenics after chronic use of these agents. It is rarely seen today. In this condition, the skin turns grayish-blue in the areas of hyperpigmentation, producing a metallic appearance. This usually occurs in areas exposed to sunlight. CPZ is usually the offending agent.

The incidence of this effect seems to be about 1%. Patients who develop this reaction sometimes have associated deposits of the pigment in the cornea and lens. For this reason, any patient with such manifestations should have periodic eye examinations. It has been postulated that the hyperpigmentation may be a result of an interaction between pigmentary proteins and a metabolite of CPZ. If this reaction occurs, the causative drug should be discontinued, and exposure to the sun should be avoided. Some mild cases of this reaction may diminish over time. In susceptible patients, potent antipsychotics are preferable.

Pregnancy and Lactation

As a general rule, medications should be avoided during pregnancy, especially during the first trimester. In some psychiatric patients, however, symptoms can become severe enough to jeopardize the safety of the mother and the fetus. This is especially true in pregnant women who become psychotic from any cause. In this situation, the benefits of antipsychotic medications often outweigh the risks, even during the first trimester.

There have been reports of adverse effects of phenothiazines and butyrophenones on the development of the human fetus, but these effects have not been confirmed by controlled studies. Some reported side effects include chromosomal abnormalities, jaundice, agitation, and central nervous system depression (42). Extrapyramidal symptoms have been reported in newborns where the mother has taken antipsychotic drugs 1 to 2 weeks before delivery (42). These symptoms have included tremors, hypertonia, weakness, and poor reflexes.

A French study of women taking phenothiazines during the first trimester reported an increased incidence of fetal malformations in almost every major organ system including the central nervous, cardiovascular, digestive, musculoskeletal, and genitourinary systems (43). Other defects reported were microcephaly, ventricular septal defect, cleft lip, hypospadias, polydactylia, and syndactyly. A more recent study by Edlund and Craig reported that children exposed to neuroleptics between 8 and 10 weeks gestation demonstrated a 5.4% incidence of congenital anomalies, compared to 3.2% in a control group not exposed to drugs (44).

Butyrophenones and haloperidol have also been associated with the presence of congenital abnormalities in children whose mothers had taken this agent during the first trimester of pregnancy (42). In addition to phenothiazines and butyrophenones, drugs from other major antipsychotic families such as loxipine, molindone, and thiothixene have not been well studied with regard to teratogenicity.

In summary, because of the troublesome reports of congenital defects related to the major antipsychotics, it is best to avoid these agents during the first trimester of pregnancy. In the psychotic pregnant patient who suffers from schizophrenia and for whom no other therapy is efficacious, the clinician is forced to use these agents to protect the mother and the fetus. In psychotic women who suffer from affective disorders, the antipsychotics are probably safer than lithium, although the use of ECT in these patients may be safer than antipsychotics in the first trimester of pregnancy (45).

Most antipsychotics are found in the breast milk of mothers who are taking these agents while nursing their infants. Sedation may occur in the infant, but most authors agree that the quantities of antipsychotics secreted in the breast milk are small and have not been observed to cause harm to infants (46). There are no studies on long-term effects of these agents on the developing child or adult who has been breast fed by a mother taking antipsychotics.

Endocrine Effects

Antipsychotic drugs can cause gynecomastia in both men and women, and galactorrhea in women either in the presence or absence of gynecomastia. Ten to fifteen percent of females taking these medications may experience lactation or secretion of colostrum. Amenorrhea can also occur and is usually associated with lactation. The cause of these breast changes seen with the use of antipsychotic drugs is probably related to their dopamine-blocking properties which cause an increased secretion of prolactin from the pituitary gland. All antipsychotic agents have this property. This effect is reversible with discontinuation of the antipsychotic drugs and usually takes from 48 to 96 hours to normalize. This problem can sometimes be resolved by changing to another family of antipsychotics.

Almost every menstrual abnormality has been reported with the use of antipsychotic drugs. Amenorrhea is probably the most common abnormality associated with these agents. For obvious reasons, well-controlled studies addressing this topic are lacking. Reduction of the dose of antipsychotic drugs can sometimes ameliorate this problem. In some patients, menstrual periods will return to normal over time even with the continued use of the offending antipsychotic. Some patients may require a change to another family of antipsychotics.

Weight gain is a common side effect with antipsychotic medications, especially with the low-potency drugs, such as chlorpromazine and thioridazine. The reason for this weight gain is not known. A hypothalamic effect is possible. Recent claims indicate that molidone may be unique as an antipsychotic because it has not been associated with weight gain.

Antipsychotic drugs can also reduce inappropriate secretion of antidiuretic hormones. This in turn can cause water intoxication. A "psychogenic" cause of excessive water consumption has also been associated with this syndrome which includes irritability, lethargy, confusion, seizures, and even death.

Glucose metabolism can be affected by antipsychotic drugs. A hyperglycemic effect can be seen in some patients taking these medicines. This can even result in glycosuria. This effect is reversible when the drug is discontinued. There have been reports of worsening of diabetes in known diabetics after administration of CPZ. CPZ can also cause an abnormal glucose tolerance test result in some "prediabetic" patients. In some latent diabetics, antipsychotic therapy has been reported to cause symptoms of diabetes mellitus. It should be stressed that these drugs are not contraindicated in psychotic patients who also suffer from diabetes mellitus, and there is no definite evidence that these drugs cause diabetes clinically. At this time, the etiology of the alteration in serum glucose or glucose metabolism is unknown.

TREATMENT OF THE ACUTELY PSYCHOTIC (SCHIZOPHRENIC) PATIENT

Antipsychotic medication continues to be the mainstay in the treatment of the acutely psychotic patient. Most of the literature on this topic focuses on the acute schizophrenic, because schizophrenics were thought to comprise the majority of patients who demonstrate acute psychotic decompensation. Recent trends in diagnosing psychotic patients have produced a shift in the diagnostic practices of American psychiatrists. Previous research and clinical diagnostic criteria focused primarily on cross-sectional clinical symptoms, usually observed at the time of admission to the hospital. Current researchers in nosology and phenomenology stress the need to include other diagnostic parameters including longitudinal history, evolution of symptomatology during the present episode (including clinical course prior to hospitalization), input from collateral historians (especially from family), family psychiatric history, age of onset, and prior response to treatment. Furthermore, it is now recognized that so-called "schizophrenic" symptoms during acute episodes are not diagnostic and can be present in other disorders, especially affective disorders (47).

Thus, until recently, schizophrenia was probably over-diagnosed, and affective disorders (especially manic episodes) were probably under-diagnosed. For this reason, many research subjects in studies addressing the treatment of acute schizophrenia have probably been acute manic patients as well as those with drug-induced psychoses. Moreover, many of these studies have included a heterogeneous population of "schizophrenics" such as paranoid schizophrenics, disorganized schizophrenics, schizo-affectives, and catatonic schizophrenics. Many feel that the latter two diagnostic categories more often than not tend to be affectively disordered patients when followed longitudinally and diagnosed according to the diagnostic criteria of DSM-III. Although these studies are not without merit and have provided valuable preliminary data on the drug treatment of acutely psychotic patients, the generalization of results from these studies to the treatment of one particular acutely psychotic patient group should be made with caution.

Initially, it was felt that the treatment of acutely schizophrenic patients with antipsychotics could be conceptualized on a dose-response curve model, with the therapeutic range somewhere between 300 and 800 mg of CPZ equivalence (48). During the past decade, controlled studies with various treatment strategies have challenged this concept.

Several treatment strategies have been used to treat acutely psychotic schizophrenic patients. These include rapid tranquilization; use of increasing high doses or initial loading dose; fixed, standard dose; and megadose therapy.

Rapid Tranquilization

This technique is also called rapid neuroleptization, digitalization, or psychotolysis (49). It is characterized by the use of the potent antipsychotics (usually haloperidol) administered parenterally, usually in large doses at frequent intervals during the acute stage of symptomatology. After the patient has improved, the dose is then lowered to standard amounts and given in oral form once or twice a day. Recent control studies have shown that, except for perhaps the first initial dose, psychotic symptoms improve at no greater speed compared with the oral, standard, fixed-dose method (50). There is some indication that clinical improvement from this method may be more of a result of the rapid sedation resulting from such aggressive treatment rather than the antipsychotic properties of the medication per se. A study by Lerner and colleagues supported this theory and showed that rapid parenteral use of diazepam produced similar results with regard to improvement of acute psychotic symptoms when compared with patients given rapid tranquilization with antipsychotics (51). An advantage of rapid tranquilization in the first few doses may be due to greater bioavailability of the antipsychotic medication (especially haloperidol) when compared with the oral form (52).

Loading Dose

In another frequently used technique, antipsychotics are started at a high oral daily dose or increased to a high oral dose during the first few days of treatment until symptoms are decreased. After that time, the dose is then tapered down to standard maintenance dose, also given orally. As in the case of rapid tranquilization, this method has shown to be no more effective in reducing psychotic symptoms during the initial stages of therapy than standard, fixed-dose strategy (53,54).

Megadose Therapy

A less frequently used technique is the megadose method. In this situation, patients are given much larger-than-standard doses of antipsychotics (over 1,000 mg of CPZ equivalence) during the initial stages of treatment. This method is especially advocated for patients refractory to standard doses. In studies of this method that employ control groups, no advantage has been substantiated (48). Understandably, the use of such high doses greatly increases the risk of side effects, especially EPS.

Fixed, Standard Dose

The fixed, standard-dose method has withstood the challenge of the previously mentioned, more aggressive strategies. This method, as the name implies, involves the use of standard doses (between 300 and 800 mg of CPZ equivalence) starting from the first day of treatment and continuing until the acute symptoms have been curtailed. Antipsychotic medication is given in oral form, one or two doses per day.

Low Dose

Recently, there has been some evidence that less-than-standard therapeutic doses of antipsychotics may be effective for the acutely psychotic patient (55). Some investigators have employed antipsychotics in the dose range of 100–300 mg of CPZ. These studies have reported improvement in many acutely psychotic patients during the initial stages of therapy, even in this dose range, which was previously felt to be below the therapeutic part of the dose–response curve.

Other Potential Strategies

During the past decade, several principles have evolved regarding the treatment of the acutely psychotic patient. First of all, acute psychosis is not necessarily synonymous with acute schizophrenic decompensation. Future clinical research will probably focus on specific subcategories of schizophrenia and other major diagnostic groups, such as manic depressive disorder, which frequently present with acute psychotic symptoms. The dose–response curve concept, which gained popularity from preliminary studies of schizophrenics has since been challenged by later studies questioning this model. Moreover, better control studies have not supported the notion that "more is better": aggressive therapy of the acutely psychotic patient with large, rapid parenteral doses of potent antipsychotics does not seem to be more effective than conservative, conventional therapy with fixed, standard oral doses. Nonetheless, because of the rapid sedating effect and greater bioavailability of parenteral use of potent antipsychotics, many patients still benefit from the rapid tranquilization technique, especially if extremely agitated behavior is present.

There are several promising research possibilities that may be helpful in future studies in the treatment of acutely psychotic patients. The ability to measure dopamine blocking effect is now available in some research laboratories. This parameter may be more useful in establishing a dose–response relationship than the previous method of using plasma levels of antipsychotics. Since many of the major antipsychotics used in clinical practice have one or more active metabolites, the use of plasma levels to correlate with clinical response could only be used with antipsychotics with either no or one active metabolite.

Recently, different techniques of brain imaging have shown promise in the research involving psychiatric patients. These include the computed tomography (CT) scan, the position emission tomography (PET) scan, and the nuclear magnetic resonance (NMR) technique. This technology could provide an anatomical and physiological method of assessing dose–response relationships in the treatment of acutely psychotic patients. Lastly, attempts are being made to assess the use of agents other than antipsychotics in the treatment of acutely ill patients. This strategy may be useful in confirming the antipsychotic effect of dopamine blocking agents such as antipsychotics or may help in identifying other properties of these medications, such as sedation, which might play a role in resolving psychotic symptoms.

LONG-ACTING ANTIPSYCHOTICS

Long-acting depot antipsychotics have been available for clinical use for the past two decades. The initial clinical trials of these agents occurred in 1968 in England. Since that time, millions of patients have been administered long-acting antipsychotics. In this country, there are three available forms of the long-acting depot neuroleptics: fluphenazine enanthate, fluphenazine decanoate, and haloperidol decanoate. Although haloperidol decanoate has been available in Europe since 1978, it has only recently been approved for use in the United States.

Initially, the advent of the injectable long-acting form of antipsychotics raised the hopes that relapse rates of chronic psychotic patients who had difficulty complying with oral medications would decrease and result in decreased frequency of both chronic and acute hospitalizations as well as improvement in the functioning of these patients. Although the initial enthusiasm has been dampened somewhat as controlled studies have failed to prove, without a doubt, that these depot agents are more effective than placebos or shorter-acting oral agents in controlling relapse, most clinicians and researchers feel that these long-acting antipsychotics are still indicated with many patients. During the past decade, more sophisticated studies on the type and frequency of adverse effects from these agents as well as their pharmacokinetics have led to a better understanding of their use in the clinical setting.

Fluphenazine hydrochloride can be converted to long-acting depot form because it has an alkyl-piperazine side chain which can be esterified with long-chain fatty acids. When this molecule is dissolved in a sesame oil vehicle, the duration of action can be increased from about 24 hours (as in the oral hydrochloride form) to one to several weeks depending on the length of the carbon side chain of the esterified form. The longer effect of the ester form is a result of the slower rate of absorption of the esterified phenothiazine from the sesame oil vehicle. In general, the parent fluphenazine is quickly released from the lipid to the aqueous phase, and it is the presence of the long, fatty acid side chain made possible by esterification that slows the rate of absorption. The enanthate form possesses a 7-carbon side chain, and the decanoate form has a 10-carbon side chain. Apparently, side chains shorter than 7 carbons or longer than 10 carbons decrease the duration of action because the rate of transfer from lipid to aqueous phases is diminished.

Animal studies have shown that fluphenazine decanoate in a sesame oil vehicle is relatively quickly taken up in secondary depots in fatty tissue throughout the body. The conjugate form cannot pass the blood–brain barrier until it is hydrolyzed to the free fluphenazine. Active metabolites of fluphenazine are not known. Hydrolysis probably occurs in the secondary depots as well as in the liver. The free fluphenazine is primarily metabolized in the liver and largely excreted in the feces with smaller amounts excreted in the urine.

Long-acting antipsychotics are indicated primarily for chronic outpatient schizophrenics who have difficulty in complying voluntarily with oral antipsychotic therapy or who do not respond sufficiently to oral agents. In most cases this group of patients has already been stabilized by either oral antipsychotics or injectable short-acting antipsychotics. Although it is recommended that schizophrenics with acute exacerbations be stabilized first before maintenance therapy with depot long-acting antipsychotics is initiated, there are some patients who can be started with long-acting antipsychotics during the acute phase if they have a history of prior response with a known dose to these agents. Patients who suffer from chronic paranoid disorders can also be candidates for maintenance therapy with long-acting antipsychotics if episodes are frequent and severe and if compliance with any oral medication is difficult.

Efficacy of Long-Acting Fluphenazine in Schizophrenia

During the past two decades, there have been several studies attempting to assess the efficacy of long-acting antipsychotics in the maintenance of chronic schizophrenics. The reader is referred to the summary article by Kane for a more elaborate critique of these studies (56). Most of the studies have compared depot fluphenazine to either oral fluphenazine, placebo, or both. The two major parameters of relapse were usually re-emergence of psychotic symptoms or rehospitalization. Some studies addressed the effect of different doses of the long-acting agents while others attempted to assess the clinical parameters other than psychotic symptoms, such as social adaptation and vocational functioning. Surprisingly, many of the studies did not show significantly different rates of relapse and rehospitalization, when long-acting antipsychotics were compared to a control group. However, as Kane points out, all of the studies reviewed, except one, were too short to be expected to demonstrate statistically significant difference. The only study that did show an advantage of the depot antipsychotics was of the longer duration, and the superiority of fluphenazine decanoate was apparent in the second year of the study. Despite this lack of convincing data in past attempts to research this issue, the long-acting antipsychotics are still considered to play an important role in preventing relapse of chronic schizophrenic outpatients who are unable to comply with an oral regime.

Adverse Effects

The most common adverse effect reported from the long-acting depot antipsychotics are the extrapyramidal symptoms (EPS), which are similar in quality to those seen with oral phenothiazines of the piperazine group. These EPS include dystonia, akathisia, and parkinsonian symptoms. Several research studies indicate that the use of depot fluphenazines produce a higher incidence of EPS than oral fluphenazine treatment. Other studies show no difference. Two issues cloud this area of research. First, these symptoms may be dose related, and it is difficult to find dose equivalence of oral and depot injectable fluphenazine.

Second, the higher incidence of EPS seen in patients receiving a depot fluphenazine may be attributed to the greater percentage of compliance with the injectable versus the oral form. Several studies indicate that the decanoate form of the long-acting fluphenazine may produce less of an incidence of EPS than the enanthate form. In most studies addressing the need for antiparkinsonian medication during the use of the long-acting fluphenazines, 50–100% of the patients require antiparkinsonian coverage whether decanoate or enanthate is administered.

Although some investigators have reported a higher incidence of tardive dyskinesia associated with the use of the long-acting depot fluphenazines, this accusation has never been definitely confirmed with long-term prospective studies. It is possible that the depot antipsychotics, because of their high potency with regard to dopamine blocking activity, have a greater tendency to produce tardive dyskinesia with long-term use. This adverse effect may be a result of the long-term use of low-dose potent antipsychotics in general, rather than a result of use of the injectable potent forms per se. Moreover, since compliance in patients prescribed long-acting injectable antipsychotics is usually greater than those taking oral antipsychotics on an outpatient basis, this variable would have to be controlled closely in any definitive study addressing this issue.

There has been some speculation that long-acting injectable depot fluphenazines may increase the risk of the neuroleptic malignant syndrome (NMS). Most cases of NMS have been associated with the use of potent antipsychotics in general, especially haloperidol and fluphenazine (oral and injectable forms). It should be noted that just about every major class of antipsychotic has been incriminated in causing NMS. The culpability of the long-acting injectable form of fluphenazine may be difficult to assess, since it cannot be eliminated from the body as rapidly as the oral medications, and thus the severity and irreversibility of NMS in patients taking long-acting fluphenazine may be related more to the pharmacokinetics of the long-acting form rather than to the agent itself.

Techniques of Using Long-Acting, Injectable Antipsychotics in Clinical Practice

Fluphenazine decanoate is more commonly used than fluphenazine enanthate in clinical practice for two major reasons. First, it is felt that the decanoate form has a longer duration of effect (2–4 weeks) than the enanthate form (1–2 weeks). Furthermore, there is an indication from the research literature that the decanoate form produces a lower incidence of EPS than the enanthate form.

Recently, some authors have stressed the importance of proper intermuscular injection technique when giving the long-acting depot fluphenazines (57). The "Z-track" technique is preferred and consists of sliding the skin to the side before the injection and then backward toward the injection site after the medicine is injected. This technique can promote optimum bioavailability by preventing loss of medication at the injection site. Subcutaneous lumps, induration, abscesses, or other complications from the injection of depot antipsychotics may be prevented with this method.

Several methods of initiation of depot antipsychotic therapy have been suggested by different authors in the acutely ill psychotic patient (58–60). This process seems to be an art which must be done empirically. For the acutely psychotic schizophrenic who has never had depot antipsychotics, most experts agree that a low dose should be used initially and increases in doses be done gradually over the first few weeks of therapy. A common starting dose is 6.25 mg, and increments of 6.25–12.5 mg are recommended every few days to a week until the patient is stabilized. Most patients respond to a dose range from 12.5 to 50 mg of decanoate. In most cases, a patient should be stabilized on oral fluphenazine HCl before the decanoate form is introduced. In other cases, where time is a factor, the depot form can be given along with the oral form until the patient responds to the depot form which can take from a few days to a few weeks, depending on the dosage requirement of the individual patient. Unfortunately, there is no convenient conversion factor to facilitate the switch from the oral fluphenazine to the decanoate depot form. Since EPS reactions require treatment with the depot form, it is imperative that patients and their families be educated with regard to the various acute reactions in order to prevent discontinuation of the medication from fear after experiencing an uncomfortable, acute adverse effect.

Since the rate of EPS is so high with depot fluphenazine, many clinicians initiate antiparkinsonian agents prophylactically when the depot form is started to prevent frightening and uncomfortable EPS. This is especially true with younger male patients who are at greater risk of experiencing violent dystonic reactions. Geriatric patients should be given lower than standard doses initially with increases in doses in a more gradual, cautious manner. For acutely psychotic patients who have a history of responding to a certain dose of the depot form, this dose can be initiated at the beginning of treatment without a trial of lower doses.

Once stabilized on a dose of fluphenazine decanoate, the patient should receive treatment every 2 weeks for at least several months. After this period of time, attempts can be made to either lower the dose or increase the amount of time between injections. Several authors feel that patients stabilized on maintenance decanoate therapy can receive their injections every 3 or 4 weeks. The clinician should never feel complacent once the patient has been stabilized. Every 6–12 months, an effort should be made to gradually taper the dose. Some investigators report that low-dose maintenance decanoate therapy (ranging from 2.5 to 5 mg) can be just as effective as standard dose ranges (25–50 mg) and provide the advantage of a decreased incidence of EPS (61). The use of "megadose" therapy consisting of 100 mg and greater is effective for certain individual refractory schizophrenic patients. This dose range has been used mostly in Europe and rarely in this country. Some clinicians recommend using standard doses of decanoate on a weekly basis for patients who do not respond to treatment given at less frequent intervals. It is felt that these patients may be rapid metabolizers who show a poor response because of low serum levels of fluphenazine when treated with standard doses at the usual 2- to 4-week interval of treatment.

The decanoate conjugate of haloperidol was released in 1986 with indications for maintenance treatment of chronic schizophrenic patients. Two studies (62, 63) have established its therapeutic efficacy in chronic schizophrenia. Zissis and colleagues (62) evaluated haloperidol decanoate in 32 stabilized chronic schizophrenic patients in a double-blind randomized placebo controlled trial. None of the 16 patients assigned to the active drug group deteriorated and 5 were considered improved, whereas 13 of the patients in the placebo group required supplemental treatment with oral haloperidol due to deterioration of their condition. In the second study (63) haloperidol decanoate was studied by a crossover open design in which patients were stabilized on haloperidol oral preparation for two weeks, maintained on a constant daily dose for two more weeks, and switched to haloperidol decanoate, which they received for five months. The authors claimed that haloperidol decanoate was comparable to oral haloperidol in alleviating symptoms of schizophrenia. It was further noted that the effective therapeutic dose range for this preparation was 9.4–15 times the daily oral dose administered at monthly intervals.

Both studies noted that the decanoate preparation was essentially equivalent to oral haloperidol in safety and patient acceptance factors. Very recent anecdotal experience suggests that this preparation may result in a lower incidence of extrapyramidal symptoms than oral or intramuscular haloperidol. This observation is still awaiting confirmation by controlled studies.

Pharmacokinetic characterization of haloperidol decanoate has indicated that peak concentrations are attained at about 6 days after injection and that the elimination half-life of this preparation is about 3 weeks. Steady-state levels are attained after about 3 dose intervals (3 months if administered once a month) (64). Nair and colleagues (63) and Nayak and colleagues (65) studied haloperidol plasma concentrations during the 4-week dosing interval. Both investigators noted similar results; generally lower plasma drug concentrations were observed during haloperidol decanoate treatment than during oral treatment of comparable efficacy.

It has been suggested that the appropriate dose of haloperidol decanoate can be obtained by multiplying the daily oral dose by 10–15 and then administering that dose in milligrams of haloperidol decanoate at monthly intervals. An alternative is to begin with a low starting dose, usually 50 mg per month, and titrate upwards as necessary. Haloperidol oral preparation can then be used if the initial starting dose proves too low and additional medication is required. The usual maintenance dosage will lie between 50–500 mg/month (64). The technique of injection that is recommended for haloperidol decanoate is the same as the Z-track technique recommended above for fluphenazine decanoate and enanthate.

Reasons for Choice of Antipsychotics

Although all antipsychotic preparations are equal in clinical efficacy, there are reasons to choose one agent over another. Several variables need to be considered in making this choice. In general, the clinician should use an antipsychotic with which he or she is most familiar. Experience with a few of the major families of antipsychotics enables one to recognize adverse effects and manipulate dosages with greater confidence. It is usually recommended that one learn to use at least two antipsychotics in different ranges of potencies (high potency, mid potency, low potency). Furthermore, it is useful to be familiar with at least two antipsychotics outside of the phenothiazine family in case the patient is allergic to this family of antipsychotics. If the patient has a history of treatment with antipsychotics, its success or failure may prove to be a useful guide to the present treatment. Family history of response to antipsychotic treatment can also be useful in the choice of antipsychotics in a particular patient.

It is also helpful to consider the patient's personality style, especially with regard to medication compliance and interactions with health care professionals. A persistent history of irresponsibility or difficulty following treatment plans can predict future noncompliance on an oral regime, and long-acting depot antipsychotics might be preferable with this type of patient. Some patients who have been treated with several different antipsychotics in the past may have already developed preferences to one agent, and their requests should be respected because, although the physician may prefer another agent, patients will often sabotage treatment in order to get the medication of their choice. In some instances the patient's aversion to one antipsychotic may be based on erroneous conclusions about side effects or clinical folklore. In this situation the clinician may wish to make an attempt to re-educate the patient if another antipsychotic drug is preferable. Unless there is some strong contraindication for the patient's choice, it is probably best to respond to his or her request since antipsychotics are interchangeable in efficacy, and the clinician may risk alienating the patient by pursuing the change with excessive zeal.

The rate and form of administration can also be an important factor in choosing an antipsychotic. For example, parenteral haloperidol has been well studied in the use of acutely agitated psychotic patients. It is considered to be quite safe when given in this form. Higher doses can also be given since it is a potent antipsychotic. Chlorpromazine has also been given intramuscularly (IM) to acutely agitated patients, but large doses can cause postural hypotension and occasional serious arrythmias when given as injections. Thioridazine cannot be given parenterally. Sometimes oral liquid antipsychotics are indicated in patients who refuse injections but in whom rapid absorption is required. This form of administration is also given to patients suspected of "cheeking" their medications. Some liquid forms of antipsychotics such as chlorpromazine are tolerated poorly because of the taste.

In some patients, the sedating property of an antipsychotic becomes an issue. Acutely psychotic patients who need prompt relief of agitation for their own safety and those staff involved in their care probably should be given more sedating antipsychotics. Withdrawn patients with decreased psychomotor activity and social interaction may be candidates for nonsedating antipsychotics.

The presence of medical problems in psychotic patients is another consideration in choosing an antipsychotic drug. For example, if the patient is significantly dehydrated, CPZ or thioridazine may not be the best choice because of the potential of aggravating postural hypotension. Antipsychotics high in anticholinergic properties should be used cautiously in patients with angle closure glaucoma or prostatic hypertrophy.

If the patient is taking other medications, this may also play a role in the choice of antipsychotic agents. For example, if a patient is already being prescribed an agent with anticholinergic properties, it would be prudent to avoid antipsychotics with similar anticholinergic affects. In this situation, even a potent antipsychotic may be contraindicated if the patient will require anticholinergic coverage for adverse effects. Some patients with cardiac problems may be taking medications that have postural hypotension as an adverse affect. The use of sedating nonpotent antipsychotics should be avoided in patients who are already on other central nervous system (CNS) depressants.

The age of the patient can be an important influence on the choice of an antipsychotic agent. Younger patients, especially males, seem to be a greater risk to developing severe acute EPS, especially dystonic reactions from potent antipsychotics. Although these symptoms can frequently be controlled by anticholinergic agents, the clinician may wish to avoid even the possibility of such a reaction if the discomfort will produce a strong aversion to antipsychotics in general. Also, in young males, antipsychotics that have a higher frequency of causing sexual dysfunction should probably be avoided. Some older patients tolerate EPS rather poorly and probably should be tried on low-potent agents initially. Anticholinergic adverse affects may be more dangerous in some elderly patients because of the risk of such adverse effects as urinary retention, constipation, and postural hypotension. In this age group, mid-potency neuroleptics, such as thiothixene or perphenazine, may be preferable.

Other miscellaneous factors in choosing an antipsychotic include: differential cost of different agents, presence of a particular antipsychotic on a mandated formulary, size of the pill (in the elderly patient), or the availability of "new generation" antipsychotics for the patients who have strong preferences for the most recent drugs on the market.

In general, the factors listed above make the choice of antipsychotics somewhat more complex than expected for a class of medications that are no different in producing the desired clinical effect. In most situations, an antipsychotic is chosen to avoid certain adverse affects. However, the clinician must be aware of other clinical factors listed that may make a significant difference in successful treatment with antipsychotic medications.

REFERENCES

1. Holley, F. O., Magliozzi, J. R., Stanski, D. R., Lombrozo, L., and Hollister, L. E. (1983). Haloperidol kinetics after oral and intravenous doses. *Clinical Pharmacology and Therapeutics* 33:477–484.
2. Richelson, E. (1984). Neuroleptic affinities for human brain receptors and their use in predicting adverse effects. *Journal of Clinical Psychiatry* 45:331–336.
3. Davis, J. M. (1976). Recent developments in the drug treatment of schizophrenia. *American Journal of Psychiatry* 133:208–214.
4. Hollister, L. E. (1973). *Clinical Use of Psychotherapeutic Drugs.* Springfield, IL: Charles C Thomas, 13–55.
5. Davis, J. M. (1976). Comparative doses and costs of antipsychotic medication. *Archives of General Psychiatry* 33:858–861.
6. Hollister, L. E. (1976). Psychiatric disorders. In *Drug Treatment*, ed. G. S. Avery, p. 808. Seaforth, Australia: ADIS Press.
7. Andreason, N. C. (1982). Negative symptoms in schizophrenia: definition and reliability. *Archives of General Psychiatry* 39:784–788.
8. Crow, T. J. (1980). Positive and negative schizophrenic symptoms and the role of dopamine. *British Journal of Psychiatry* 137:383–386.
9. Crow, T. J. (1980). Molecular pathology of schizophrenia: more than one disease process? *British Medical Journal* 280:66–68.
10. Itil, T. M., Keskiner, A., and Fink, M. (1966). Therapeutic studies in "therapy-resistant" schizophrenic patients. *Comprehensive Psychiatry* 7:488–493.
11. Angrist, B., Rotrosen, J., and Gershon, S. (1980). Differential effects of amphetamine and neuroleptics on negative vs. positive symptoms in schizophrenia. *Psychopharmacology* (Berlin) 72:17–19.

12. Johnstone, E. C., Crow, T. J., Frith, C. D., et al. (1978). Mechanism of the antipsychotic effect in the treatment of acute schizophrenia. *Lancet* 1:848-851.
13. Csernansky, J. G., Lombrozo, L., Gulevich, G. D., and Hollister, L. E. (1984). Treatment of negative schizophrenic symptoms with alprazolam: a preliminary open-label study. *Journal of Clinical Psychopharmacology* 4:349-352.
14. NIMH-PSC Collaborative Study Group. (1964). Phenothiazine treatment in acute schizophrenia. *Archives of General Psychiatry* 10:528-533.
15. Branchey, M. H., Lee, J. H., Amin, R., and Simpson, G. M. (1978). High- and low-potency neuroleptics in elderly psychiatric patients. *Journal of the American Medical Association* 239:1860-1862.
16. Hollister, L. E. (1980). Transient psychoses and personality disorders. Presented at the 133rd Annual Meeting of the American Psychiatric Association, San Francisco.
17. Gunderson, J. G. (1980). Psychotic regressions in borderline patients. Presented at the 133rd Annual Meeting of the American Psychiatric Association, San Francisco.
18. Shopsin, B., Gershon, S., Thompson, H., and Collins, P. (1975). Psychoactive drugs in mania. *Archives of General Psychiatry* 32:34-42.
19. Lerer, B. (1985). Alternative therapies for bipolar disorder. *Journal of Clinical Psychiatry* 46:309-316.
20. Spiker, D. G., Weiss, J. C., Dealy, R. S., et al. (1985). The pharmacological treatment of delusional depression. *American Journal of Psychiatry* 142:430-436.
21. Gelenberg, A. J. (1976). The catatonic syndrome. *Lancet* 1339-1341.
22. Abrams, R., and Taylor, M. A. (1976). Catatonia: A prospective clinical study. *Archives of General Psychiatry* 33:579-581.
23. Schaffer, C. B., Campbell, R., and Tupin, J. P. (1984). Assessment and treatment of the catatonic patient. In *Transient Psychosis*, ed. J. P. Tupin, U. Halbreich, and J. J. Pena, p. 265. New York: Brunner/Mazel.
24. Lindsay, P., and Wyckoff, M. (1981). The depression-pain syndrome and its response to antidepressants. *Psychomatics* 22:571-577.
25. Sigwald, J., Herbert, H., and Quetin, A. (1957). Traitment du zone et des aigies zosteriennes—ainsi que de certaines aigies rebelles—par les phenothiazines. *Semaine des Hopitaux de Paris* 33:1137-1139.
26. Hakkarainen, H. (1977). Fluphenazine for tension headache: a double-blind study. *Headache* 17:216-218.
27. Caviness, V. S., and O'Brian, P. (1980). Cluster headache: response to chlorpromazine. *Headache* 22:128-131.
28. Shapiro, A. K., Shapiro, E., Brunn, R. D., and Sweet, R. D. (1978). *Gilles de la Tourette Syndrome*. New York: Raven Press.
29. Shapiro, A. K., and Shapiro, E. (1981). The treatment and etiology of tics and Tourette syndrome. *Comprehensive Psychiatry* 22:193-205.
30. Brockington, I. F., Cernik, K. F., Schofield, E. M., et al. (1981). Puerperal psychosis. *Archives of General Psychiatry* 38:829-833.
31. Cassem, N. H., and Sos, J. (1978). Intravenous use of haloperidol for acute delirium in intensive care settings. Presented at the 131st Annual Meeting of the American Psychiatric Association, Atlanta, May.

32. Dudley, D. L., Rowlett, D. B., and Loebel, P. J. (1979). Emergency use of intravenous haloperidol. *General Hospital Psychiatry* 3:240–247.
33. Rifkin, A., Quitkin, F., Kane, J., et al. (1978). Are prophylactic anti-Parkinsonian drugs necessary? A controlled study of procyclidine withdrawal. *Archives of General Psychiatry* 35:483–489.
34. Simpson, D. M., and Davis, G. C. (1984). Case report of neuroleptic malignant syndrome associated with withdrawal from amantadine. *American Journal of Psychiatry* 141:796–797.
35. Zubenko, G., and Pope, H. G., Jr. (1983). Management of a case of neuroleptic malignant syndrome with bromocriptine. *American Journal of Psychiatry* 140:1619–1620.
36. VanPutten, T. (1975). The many faces of akathisia. *Comprehensive Psychiatry* 16:43–47.
37. Mueller, P. S. (1985). Neuroleptic malignant syndrome. *Psychomatics* 16:654–662.
38. American Psychiatric Association Task Force on Late Neurological Effects of Antipsychotic Drugs. (1979). Epidemiology of tardive dyskinesia. In *APA Task Force Report #18—Tardive Dyskinesia*, pp. 43–56. Washington, DC: American Psychiatric Association.
39. Casey, D. E., and Gerlach, J. (1984). Tardive dyskinesia: management and new treatment. In *Guidelines for the Use of Psychotropic Drugs: A Clinical Handbook*, ed. C. Stancer, P. E. Garfinkel, and V. M. Rahoff, pp. 183–203. New York: SP Medical and Scientific Books.
40. Baldessarini, R. J. (1985). Clinical and epidemiologic aspects of tardive dyskinesia. *Journal of Clinical Psychiatry* 46(4, Sect. 2): 8–13.
41. American Psychiatric Association Task Force on Late Neurological Effects of Antipsychotic Drugs. (1979). Prevention and treatment. In *APA Task Force Report #18—Tardive Dyskinesia*, pp. 137–159. Washington, DC: American Psychiatric Association.
42. Hauser, L. A. (1985). Pregnancy and psychiatric drugs. *Hospital and Community Psychiatry* 36:817–818.
43. Rumeau-Roquette, C., Goujard, J., and Heul, G. (1977). Possible teratogenic effect of phenotiazines in human beings. *Teratology* 15:57–64.
44. Edlund, M. J., and Craig, T. J. (1984). Antipsychotic use and birth defects: an epidemiologic reassessment. *Comprehensive Psychiatry* 25:32–37.
45. Nurnberg, H. G., and Prudic, J. (1984). Guidelines for treatment of psychosis during pregnancy. *Hospital and Community Psychiatry* 35:67–71.
46. Baldessarini, R. J. (1985). Antipsychotic agents. In *Chemotherapy in Psychiatry*, p. 86. Cambridge, MA: Harvard University Press.
47. Pope, H. G., Jr., and Lipinski, J. F. (1978). Diagnosis in schizophrenia and manic-depressive illness: a reassessment of the specificity of schizophrenic symptoms in the light of current research. *Archives of General Psychiatry* 35:811–828.
48. Davis, J. M., Schaffer, C. B., Killian, G. A., et al. (1980). Important issues in the drug treatment of schizophrenia. *Schizophrenia Bulletin* 6:70–82.
49. Donlon, P. T., Hopkin, J., and Tupin, J. P. (1979). Overview: efficacy and safety of the rapid neuroleptization method with injectable haloperidol. *American Journal of Psychiatry* 136:273–278.

50. Donlon, P. T., Meadow, A., Tupin, J. P., and Wahba, M. (1978). High vs. standard dosage fluphenazine HCl in acute schizophrenics. *Journal of Clinical Psychiatry* 39:800–804.
51. Lerner, Y., Lwow, E., Levitan, A., et al. (1979). Acute high-dose parenteral haloperidol treatment of psychosis. *American Journal of Psychiatry* 136:1061–1064.
52. Schaffer, C. B., Shadid, A., Javaid, J., et al. (1982). Bioavailability of intramuscular vs. oral haloperidol in schizophrenic patients. *Journal of Clinical Psychopharmacology* 2:274–277.
53. Donlon, P. T., Hopkin, J., Tupin, J. P., et al. (1980). Haloperidol from acute schizophrenic patients: an evaluation of three oral regimens. *Archives of General Psychiatry* 37:691–695.
54. Ericksen, S., Hurt, S. W., and Chang, S. (1978). Haloperidol dose, plasma levels and clinical response: a double-blind study. *Psychopharmacology Bulletin* 14:15–16.
55. Cohen, B. M., Lipinski, J. F., Pope, H. G., et al. (1980). Neuroleptic blood levels and therapeutic effects. *Pharmacology* 70:191–194.
56. Kane, J. M. (1984). The use of depot neuroleptics: clinical experience in the United States. *Journal of Clinical Psychiatry* 45:5–12.
57. Kinnes, C. F. (1981). Oily injections that ooze (letter). *British Journal of Psychiatry* 138:178.
58. (1983). Doing decanoate. *Biological Therapies in Psychiatry* 6:25–26.
59. Ayd, F. J. (1978). The depot fluphenazines: twelve years' experience—an overview. In *Depot Fluphenazines: Twelve Years of Experience*, ed. F. J. Ayd, pp. 138–144. Baltimore, MD: Ayd Medical Communications.
60. Mason, A. S., and Granacher, R. P. (1980). *Clinical Handbook of Antipsychotic Drug Therapy*. New York: Brunner/Mazel, 171–181.
61. Kane, J. M., Woerner, M., and Sarantakos, S. (1986). Depot neuroleptics: a comparative review of standard, intermediate and low-dose regimens. *Journal of Clinical Psychiatry (Suppl.)* 47:30–33.
62. Zissis, N. P., Psaras, M., and Lyketsos, G. (1982). Haloperidol decanoate, a new long-acting antipsychotic in chronic schizophrenics: double-blind comparison with placebo. *Current Therapeutic Research* 31:650–655.
63. Vasavan Nair, N. P., Suranyi-Cadotte, B., Schwartz, G., et al. (1986). A clinical trial comparing intramuscular haloperidol decanoate and oral haloperidol in chronic schizophrenic patients: efficacy, safety and dosage equivalence. *Journal of Clinical Psychopharmacology* 6:30S–37S.
64. Gelenberg, A. J., ed. (1987). Haloperidol (Haldol) decanoate. *Biological Therapies in Psychiatry* 10:3.
65. Nayak, R. K., Doose, D. R., and Nair, N. P. (1987). The bioavailability and pharmacokinetics of oral and depot intramuscular haloperidol in schizophrenic patients. *Journal of Clinical Pharmacology* 27:144–150.

2

Depressive Disorders

Alan F. Schatzberg, M.D.

Depressive disorders are among the most common of psychiatric disorders with approximately 10% of the general adult population being at risk for experiencing a depressive episode in their lifetime (1). In the past three decades, the development of effective antidepressant agents has revolutionized the treatment of patients with serious depressive illnesses. Whereas, thirty years ago, the treatment of depression revolved primarily around electroconvulsive treatment (ECT) and psychoanalytically oriented psychotherapy, a wide range of alternative psychopharmacological and psychotherapeutic approaches now exists. This chapter reviews aspects of the psychopharmacological treatment of depressive disorders and develops a framework for treating both the acutely and chronically depressed patient. Emerging treatments are also discussed.

DIAGNOSIS AND CLASSIFICATION

Medical Evaluation

Obviously, a comprehensive psychiatric and medical assessment of any patient must precede any treatment decisions. Although a full discussion of diagnosis is beyond the scope of this chapter, a number of areas are worthy of brief review.

The clinician should first assess whether the patient's depression is due to or accompanied by a significant medical condition. A whole host of conditions can be associated with depressive symptoms, although the following list shows a number that are relatively more common than are others:

1. Endocrine disorders
   - thyroid disease (hypothyroid and hyperthyroid states)
   - parathyroid disease (hypoparathyroid and hyperparathyroid states)
   - adrenal disease (hypoadrenal and hyperadrenal states)
2. Neurological disorders
   - parkinsonism
   - dementia–Alzheimer's disease
   - cerebrovascular insults
   - covert seizure disorders
3. Other disorders
   - myocardial insults
   - secondary effects of chemical dependence/abuse
   - diabetes mellitus

For example, the clinician should consider thyroid disease (either hyperthyroid or hypothyroid states), presenile dementia, infectious diseases (e.g., hepatitis), parathyroid disease, diabetes mellitus, seizure disorders (typical or atypical), alcoholism, parkinsonism, and so forth.

In addition, clinicians should ascertain whether their patients are taking any medications that could result in depressive symptoms. Again, an examination of a *Physicians' Desk Reference* (PDR) reveals that many, if not most, medications can result in depressive symptoms. Here, too, are some more commonly thought of as being involved:

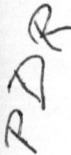

Diagnosis and Classification

1. Probable
   - catecholamine-receptor blockers: propranolol, clonidine
   - catecholamine depleters or "inhibitors": methyldopa, reserpine
   - other antihypertensives: chlorthiazide, hydrochlorthiazide
   - sedative hypnotics: barbiturates, glutethimide, and so forth
   - anesthetic/surgical procedures
2. Possible
   - oral contraceptives

Although both medical illnesses and pharmacological treatments can cause depression, most of these are relatively infrequently implicated in patients' illnesses, as seen by the psychiatrist in general practice. (Obviously, some factors—for example, alcoholism and thyroid disease—are more common.) Moreover, in many patients in whom serious medical factors play a role, the presenting picture is frequently one of fatigue and being "washed out," rather than of classic neurovegetative signs and symptoms. Still, there are some medical and neurological patients who may present with symptoms similar to the more traditional depressive, and physicians working in acute care or general hospital settings need to be particularly alert to this possibility. A review of medical symptoms should be undertaken in all patients, particularly in patients older than 50 years of age, and follow-up examinations by internists should be employed as needed.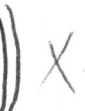

Diagnostic Standards

The classification of depressive disorders has been an area of great debate for some seventy years. Numerous classification schema have been proposed by various groups of investigators, each offering unique definitions, criteria, and so forth, and these have been reviewed elsewhere in great detail (2,3). DSM-III (4) attempted to meld a number of approaches to classification, and with its revised versions represents a major step forward in categorizing depressed patients. Principal DSM-III and III-R (5) categories of depression addressed in this chapter include: bipolar disorder (depressed phase), major depression (with or without melancholia or psychotic features), and dysthymic disorder.

Major depression and bipolar disorder, depressed phase, are discriminated on the basis of previous hypomania or mania. If present, the patient is bipolar; if not, major depression is used. The 6-month prevalence of major depression (about 3%) is some four to five times more common than is bipolar disorder (less than 1%) (6). To meet criteria for major depression, patients must have demonstrated at least five of nine symptoms for a period of at least 2 weeks: sleep disturbance, depressed mood, diminished interest, significant weight loss or gain, psychomotor retardation or agitation, guilt, suicidal ideation, fatigue, diminished ability to think or concentrate. In addition to these criteria, a patient who was to be diagnosed as bipolar must have demonstrated a 1-week period during which three of seven symptoms of mania were present, such as pressured speech, flight of ideas, decreased need for sleep, and grandiosity.

A major criticism of both DSM-III and III-R has been that the time constraints for these disorders may be too brief and the numbers of requisite symptoms too few so that patients who meet the same criteria may actually suffer from different disorders. For example, one patient who meets criteria for major depression may be typical of what others have over the years called "endogenous depression" (i.e., have classic vegetative signs); another may not. The updated DSM-III-R, (5) requires a bit more in the way of symptoms: five of nine symptoms for major depression and four of seven manic symptoms, if the patient's mood is irritable and not elated. Although this may help to tighten diagnoses, the time constraints may still be too brief.

DSM-III and III-R do define a syndrome—major depression with melancholic features—that is more akin to endogenous depression. The DSM-III-R calls for five of nine features. Additional features include: lack of significant personality problems prior to initial episode, one or more major depressive episodes followed by complete recovery, and prior good response to antidepressant therapy. In addition, DSM-III-R provides specific criteria for determining severity of major depressive and manic episodes.

Major depressed patients with delusions or other psychotic symptoms are designated as "major depression with psychotic features." Specific criteria were not detailed in DSM-III. DSM-III-R provides more detailed criteria for both mood-congruent and mood-incongruent psychotic features. Such patients generally also meet criteria for melancholia, and many investigators have used the rubric, "delusional depression" (7). Approximately 10-15% of patients with major depression may also be delusional.

Dysthymic disorder is a more chronic and milder condition than is major depression. The syndrome has a course of at least 1 year (although the patient may demonstrate brief periods of euthymia). In DSM-III, patients must also demonstrate at least four of some eleven symptoms, some of which traditionally have been associated with anxiety or nonendogenous depressive disorders, for example, irritability, anxiety, and obsessiveness. DSM-III-R calls for two of six symptoms in addition to chronic depression for at least 2 years. The 6-month prevalence of this disorder is similar to that of major depression.

TREATMENT: GENERAL PRINCIPLES

The first class of antidepressants introduced into the U.S. market were the monoamine oxidase inhibitors (MAOIs) (8,9) followed by the tricyclic antidepressants (TCAs) (10). Until the 1980s, when two 4-ringed structures—amoxapine and maprotiline—were introduced (11,12) these two classes represented the bulk of the pharmacological treatments available in the United States. Subsequently, two antidepressant compounds with radically different structures (trazodone and nomifensine) were released in the United States; however, nomifensine has recently been withdrawn by the manufacturer. There is little or no evidence that any of the new drugs are more effective overall than are the more traditional TCAs or MAOIs, although they may offer some advantages in terms of side effects, and speed of onset of action.

Traditionally, endogenous depressive syndromes (similar to major depression with melancholia) have been thought to be far more responsive to somatic treatments than are nonendogenous depressions or dysthymia. For example, in their classic review, Bielski and Friedel (13) concluded that the following symptoms predicted positive responses to TCAs: insidious onset, middle and late insomnia, psychomotor disturbances, anorexia, and weight loss. In contrast, a number of symptoms predicted poor responses: delusions, multiple prior episodes, and neurotic, hypochondriacal, and hysterical traits.

Much has been made of whether a different set of symptoms predicts differential responses to MAOIs as opposed to TCAs. A number of years ago, West and Dally (14) and Sargant (15) noted that patients with atypical symptoms, such as anxiety, hypochondriasis, obsessionality, reversed diurnal variation, respond more favorably to MAOIs than to TCAs. More recently, studies in anxious and atypical depressives point to marked interpersonal sensitivity and panic attacks as predicting MAOI, rather than TCA response (16, 17). Although anxiously depressed patients do appear to respond (preferentially) to MAOIs, many experienced physicians now believe that many patients with endogenous depressions *also* respond to MAOIs when these drugs are prescribed in sufficiently high doses (18–20). Early studies on MAOIs involved relatively low doses (e.g., 45 mg of phenelzine) (20,21).

TRICYCLIC ANTIDEPRESSANTS (TCAS) AND RELATED DRUGS

For patients with major depression without psychotic features, a trial first on TCAs seems warranted. (For delusional patients, see later section in this chapter.) Although the newer antidepressants may offer certain advantages vis-à-vis side effects, they are not more effective than the TCAs. The MAOIs are effective agents; however, the increased risk of serious untoward effects (e.g., hypertensive crises), particularly when one considers that maintenance therapy has become increasingly common, generally render them as second-line treatments.

Bipolar depressed patients also respond favorably to TCAs as well as other antidepressants. However, because of the risk of becoming hypomanic or manic, bipolar patients require simultaneous treatment with lithium carbonate or another mood stabilizer. Since lithium is an effective antidepressant in only about 50% of patients (22), a tricyclic or other antidepressant is often required in conjunction with lithium carbonate, even though some investigators recommend great caution overall in using TCAs in bipolar patients because of the possible risk of intensifying cycling.

Seven TCAs and two related 4-ring compounds are now available on the U.S. market. These agents are more similar than they are dissimilar. They all exert some effect on norepinephrine (NE) and serotonin (5-HT) reuptake although they differ in their relative NE and 5-HT effects (23) (see Table 2-1). In addition, all or virtually all antidepressants cause down-regulation of post-synaptic beta receptors. At one time, the relative NE versus 5-HT effects were invoked to explain the relative energizing versus sedating properties. Thus, desipramine would be more energizing; amitriptyline, more sedating (Table 2-1). In recent years, increasing attention has been paid to the other neurochemical receptor-blocking properties of these drugs—particularly anticholinergic and antihistaminic—and these properties may also account for both beneficial effects and side reactions. (It must be noted that 1:1 correlations do not exist between neurochemical effects and side reactions.) For example, the anticholinergic and antihistaminic (H_1) properties may both be involved in inducing sleepiness (as can be the relative serotonin effects); see Table 2-2. In addition, anticholinergic effects account for patients experiencing dry mouth, constipation, urinary hesitance, confusion, and so on. Another antihistaminic side effect is thought to be weight gain. The relative H_1 and H_2 effects suggest these drugs may produce analgesia, counteract allergic reactions, and promote healing of gastrointestinal ulcers.

The relative NE and acetylcholine (ACH) effects of these drugs largely account for their cardiovascular effects. Some patients demon-

TABLE 2-1 Relative Reuptake Blocking Effects of TCAs and Related Drugs

	NE	5-HT	DA
Desipramine	+++	±	0
Imipramine	++	+	0
Nortriptyline	++	±	0
Amitriptyline	++	++	0
Trimipramine	±	±	0
Protriptyline	++	±	0
Doxepin	+	±	0
Maprotiline	+++	0	0
Amoxapine	++	+	++[a]

Based on various studies in animals.
[a]In some patients, drug metabolism may result in formation of a neuroleptic-like metabolite with dopamine antagonist properties, potentially neutralizing DA reuptake effects of amoxapine.
Legend: +++ = Strong, ± = weak/equivocal, 0 = none.

TABLE 2-2 Relative ACH, H₁ and H₂ Receptor Blocking Effects of TCAs and Related Drugs

	ACH	H$_1$	H$_2$
Desipramine	+	0	0
Imipramine	++	±	±
Nortriptyline	+	±	±
Amitriptyline	+++	+++	++
Trimipramine	++	++	?
Protriptyline	+++	0	0
Doxepin	++	+++	+
Maprotiline	+	?	?
Amoxapine	+	?	?

Legend: +++ = Strong, ± = weak/equivocal, 0 = none, ? = unknown.

strate a tachycardia on TCAs; others may demonstrate prolonged intracardiac conduction. The latter effect can be utilized to decrease ventricular premature beats, but presents a potential problem—if not a contraindication in patients with conduction delays. TCAs and related compounds are all potentially lethal if taken in overdoses.

Clinically, the relative sedating versus activating properties are important features in drug selection. Desipramine, maprotiline, protriptyline, and amoxapine are relatively more stimulating than are amitriptyline and doxepin, which are more sedating. Imipramine, nortriptyline, and trimipramine are more intermediate in their effects, although trimipramine does appear to have a pronounced effect on inducing sleep at night.

The general rule of thumb has been to use sedating TCAs for depressed patients with pronounced anxiety, agitation, and insomnia. For the more anergic patients, it is wisest to use the more stimulating or intermediate drugs. (Nomifensine was quite stimulating and was another option, until recently; see page 59.) Generally, I begin with imipramine because of a relatively favorable side-effect profile, mild calming effect, and lack of pronounced sedative effects. In some instances where anticholinergic effects are to be particularly avoided (e.g., in older men where the prostate may be enlarged), a trial on nortriptyline or desipramine often may make the most sense.

For imipramine, beginning in adult patients with a 25-mg test dose with a repeat of one dose on day 1 is a common approach. The dose can then be increased at a rate of 25 mg every 2 days or 50 mg every 3–4 days until a daily dose of 150 mg is achieved. Since clinical responses to TCAs generally unfold over several weeks, the patient should remain at 150 mg/day for 10–14 days. Thereafter, the dosage of imipramine can be increased at a rate of 50 mg every 3–4 days until 300 mg/day is achieved. It is important to increase dosage to maximally allowable range if the patient has not responded and is tolerating the medication. Similar dosaging schedules can be used for doxepin, amitriptyline, and desipramine.

For the other drugs, dosage ranges are quite different (Table 2–3). Maprotiline, when first released, had a starting dose of 150 mg/day and a maximum dosage of 300 mg/day. Because of the number of seizures observed with aggressive dosing, the recommended dosage regimen was changed to initiation at 75 mg/day for 2 weeks with a maximum of 225 mg/day and maintenance at less than 200 mg/day. At one time, a 4-week trial was often considered adequate. Currently, most experienced clinicians and investigators recommend a 6-week trial before determining whether a given drug is effective (24).

If the patient has not responded to a 6-week trial of imipramine or similar drug, the clinician has a number of options available to him. First, he can obtain a TCA plasma level to determine whether the patient is developing adequate plasma levels. The ability to

TABLE 2–3 Starting and Therapeutic Dosages of TCAs and Related Drugs

	Starting Dose (mg/day)[a]	Therapeutic Dosage Range (mg/day)[b]
Desipramine	75	150–300
Imipramine	75	150–300
Nortriptyline	50	50–150
Amitriptyline	75	150–300
Trimipramine	75	150–300
Protriptyline	20	30–60
Doxepin	75	150–300
Maprotiline	75	150–225[b]
Amoxapine	150	150–450

[a]Some patients require lower-starting and therapeutic dosages.
[b]Maintenance dosage: 200 mg/day or less.

measure extremely low concentrations of TCAs and their metabolites (billionths of a gram per milliliter) in the laboratory opened up new vistas on determining adequacy of treatment. In the 1970s, Glassman and colleagues and Asberg and colleagues in their classic studies reported that there were relationships between imipramine/desipramine and nortriptyline levels and clinical response in patients with endogenous-type depression (25,26). For clinicians who have reliable laboratories available to them, checking a TCA level is reasonable. If the patient who has not responded by 6 weeks has a low plasma level, and side effects are not pronounced, dosages can be increased to push levels into so-called therapeutic range. If, on the other hand, the patient's plasma level is in the so-called therapeutic range at the 6-week point, the clinician can reasonably conclude that the patient is unlikely to respond to this agent. (Some individuals were reported to have responded to further increases to achieve very high plasma levels, although this is the exception rather than the rule.) Each drug has its own therapeutic range of plasma levels (for treatment of severely depressed patients) and these can be obtained from the specific laboratory employed. Of particular importance is that nortriptyline has a clear therapeutic window, that is, levels below or above the window are associated with poor responses; those within the window are associated with higher response rates. Clear therapeutic windows do not exist for the other antidepressants.

What other options are available to the treater? At one time, it was common to switch a patient from one TCA to another, usually from a relatively more serotoninergic agent (e.g., amitriptyline) to a more noradrenergic compound (e.g., desipramine). This approach was based largely on the hypothesis that there were two major biological types of depression: a low NE and a low 5-HT depression (27). Our experience with this approach has not been favorable. It is our current opinion that if a patient has tolerated an adequate trial of a TCA, switching to another TCA is unlikely to be fruitful since there is too wide an overlap in biochemical effects among these drugs to offer much hope that such a manuever will promote a response.

Instead, the clinician should consider a number of other options. The addition of 25–50 µg of L-triiodothyronine may bring out a clinical response to a TCA within 7–10 days (28). Another option has been the addition of relatively low doses (900–1200 mg/day) of lithium carbonate which may bring out a clinical response within 7–

14 days (29,30). If a patient responds to the addition of either of these, maintaining the dosage of either the lithium or the thyroid preparation for at least 2 months seems quite reasonable. Thereafter, the added agent may be tapered and the patient maintained on the original drug if possible. Should symptoms re-emerge, the adjunctive therapy should be restarted.

If such adjunctive agents fail, clinicians should begin to taper the TCA and consider switching to another class of antidepressant. Tapering is important to avoid an "acetylcholine-rebound" syndrome, characterized by such symptoms as marked nausea, vomiting, shakiness, and headaches (31). Some patients who abruptly stop their antidepressants may also become hypomanic or manic (32).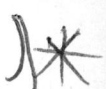

Which class of antidepressant should one switch to? Here there are some general rules of thumb. If the patient demonstrates anergia and marked psychomotor retardation, nomifensine—if and when available—may be effective. Another option is the MAOI tranylcypromine. For the more anxious, insomniac, and perhaps more mildly depressed patient, trazodone is a good choice. If the patient demonstrates anxiety, agitation, and even pronounced depression with vegetative signs, MAOIs (particularly phenelzine) should also be considered.

NOMIFENSINE

Although recently released in the United States, Nomifensine is no longer manufactured here. It had been on the market in West Germany for many years and had been available in Canada for the past few years. The drug differed from the TCAs both in its quinolone structure and in its having a pronounced effect on dopamine reuptake as well as being a potent norepinephrine reuptake blocker (Table 2–4). It had been touted as being particularly effective in the more anergic and psychomotor retarded patients and our experience had been favorable in such patients.

Available in 50-mg capsules, the recommended starting dose was 100 mg/day with increases to 200–250 mg/day. The drug had an extremely short half-life (2 hours) but could be given once daily, suggesting that it has active metabolites. Although one might expect rather prompt responses to this agent (similar to amphetamines), studies in the United States pointed to a response pattern parallel to the more traditional TCAs (33). Occasional patients would show

TABLE 2–4 Relative Reuptake Blocking Effects
of Newer Non-TCA Agents

	NE	5-HT	DA
Nomifensine	++	0	++
Trazodone	0	+	0
Fluoxetine	0	+++	0
Bupropion	0	0	+

Legend: +++ = Strong, ± = weak/equivocal, 0 = none.

some increases in energy within 7–10 days, but fuller responses would generally unfold over 2–4 weeks.

The drug offered a number of advantages. It exerted little or no anticholinergic effects, making it relatively tolerable to most patients. In addition, the drug appeared much safer than TCAs in the case of overdoses. As with all psychotropic medications, there were potential problems. Since the drug was often stimulating, the manufacturer recommended that patients not take the drug after 3 P.M. More importantly, the drug was associated with hyperpyrexic, flu-like allergic responses, which generally abated with cessation of the drug. The exact prevalence of this response was unclear; however, in our limited experience to date, as many as 10% of patients may have demonstrated this reaction. We had not observed serious sequelae to this reaction. Some patients, particularly in Great Britain, developed hemolytic anemias and eventually died, resulting in the manufacturer withdrawing the drug worldwide.

TRAZODONE

Trazodone, a multiringed complex structure with a complicated and mixed pharmacology, exerts little NE reuptake blocking effect but is thought to possibly act via serotonergic systems, blocking reuptake of serotonin (5-HT) in the brain (Table 2–4). Its central 5-HT effect is weaker than that of the specific 5-HT reuptake blockers. Peripherally, however, it appears to act as a serotonin antagonist and may act as a central antagonist as well. The drug is a potent hypnotic and is also calming when taken during the day. Its efficacy as an antidepressant in the more endogenously depressed patient has at times been questioned, and generally we recommend it for the more anxious, insomniac patient with or without pronounced vegetative symptomatology. It exerts little anticholinergic side effects and is also relatively safe in overdosages. The drug does produce dry mouth, presumably via an NE effect.

At one time, trazodone was purported to not induce manic or schizophrenic reactions. Our experience has been that the drug may be less likely to do so than the TCAs; however, we have seen patients develop such reactions on the drug.

Trazodone (Desyrel) is available in 50- and 100-mg tablets. The manufacturer recommends beginning at 150 mg/day with increases to a maximum of 600 mg/day. Our experience has been that most patients cannot tolerate starting at 150 mg/day because they frequently experience pronounced sedation. Rather, we recommend 50 mg at bedtime on day 1 with increases to 150 mg/day over a 5- to 7-day period. In our hands, patients rarely require over 300 mg/day. Indeed, most of our patients do far better on relatively lower doses (less than 250 mg/day) than they do on higher doses (more than 400 mg/day). Some investigators have postulated that the drug may have a therapeutic window, that is, an optimal range of blood levels, below or above which patients do relatively poorly. Studies on blood levels have, however, failed to demonstrate a clear therapeutic range or so-called window.

Although generally well tolerated, trazodone can pose a number of potential difficulties. When taken on an empty stomach, particularly in large dosages, the drug may produce acute drops in blood pressure with dizziness, fainting, and, at times, nausea. Thus, patients need to be counseled to take the medication on a full stomach. In addition, in our experience, the drug may be somewhat more commonly associated with headaches than are TCAs. Last, there have been a number of reports of serious priapism on this medication, and men should be warned to stop the drug immediately if this side reaction occurs. Although the prevalence of this reaction is fortunately low, it is so potentially problematic when it does occur that clinicians and patients should be on guard. Surgical intervention has been required for a few patients with priapism. The reaction can be relieved immediately by intrapenile injection of adrenergic agonists.

MONOAMINE OXIDASE INHIBITORS (MAOIs)

MAOIs were originally discovered by serendipity when iproniazid was found to elevate mood in patients with tuberculosis. These drugs, from their earliest use, have been thought particularly effective in depressed patients with pronounced anxiety or with atypical features [e.g., reversed diurnal variation (14,15)]. More recently, as listed above, clinicians and investigators have re-emphasized their use in endogenous or melancholic depressives, particularly when prescribed in sufficiently high dosages (18,20).

There are currently three MAOIs that enjoy "approved" indications in the United States for the treatment of depression. Two are nonhydrazine in structure (phenelzine and isocarboxazid) and one (tranylcypromine) is a hydrazine derivative. Tranylcypromine is more similar to d-amphetamine than the other two and has more in the way of stimulant properties. It thus may offer some advantage in the more retarded patient.

Starting doses of the three compounds are: tranylcypromine, 20 mg; isocarboxazid, 30 mg; and phenelzine, 45 mg. Gradual titration upward is reasonable to approximate maximal dosages: tranylcypromine, 40–60 mg; isocarboxazid, 40–50 mg; and phenelzine, 90 mg. The PDR recommended maximum dose of isocarboxazid (30 mg) is the same as its recommended starting dose, and this is probably erroneous. There is less known about the "true" dosage range of isocarboxazid since this drug has been used less frequently in clinical practice than the others. The response to MAOIs is, if anything, slower than with other medications, with patients frequently requiring 4–6 weeks to respond.

Plasma levels of MAOIs are not available for routine clinical use. In some settings, platelet MAO activity levels may be determined before and during treatment to assess adequacy of treatment. Several years ago, Robinson and colleagues (34) reported that response to treatment with phenelzine was associated with an 80% reduction in platelet MAO activity. Similar findings have been reported for isocarboxazid (35) but not for tranylcypromine which produces marked inhibition of activity at relatively low dosages.

For patients who do not respond fully to an MAOI, the addition of lithium carbonate may be helpful. There are several reports in the literature that the combination of lithium carbonate with an

MAOI is frequently effective, particularly in refractory or "atypical" patients with hyperphagia and hypersomnia (36).

Common side effects with these drugs include insomnia, daytime sedation (perhaps related to insomnia), orthostatic hypotension, anorgasmia, myalgia/myositis, constipation, weight gain, and dry mouth. Of particular importance in using MAOIs are untoward interactions with certain foodstuffs and medications, resulting in hypertensive and hyperpyrexic reactions. Medications to be avoided include meperidine, sympathomimetic decongestants, antihistamines (particularly long-acting preparations and those containing sympathomimetics), as well as local anesthetics containing sympathomimetics.

In spite of the concern for such reactions as foodstuffs, there is considerable reason to believe that the list of proscribed foods that appears in the package inserts is too inclusive. More recently, a number of investigators have argued that many foods can in fact be ingested in usual or in moderate amounts by patients taking MAOIs with little risk of untoward interactions. For example, in reviewing the literature, McCabe and Tsuang (37) concluded that chocolate, sour cream, and yogurt could probably be ingested in small-to-moderate amounts with little risk of interactions. Dietary preparations produced through the aging process are to be particularly avoided, for example, red wine, beer, sausage, liver, aged cheeses, and pickled herring.

The use of TCAs with MAOIs has been another area of controversy for many years. Many clinicians have advocated the combination in refractory patients. To date, there is little evidence that the combination is more effective than using either of its components alone (38). However, most studies have used relatively low dosages of a TCA and an MAOI, so that one cannot rule out that combining higher dosages of both could prove more effective. Interestingly, the combination of TCAs and MAOIs does not appear to be more dangerous, that is, hypertensive crises are not more common with the combination than with MAOIs alone. In fact, the use of a tricyclic may protect patients from hypertensive crises resulting from interactions with foods. Moreover, recent experience suggests that low doses of the stimulants (starting at 2.5 mg/day) methylphenidate and amphetamine can be added to an MAOI or to a TCA/MAOI combination without untoward effects (39). Although this approach is somewhat counterintuitive in view of a general proscription of sympathomimetics with MAOIs, this strategy has been recommended as a possible way of dealing with orthostatic hypotension produced by the MAOI or the TCA/MAOI combination or of bringing out a clinical response. Maximum doses of methylphenidate or amphetamine should not exceed approximately 15 mg/day when given with MAOIs (39).

INVESTIGATIONAL DRUGS

Serotonin (5-HT) Reuptake Blockers

Rapidly nearing release in the United States are the 5-HT reuptake blockers. Zimelidine, for example, was extensively studied in the United States and Europe a number of years ago. However, the emergence of serious side reactions resulted in the drug being withdrawn both here and abroad. At least three compounds, fluoxetine, fluvoxamine, and setraline, are currently being studied in the United States. Of these, fluoxetine appears to be furthest along in its development.

In recent years, there has been renewed interest in the United States in 5-HT as a key neurotransmitter in the pathophysiology of depressive disorders. More than 15 years ago, British investigators were arguing that 5-HT played a key role in depression while Americans emphasized NE. Although this debate is likely to continue, recent studies do point to an important role for 5-HT. Most notably, imipramine binding sites in blood components also bind to 5-HT, and reuptake of 5-HT in platelets has been reported to be low in depressed patients (40). Further, low cerebrospinal fluid (CSF) levels of 5-hydroxyindoleacetic acid (5-HIAA) have been associated with an increased risk for suicide (41). These findings suggest that low serotinergic activity may be involved in some depressed patients. Understandably, 5-HT reuptake blockers could prove particularly effective in some depressed patients.

In contrast to TCAs, fluoxetine exerts little or no effect on noradrenergic or dopaminergic reuptake. Instead, it is a potent blocker of 5-HT reuptake (Table 2-4). In addition, the drug does not block NE, dopamine, ACH or histamine. Recent reports suggest it may weakly block some 5-HT receptors.

Fluoxetine has been shown to be as effective as TCAs in the treatment of major depression (42). Studies indicate that there is a strong positive correlation between fluoxetine plasma level and 5-HT reuptake blockade in humans (43). Still, as with other antidepressants, the drug is effective in only some 70–80% of patients, suggesting the 5-HT story may not be the complete answer to the biology of depression question.

The drug appears to have a relatively favorable side-effect profile. Principal side effects include nausea, tremor, sweating, dyspepsia, and drowsiness. However, the prevalence of many of these side effects appears relatively low (44), and overall the drug appears to be better tolerated than are the TCAs. Of particular importance is the absence of anticholinergic side effects and prominent weight gain on drug. In fact, many patients lose weight on the drug.

The starting dose of fluoxetine is 20 mg/day and when released, maintenance of the starting dose for 3 weeks will be recommended. Thereafter, dose can be increased to 60–80 mg/day. Most patients will respond to 20 mg/day, although, some will require higher doses. It can be given once a day or in divided (b.i.d.) doses. Maintenance studies indicate the drug is both effective and well-tolerated (45). Obviously, the full scope of efficacy and potential untoward effects cannot be determined until the drug is in widespread clinical use; however, this class of drugs may represent the next important breakthrough in the treatment of depression.

Bupropion

Bupropion has been well studied in this country and was about to be released when it was taken out of production by the U.S. FDA because of seizures in bulimic patients. It appears effective in patients with major depression and continues to have research programs associated with it (46). Its mode of action is unclear; it does not block the reuptake of NE and 5-HT, although it does block the reuptake of dopamine (Table 2–4). This has, at times, been inferred to be the mechanism of action; however, this effect occurs only at high dosages and high plasma levels. Indeed, the dopaminergic effects may relate more to side effects than to clinical response.

The drug is produced in 75-mg tablets and the recommended starting dose is 150–225 mg/day with the usual therapeutic dose being 300–450 mg/day. Side effects are mild. Some patients complain of headaches, and occasional seizures have been reported in depressed patients. A large-scale study on the prevalence of seizures in bupropion is currently being planned.

Of particular interest is the potential use of the drug to stabilize cycling manic-depressive patients. A number of investigators have reported favorable results in preventing recurrences in patients with rapid-cycling disorders (47,48), an interesting observation worthy of further study.

PSYCHOTIC (DELUSIONAL) DEPRESSION

In recent years, increasing attention has been given to delusional depression, a severe depressive subtype with increased morbidity and increased risk for suicide. A number of studies have indicated that delusional (or psychotic) depressives respond less favorably to TCAs than do their nondelusional counterparts (26,49,50). Instead, delusional depressives respond to combined tricyclic-neuroleptic treatment or to ECT (51,52).

For example, Spiker and colleagues reported that a combination of perphenazine and amitriptyline was superior to either drug given alone in psychotic depressives. These two drugs were relatively ineffective when given individually (51). Daily dosages of both drugs appeared to be quite adequate (approximately 64 mg of perphenazine and 250 mg amitriptyline), and the greater efficacy did not appear to be due to perphenazine causing a relative increase in plasma levels of amitriptyline. In treating a delusionally depressed patient, the clinician must choose between ECT and combined treatment. If the latter is tried and fails to produce a response, the addition of lithium carbonate may facilitate a response (53).

The additive beneficial effects of antipsychotics in the treatment of this disorder suggest a possible role for dopamine in the condition. Recently, our group has hypothesized that corticosteroid–dopamine interactions may play a role in the disorder (54). Briefly, delusional depressives have markedly elevated cortisol activity (55). Our group and others have also reported that the acute administration of dexamethasone in humans significantly increases plasma-free dopamine and homovanillic acid (HVA) levels in normal control subjects (56,57). Moreover, dexamethasone and corticosteroids increase dopamine levels in the brains of rats and other species (58,59). These various findings have led us to hypothesize that the marked hypercortisolemia observed in deluded depressives could play a role in increasing brain dopamine activity and in leading to the development of delusional thinking. At any rate, these findings all suggest that enhanced steroidal and dopamine activity could be key factors in deluded depressives and may ultimately explain the need for combined neuroleptic-antidepressant treatment.

TREATMENT-RESISTANT DEPRESSION

Fortunately, most depressed patients respond to treatment with antidepressant medications. However, a substantial number (some 20%) do not. At one time, it was common to ascribe a failure to respond to an underlying neurotic or personality disorder, but it has become quite apparent that some endogenously depressed patients also fail to respond to medication and may become chronic.

In evaluating any depressed patient who has failed to respond, it is important to reassess the patient's clinical presentation, course, specific responses to specific treatments (dosage, duration, etc.) as well as his/her medical and neurological condition. We have already described our experience with patients who had previously failed to respond to antidepressant treatment (18,60). Two important factors that contributed to nonresponse were inadequate treatment (low dosages prescribed for too brief periods) and intolerance to antidepressants, particularly with TCAs, which often resulted in inadequate trials. The latter factor is often unappreciated. Some patients have great difficulty tolerating the stimulating, agitating, or anticholinergic effects of the TCAs. For such patients, MAOIs or the addition of lithium carbonate may be particularly helpful.

More recently we have become impressed that some refractory depressives may not have primary depression but rather a variant of temporal lobe epilepsy of dysfunction. Himmelhoch (61) has reported that some 10% of chronically depressed patients in his affective disorder clinic suffer from a variant of temporal lobe epilepsy. Our experience has been that some chronic depressives complain of periods of confusion, episodic dysphoria, and perceptual distortion (micropsia, depersonalization, etc.). Such patients often have normal routine electroencephalographic (EEG) studies but abnormal computer-enhanced spectral studies (62). We have found that carbamazepine and valproic acid may be helpful in these patients, either alone or in combination with more traditional antidepressant drugs. At any rate, the clinician should be alert to alternative diagnoses in evaluating chronic and atypical patients.

REFERENCES

1. Robins, L. N., Helzer, J. E., Weissman, M. M., et al. (1984). Lifetime prevalence of specific psychiatric disorders in three sites. *Archives of General Psychiatry* 41:949–958.
2. Schatzberg, A. F. (1978). Classification of depressive disorders. In *Depression: Biology, Psychodynamics and Treatment*, ed. J. O. Cole, A. F. Schatzberg, and S. H. Frazier. New York: Plenum.
3. Schatzberg, A. F. (1984). Classification of affective disorders. In *The Brain, Biochemistry, and Behavior. Proceedings of the Sixth Arnold O. Beckman Conference in Clinical Chemistry*, ed. R. L. Habig. Washington, DC: American Association for Clinical Chemistry.
4. *Diagnostic and Statistical Manual of Mental Disorders*, 3rd ed. (1980). Washington, DC: American Psychiatric Association.
5. *Diagnostic and Statistical Manual of Mental Disorders*, rev. 3rd ed. (1987). Washington, DC: American Psychiatric Association.
6. Myers, J. K., Weissman, M. M., Tischler, G. L., et al. (1984). Six-month prevalence of psychiatric disorders in three communities. *Archives of General Psychiatry* 41:959–967.
7. Charney, D. S., and Nelson, J. C. (1981). Delusional and nondelusional unipolar depression: further evidence for distinct subtypes. *American Journal of Psychiatry* 138:328–333.
8. Kline, N. S. (1958). Clinical experience with iproniazid (marsilid). *Journal of Clinical and Experimental Psychopathology* 19:72–78.
9. Crane, G. E. (1957). Iproniazid (marsilid) phosphate: a therapeutic agent for mental disorders and debilitating diseases. *Psychiatric Research Reports* 8:142–152.
10. Kuhn, R. (1957). Uber die benhandlung depressiver zustande mit einem iminodibenzylderivat (G22355). Schweizer Medizinische Wochenschruft. *Journal Suisse de Medecine* 87:1135–1140.
11. Schatzberg, A. F., and Cole, J. O. (1984). Biochemical and pharmacologic properties of maprotiline: a selective norepinephrine uptake inhibitor. *Journal of Clinical Psychiatry Monograph Series* (5):7–11.
12. Ayd, F. (1980). Amoxapine: A new tricyclic antidepressant. *International Drug Therapy Newsletter* 15:33–40.
13. Bielski, R. J., and Friedel, R. O. (1976). Prediction of tricyclic antidepressant response: a critical review. *Archives of General Psychiatry* 33:1479–1489.
14. West, E. D., and Dally, P. J. (1959). Effects of iproniazid in depressive syndromes. *British Medical Journal* 1:1491.
15. Sargant, W. (1962). The treatment of anxiety states and atypical depressions by

the monoamine oxidase inhibitor drugs. *Journal of Neuropsychiatry* 3(Suppl. 1):96–103.
16. Liebowitz, M. R., Quitkin, F. M., Stewart, J. W., et al. (1984). Phenelzine v. imipramine in atypical depression. *Archives of General Psychiatry* 41:669–677.
17. Robinson, D. S., Kayser, A., Corcella, J., et al. (1983). Hyperphagia, hypersomnia, panic attacks, hysterical traits, and somatic anxiety predict phenelzine response in depressed outpatients. Presented at the Annual Meeting of the American College of Neuropsychopharmacology, San Juan, Puerto Rico, December.
18. Schatzberg, A. F., Cole, J. O., Cohen, B. M., et al. (1983). Survey of depressed patients who have failed to respond to treatment. In *The Affective Disorders*, ed. J. Davis and J. Maas. Washington, DC: American Psychiatric Press.
19. McGrath, P. J., Quitkin, F. M., Harrison, W., and Stewart J. W. (1984). Treatment of melancholia with tranylcypromine. *American Journal of Psychiatry* 141:288–289.
20. Quitkin, F., Rifkin, A., and Klein, D. F. (1979). Monoamine oxidase inhibitors. *Archives of General Psychiatry* 36:749–760.
21. Spear, F. G., Hall, P., and Stirland, J. D. (1964). A comparison of subjective responses to imipramine and tranylcypromine. *British Journal of Psychiatry* 110:53–54.
22. Ramsey, T. A., and Mendels, J. (1980). Lithium in the acute treatment of depression. In *Handbook of Lithium Therapy*, ed. F. N. Johnson. Lancaster, England: MTP Press.
23. Richelson, E. (1982). The use of tricyclic antidepressants in chronic gastrointestinal pain. *Journal of Clinical Psychiatry* 43:50–55.
24. Quitkin, F. M., Rabkin, J. G., Ross, D., et al. (1984). Duration of antidepressant drug treatment: what is an adequate trial? *Archives of General Psychiatry* 41:238–245.
25. Asberg, M., Crönholm, B., Sjöqvist, F., and Tuck, D. (1971). Relationship between plasma level and therapeutic effect of nortriptyline. *British Medical Journal* 3:331–334.
26. Glassman, A. H., Perel, J. M., Shostak, M., et al. (1977). Clinical implications of imipramine plasma levels for depressive illness. *Archives of General Psychiatry* 34:197–204.
27. Maas, J. W. (1975). Biogenic amines and depression: biochemical and pharmacological separation of two types of depression. *Archives of General Psychiatry* 32:1357–1361.
28. Goodwin, F. K., Prange, A., Post, R., et al. (1982). Potention of antidepressant effects by L-triiodothyronine in tricyclic nonresponders. *American Journal of Psychiatry* 139:34–38.
29. de Montigny, C., Grunberg, F., Mayer, A., and Deschenes, J. P. (1981). Lithium induces rapid relief of depression in tricyclic antidepressant drug nonresponders. *British Journal of Psychiatry* 138:252–255.
30. de Montigny, C., Cournoyer, G., Morissette, R., et al. (1983). Lithium carbonate addition in tricyclic antidepressant-resistant unipolar depression. *Archives of General Psychiatry* 40:1327–1334.
31. Dilsaver, S. C., and Greden, F. J. Antidepressant withdrawal phenomena. *Biological Psychiatry* 19:237–256.

32. Mirin, S. M., Schatzberg, A. F., and Creasey, D. E. (1981). Hypomania and mania after tricyclic withdrawal. *American Journal of Psychiatry* 138:87–89.
33. Cohn, J. B., Varga, L., and Lyford, A. (1984). A two-center double-blind study of nomifensine, imipramine, and placebo in depressed geriatric outpatients. *Journal of Clinical Psychiatry* 45(4, Sect. 2):68–72.
34. Robinson, D. S., Nies, A., Ravaris, C. L., et al. (1973). The monoamine oxidase inhibitor, phenelzine in the treatment of depressive-anxiety states. *Archives of General Psychiatry* 29:407–413.
35. Giller, E., and Lieb, J. (1980). MAO inhibitors and platelet MAO inhibition. Presented at the Annual Meeting of the American Psychiatric Association, San Francisco, May.
36. Himmelhoch, J. M., Detre, T., Kupfer, D. J., et al. (1971). Treatment of previously intractable depressions with tranylcypromine and lithium. *Journal of Nervous and Mental Diseases* 155:216–220.
37. McCabe, B., and Tsuang, M. T. (1982). Dietary consideration in MAO inhibitor regimens. *Journal of Clinical Psychiatry* 43:178–181.
38. White, K., and Simpson, G. (1981). Combined MAOI-tricyclic antidepressant treatment: a re-evaluation. *Journal of Clinical Psychopharmacology* 1:264–282.
39. Feighner, J. P., Aden, G. C., Fabre, L. F., et al. (1983). Comparison of alprazolam, imipramine, and placebo in the treatment of depression. *Journal of the American Medical Association* 249:3056–3064.
40. Paul, S. M., Rehavi, M., Skolnick, P., et al. (1981). Depressed patients have decreased binding of tritiated imipramine to platelet serotonin "transporter." *Archives of General Psychiatry* 38:1315–1317.
41. Asberg, M., Traskman, L., and Thoren, P. (1976). 5-HIAA in the cerebrospinal fluid: a biochemical suicide predictor? *Archives of General Psychiatry* 33:1193–1197.
42. Chouinard, G. (1985). A double-blind controlled clinical trial of fluoxetine and amitriptyline in the treatment of outpatients with major depressive disorder. *Journal of Clinical Psychiatry* 46(3, Sect. 2):32–37.
43. Lemberger, L., Bergstrom, R. J., and Wolen, R. L. (1985). Fluoxetine: clinical pharmacology and physiologic disposition. *Journal of Clinical Psychiatry* 46(3, Sect. 2):14–19.
44. Stark, P., and Hardison, C. D. (1985). A review of multicenter controlled studies of fluoxetine vs. imipramine and placebo in outpatients with major depressive disorder. *Journal of Clinical Psychiatry* 43(3, Sect. 2):53–58.
45. Feighner, J. P., and Cohn, J. B. (1985). Double-blind comparative trials of fluoxetine and doxepin in geriatric patients with major depressive disorder. *Journal of Clinical Psychiatry* 46(3, Sect. 2):20–25.
46. Preskorn, S. H., and Othmer, S. C. (1984). Bupropion: a monocyclic antidepressant. *Journal of Clinical Psychiatry Monograph* 2(5):23–26.
47. Shopsin, B. (1983). Bupropion's prophylactic efficacy in bipolar affective illnesses. *Journal of Clinical Psychiatry* 44:163–169.
48. Wright, G., Galloway, L., Kim, J., et al. (1985). Bupropion in the long-term treatment of cyclic mood disorders: mood stabilizing effects. *Journal of Clinical Psychiatry* 46:22–25.

49. Frances, A., Brown, R. P., Kocsis, J. H., and Mann, J. (1981). Psychotic depression: a separate entity? *American Journal of Psychiatry* 138:831–833.
50. Hordern, A., Holt, N. F., Burt, C. G., and Gordon, W. F. (1963). Amitriptyline in depressive states: phenomenology and prognostic considerations. *British Journal of Psychiatry* 109:815–825.
51. Spiker, D. G., Hamin, I., Cofsky, J., et al. (1981). Pharmacological treatment of delusional depressives. *Psychopharmacology Bulletin* 17:201–202.
52. Monter, R. E., and Mandel, M. R. (1979). The treatment of psychotic major depressive disorder with drugs and electroconvulsive therapy. *Journal of Nervous and Mental Diseases* 167:726–733.
53. Price, L. H., Conwell, Y., and Nelson, J. C. (1983). Lithium augmentation of combined neuroleptic-tricyclic treatment in delusional depression. *American Journal of Psychiatry* 140:318–322.
54. Schatzberg, A. F., Rothschild, A. J., Langlais, P. J., et al. (1985). A corticosteroid/dopamine hypothesis of psychotic depression and related states. *Journal of Psychiatric Research* 19:57–64.
55. Schatzberg, A. F., Rothschild, A. J., Bond, T. C., and Cole, J. O. (1984). The DST in psychotic depression: diagnostic and pathophysiologic implications. *Psychopharmacology Bulletin* 20:362–364.
56. Rothschild, A. J., Langlais, P. J., Schatzberg, A. F., et al. (1984). Dexamethasone increases plasma free dopamine in man. *Journal of Psychiatric Research* 18:217–223.
57. Wolkowitz, O. M., Sutton, M. E., Doran, A. R., et al. (1985). Dexamethasone increases plasma HVA but not MHPG in normal humans. *Psychiatry Research* 16:101–109.
58. Rothschild, A. J., Langlais, P. J., Schatzberg, A. F., et al. (1985). The effects of a single acute dose of dexamethasone on monoamine and metabolite levels in rat brain. *Life Sciences* 36(26):2491–2501.
59. Iuvone, P. M., Morasco, J., and Dunn, A. J. (1977). Effect of corticosterone on the synthesis of (^{3}H)catecholamines in the brains of CD-1 mice. *Brain Research* 120:571–576.
60. Schatzberg, A. F. (1984). Evaluation and treatment of the refractory depressed patient. In *Clinical Psychopharmacology*, 2nd ed., ed. J. G. Bernstein. Littleton, MA: John Wright, PSG.
61. Himmelhoch, J. M. (1984). Major mood disorders related to epileptic changes. In *Psychiatric Aspects of Epilepsy*, ed. D. Blumer. Washington, DC: American Psychiatric Press.
62. Schatzberg, A. F., Elliott, G. R., Lerbinger, J. E., and Duffy, F. H. (1986). Topographic mapping in depressed patients. In *Topographic Mapping of Brain Electrical Activity*, ed. F. H. Duffy, pp. 389–391. Boston: Butterworth.

3

Stress, Fear, and Anxiety

Richard I. Shader, M.D.

New findings from research on anxiety states and disorders emerged at an exponential pace in the 1980s. Despite the growth in and value of these data and perspectives, the "problem of anxiety," as Freud called it in his 1926 monograph (1), is very much with us. Anxiety is a familiar, universal experience. Yet, we all know our anxiety uniquely, have our own particular strategies for coping, and even our own semantics for describing this very subjective experience: "I feel scared," says one; "I'm nervous," says another; "I'm tense," says yet another—the list is lengthy and includes such descriptors as apprehensive, fearful, anxious, uptight, and stressed out.

To assist in the task of moving forward the scientific study and treatment of anxiety states, DSM-III (1980) and, more recently, DSM-III-R diagnostic criteria were promulgated (2). In this chapter, these latter criteria are examined, along with a discussion of three interacting yet somewhat independent concepts: stress, fear, and anxiety. Ambiguity about these terms and their definitions has contributed to the confusion in solving the problem of anxiety. Working definitions are offered here, not as definitive answers to the puzzle of anxiety but rather as fertilizer to stimulate the growth of each reader's thinking. Also, briefly reviewed are selected behavioral approaches, beta blockers, benzodiazepines, buspirone, and monoamine oxidase inhibitors and antidepressants as treatments for stress, fear, and anxiety, and their dynamic interplay in patients.

The focus here is on providing a framework so that the clinician can think about these disorders. I made a deliberate decision not to provide extensive referencing, since so much of what is done to help these patients is still the art of psychopharmacology and clinical therapeutics. Hopefully, as definitions, diagnoses, and treatments evolve and become more precise and specific, a detailed chapter on how to recognize and understand these states and when and how to intervene can be written. For those readers who wish specific psychopharmacologic reviews of this topic, there are several recent publications.

Stress, fear, and anxiety are experiences and states that are at least as old as humankind. They are probably not unique to humans, although it is easier to anthropomorphize and delineate animal models for stress and fear than for anxiety. In the nineteenth and early twentieth centuries, these concepts were merged in the diagnostic entity, neurasthenia or nervous prostration. Neurasthenia was viewed as a breakdown of the nervous system, "nature's rebellion," after a period of excessive fear, arousal, overwork, or strain. It was seen as the inevitable result of the conditions of the day, both domestic and business. Such causal notions as unreasonable or excessively lofty ambitions or aspirations beyond one's mediocre abilities were frequently implicated when physicians discussed their cases. However, not all causes were seen in this light, and a hereditary nervous temperament was considered by many as an important factor.

Treatment was quite straightforward, and the "rest cure" of S. Weir Mitchell subsumed most of the ideas of the era (3). The key treatment elements were rest, sleep, change of air and scene, removal from customary associations and surroundings, the availability of cheerful and sympathetic companions, keeping regular hours, taking soothing baths, alternating massages with electrical treatments (slowly interrupted faradic currents), elimination of alcohol and tobacco, and following a good diet. Pharmacotherapy was sometimes prescribed. The usual remedy involved a nerve tonic made from extract of coca, phosphoric acid, syrup of ginger, peppermint water, and nux vomica, a potion sounding somewhat like an uncarbonated, perhaps poisonous, variant of the early formula of Coca-Cola. Nux vomica contains strychnine and was used as a heart and nerve stimulant. Neurasthenia represented the consequences and manifestations of an overstressed life.

DEFINITIONS

Stress

Stress itself is not a disorder or an affective state. It can be defined as any perturbation of, or influence on, an organism in which the rate, intensity, duration, or nature of the input temporarily strains, exceeds, or overwhelms adaptive capacities, thus disturbing homeostasis. Both positive and negative changes can produce stress. Stress is ipsetive rather than normative. What is stressful to an organism varies and depends, in part, on the state of the organism at the time of the stimulus, as well as on its appraisal of the input. One person's stressor may be another person's fun.

Fear

Fear is also a universal experience. It is apparent in the very young in response to changes in environment, the presentation of novel stimuli, the presence of unfamiliar persons or faces, or pain. Fear is an appropriate, adaptive, and normal response to perceived threats to survival and to danger. There is much individual variation in the experience of fear, both in response intensity and in the types of external and internal stimuli which elicit it. Fear has both innate and experiential determinants and most often is self-limiting, abating when the threat to safety has passed. When the danger is not overwhelming, cautious adaptation, preparation for action, and coping should follow. Learning and planning promote mastery of fear, although avoidance is perhaps the most common response.

With intense and potentially disabling fear-inducing situations, the familiar responses of "flight" or "fight" frequently come into play. Other responses are common, however, which frequently do not receive comparable attention, including "freezing" and "fragmentation." The animal who freezes to avoid danger is a familiar image (e.g., the still, crouched rabbit). This form of hiding is less familiar in humans; rather, humans seem to hide to protect their sense of self (ego) more than to protect their bodies. Freezing and fragmentation are ego-protective responses to fear and include such experiences as denial, distortion, displacement, and disconnection in various ways. A person may respond to fear as if pulling the covers over his or her head somewhat like the ostrich is alleged to do—with its head in the sand (actually, the ostrich may be putting its ear to the ground to judge the closeness of the danger). Dissociation in various forms may ensue, particularly when the danger has come from a trusted relationship.

Anxiety

Anxiety is a highly individualized disturbance of affect which is experienced subjectively (e.g., apprehension or dread) and physiologically (e.g., tachycardia, difficult breathing, muscle tension, or shakiness). It may be situational, intermittent or attack-like, or persistent. In addition to anxious or apprehensive mood and fear-like physiological signs and symptoms, patients often experience intrusive ideations (e.g., images, ruminations, impulses, or dreams), vigilance or trouble concentrating, or an altered awareness of the self or environment (e.g., depersonalization or derealization).

Although anxiety involves emotional and physiological experiences similar to those felt during fear, in anxiety the threat to survival is either not apparent or the response to the perceived danger is disproportionate to the intensity of the stimulus. Anxiety may also be a conditioned response in which the linkages to the original stimulus or situation are now suppressed, repressed, forgotten, or lost.

As the reader can discern from these working (and evolving) definitions of stress, fear, and anxiety, the three concepts, while distinct from one another, are interactive in life. For example, the anxious person may become stressed by anxiety, the fearful person may become anxious or stressed, or anxiety could be more intense in the person under stress.

As defined, it is highly unlikely that any one of us has not experienced stress, fear, and anxiety at one time or another. For some, however, anxiety becomes an overwhelming condition, which is sometimes situational, sometimes recurrent, sometimes attack-like, and sometimes chronic. The following section reviews selected anxiety states of pathological proportions.

SOME DSM-III-R ANXIETY DISORDERS

Generalized Anxiety Disorder

The current DSM-III-R criteria for a number of important anxiety disorders are listed in the following tables. Those who are familiar with DSM-III (1980) will note that a major change for generalized anxiety disorder (GAD) is the lengthening of the time required from 1 month of continuous or persistent symptomatology to 6 months in which the patient has been bothered "more days than not" by worries (Table 3-1). Placing the emphasis on worries has also shifted the focus from a more mixed emphasis to a more cognitive disorder.

My clinical experience suggests that most outpatients with generalized manifest anxiety do not meet the GAD duration criterion of DSM-III-R at the time they seek consultation. In addition, many of these patients also have symptoms of depressed mood, discouragement, or occasional tearfulness intermixed with their symptoms of anxiety. DSM-III-R has left the clinician with the unfortunate choice of having to label this extremely typical patient as adjustment disorder with mixed emotional features (309.28). It is always possible, in my experience, to find at least one so-called "psychosocial stressor" that has occurred within the 3 months before the onset of the patient's distress in order to fit the patient into this diagnosis. Unfortunately, reviewers for some third-party payers raise questions about claims related to the care of patients with adjustment disorders; this results in increased paperwork, payment delays, and, at times, denials. Any workable diagnostic system must include a more credible category for these frequently seen patients (i.e., mixed anxiety-depression) than DSM-III-R now affords with 309.28. It will be regrettable if we have to wait until DSM-IV before this occurs. The author's temporary solution has been to call these patients 300.00, anxiety disorder NOS (not otherwise specified).

Panic Disorders (PD)

The DSM-III-R overall criteria for the panic disorders (PD) and for the subtypes, PD with agoraphobia (300.21) and PD without

TABLE 3-1 Generalized Anxiety Disorder (300.02)[a]

A. A period of 6 months or longer during which the individual has been bothered (more days than not) by unrealistic or excessive worry (apprehensive expectation) about two or more life circumstances, for example, worry about possible misfortune to child (who is in no danger), or worry about finances (for no good reason). In children and adolescents, this may take the form of worrying about academic, athletic, and social performance.

B. If another Axis I disorder is present, the focus of the worry in A is unrelated to it, e.g., the worry is not about having a panic attack (as in panic disorder), being contaminated (as in obsessive-compulsive disorder), or gaining weight (as in anorexia nervosa). In addition, the disturbance does not occur only during the course of a mood disorder or a psychotic disorder.

C. At least 6 of the following 18 symptoms are often present when anxious (do not include symptoms present only during panic attacks):

Motor Tension
1. feeling shaky, trembling, or twitching
2. muscle tension, aches, or soreness
3. restlessness
4. easy fatigability

Autonomic Hyperactivity
5. shortness of breath or smother sensations
6. palpitations or accelerated heart rate (tachycardia)
7. sweating or cold clammy hands
8. dry mouth
9. dizziness or lightheadedness
10. nausea, diarrhea, or other abdominal distress
11. flushes (hot flashes) or chills
12. frequent urination
13. trouble swallowing or lump in throat

Vigilance and Scanning
14. feeling keyed up or on edge
15. exaggerated startle response
16. difficulty concentrating or mind going blank because of anxiety
17. trouble falling or staying asleep
18. irritability

D. Not sustained by a specific organic factor (e.g., hyperthyroidism, caffeine intoxication).

[a]Reprinted courtesy of DSM-III-R (2).

Some DSM-III-Anxiety Disorders

TABLE 3-2 Panic Disorder[a]

A. At some times during the disturbance, one or more panic attacks (discrete periods of intense discomfort or fear) that were (1) unexpected, i.e., did not occur immediately before or on exposure to a situation that almost always caused anxiety, and (2) not triggered by situations in which the individual was the focus of other's attention.

B. Either four attacks, as defined in criterion A, occurred within a 4-week period, or one or more attacks were followed by a period of at least a month of persistent fear of having another attack.

C. At least four of the following symptoms developed during at least one of the attacks:
   1. shortness of breath (dyspnea) or smothering sensations
   2. choking
   3. palpitations or accelerated heart rate (tachycardia)
   4. chest pain or discomfort
   5. sweating
   6. dizziness, unsteady feelings, or faintness
   7. nausea or abdominal distress
   8. depersonalization or derealization
   9. numbness or tingling sensations (paresthesias)
   10. flushes (hot flashes) or chills
   11. trembling or shaking
   12. fear of dying
   13. fear of going crazy or of doing something uncontrolled

D. During at least some of the attacks, at least four of the symptoms listed in C. developed suddenly and increased in intensity within 10 minutes of the beginning of the first symptom noticed in the attack.

E. An organic etiology (e.g., amphetamine or caffeine intoxication, hyperthyroidism) has been ruled out, i.e., either there was no new organic factor (or change in a pre-existing organic factor) that precipitated the disturbance, or the disturbance has persisted for at least 1 month beyond the cessation of the precipitating organic factor.

[a]Reprinted courtesy of DSM-III-R (2).

agoraphobia (300.01), and given in Tables 3-2, 3-3, and 3-4, respectively.

Again, the reader familiar with DSM-III will notice several significant changes in these newer criteria. The duration criterion has been changed from three panic attacks within a 3-week period to either four attacks within a 4-week period or one or more attacks followed by a period of persistent anticipatory anxiety lasting at least 1 month. In addition, the old part D exclusion criterion, not asso-

TABLE 3–3 Panic Disorder with Agoraphobia (300.21)[a]

A. Meets the criteria for panic disorder.

B. Agoraphobia: Fear of being in places or situations from which escape might be difficult (or embarrassing), or in which help might not be available, in the event of a panic attack. As a result of this fear there are either travel restrictions or need for a companion when away from home, or there is endurance of agoraphobic situations despite intense anxiety. Common agoraphobic situations include being outside of the home alone, being in a crowd or standing in a line, being on a bridge, or traveling in a bus, train, or car.

[a]Reprinted courtesy of DSM-III-R (2)

ciated with agoraphobia, has been eliminated to create the two new subtypes.

There is a certain arbitrariness to the thirteen signs and symptoms (Table 3–2) listed for criterion C for PD and to the eighteen signs and symptoms (Table 3–1) listed for criterion C for GAD. While it is more likely that PD patients will fear dying or going crazy or being out of control than GAD patients, it is not so unusual for GAD patients to experience transient depersonalization or feel numbness or paresthesias when they hyperventilate. Similarly, it would not be unusual for a PD patient to have problems with concentration during or after an attack or to feel irritable or, for that matter, to have trouble falling asleep in anticipation of nocturnal panic attacks. The nature of the anticipatory anxiety of the full-blown PD patient does not receive adequate attention in either DSM-III-R or in DSM-III, and neither mentions that some patients may have their panic attacks only upon awakening during the night.

Social and Simple Phobias

Tables 3–5 and 3–6 list the DSM-III-R criteria for social and simple phobias. These conditions are relatively straightforward. Unfortunately, however, I find that neither really fits well with situational anxiety, a very common form of anxiety. For example, public-speaking anxiety, a common form of situational anxiety, is experienced very differently from anxiety about being in crowds or among strangers (more obvious forms of social phobia). Public-speaking anxiety or musical-performance anxiety is also not merely a sim-

TABLE 3–4 Panic Disorder without Agoraphobia (300.01)[a]

A. Meets the criteria for panic disorder.
B. Absence of agoraphobia, as defined previously.

[a]Reprinted courtesy of DSM-III-R (2)

ple phobia. There is no circumscribed object, and avoidance is not prominent (as with spider or dog phobia). Imagining performing rarely evokes anxiety in the way that imagining a spider will. Socially phobic patients often experience a vague sense of being ill at ease without prominent symptoms of autonomic hyperarousal. Simple phobic patients often experience autonomic hyperarousal along with a prominent cognitive component (e.g., imagining the spider). Situationally anxious performers often experience autonomic hyperarousal without a cognitive component (they are concentrating on their tone or fingering without thinking about why they are trembling).

TABLE 3–5 Social Phobia (300.23)[a]

A. A persistent fear of one or more situations (the phobic situations) in which the individual is exposed to possible scrutiny by others and fears that he or she may do something or act in a way that will be humiliating or embarrassing. Examples include: unable to continue talking while speaking in public, choking on food when eating in front of others, unable to urinate in public lavatory, hand trembling when writing in front of others, saying foolish things, or not being able to answer questions in social situations.

B. If an axis III or another axis I disorder is present, the fear in A is unrelated to it, e.g., the fear is not of having a panic attack (PD), stuttering (stuttering), trembling (Parkinson's disease), exhibiting abnormal eating behavior (anorexia nervosa or bulimia nervosa).

C. During some phase of the disturbance, exposure to the specific phobic stimulus (or stimuli) almost invariably provokes an immediate anxiety response.

D. The phobic situation(s) is avoided, or endured, with intense anxiety.

E. The fear or the avoidant behavior interferes with occupational functioning or with usual social activities or relationships with others, or there is marked distress about having the fear.

F. The individual recognizes that his or her fear is excessive or unreasonable.

[a]Reprinted courtesy of DSM-III-R (2)

TABLE 3-6 Simple Phobia (300.29)[a]

A. A persistent fear of a circumscribed stimulus (object or situation), other than fear of having a panic attack (as in panic disorder) or of humiliation or embarrassment in certain social situations (as in social phobia).

B. During some phase of the disturbance, exposure to the specific phobic stimulus (or stimuli) almost invariably provokes an immediate anxiety response.

C. The object or situation is avoided, or endured with intense anxiety.

D. The fear or the avoidant behavior interferes with occupational functioning or with usual social activities or relationships with others, or there is marked distress about having the fear.

E. The individual recognizes that his or her fear is excessive or unreasonable.

F. The phobic stimulus is unrelated to the content of the obsessions of obsessive-compulsive disorder.

[a]Reprinted courtesy of DSM-III-R (2)

Because each person's anxiety is unique and variable, treatment must be individualized. The following sections briefly cover general treatment principles for anxious and stressed individuals and review currently available psychopharmacological options.

STRESS MANAGEMENT AND CORE ASPECTS OF THE NONPHARMACOLOGICAL TREATMENT OF ANXIETY

For many individuals, stress is either chronic or recurrent. The strain produced can lead to significant impairment of functioning, particularly in the forms of headache, muscle and mental tension, or fatigue. Stress-reduction strategies include identification of the sources and causes of the stress (the "stressors"); support; reassurance; removal, whenever possible, of (or from) the stressors; techniques for relaxation; efforts to increase feelings of being able to manage and cope; and efforts to maintain or raise self-esteem. These same elements are basic to any psychotherapeutic strategy for the treatment of anxiety, and the essentials (which I call the five Rs) are listed in Table 3–7.

When stress is job-related, certain techniques (see Table 3–8) may directly promote a reduction in stress (4). (The reader is encouraged to consult reference 4 for greater detail and references.)

Nonpharmacological Treatment of Anxiety

TABLE 3-7 Five Rs: Core Concepts of Care for Stress and Anxiety

---

Recognition of the sources and causes of distress: consciousness raising and education

Relationships: identifying sources of help and reassurance, support systems

Removal of or from the stressors or source of anxiety or danger: managing the stimulus

Relaxation techniques: meditation, breathing exercises, and imagery

Re-engagement: deconditioning, counter-conditioning, managed re-exposure

---

To further reduce the effects of stress, simple exercises should be incorporated into the daily routine. They can be adapted to any setting, including the office chair. The aim is to relax tensed muscles through further stretching of the muscles followed by relaxation of the affected muscle groups [see (4)]. Since the head, neck, and shoulder muscles are most often involved, focusing on these muscle groups is the place to start, and a systematic effort at relaxation for 5-10 minutes a day may be sufficient. Other muscles may be involved

TABLE 3-8 LESS STRESS: A Job-Related Stress-Reduction Strategy

---

List goals, both short- and long-range, and eliminate those not attainable.

Establish a hierarchy of tasks or assignments based on realistic priorities and time requirements.

Subdivide remaining tasks into manageable projects or units.

Start with "do-able" tasks; starting with the most difficult tasks usually leads to avoidance or procrastination.

Simplify your work environment; have good lighting and avoid clutter.

Tell yourself to say "no" to additional work when you are already doing more than you can handle.

Remember to interrupt stressful periods with breaks for relaxation strategies (e.g., take six to ten deep breaths, trying to fill the chest, while sitting in a relaxed way and having adequate support for the arms, shoulders, and neck).

Envision, in conjunction with the above relaxation strategy and with your eyes closed, your favorite place, trying to capture the sounds, smells, sights, and texture of the place.

Share and discuss with others.

Structure nonwork hours to provide for adequate exercise, distraction, nutrition, and sleep.

---

and techniques can be worked out to deal with each appropriately (e.g., squeezing a tennis ball to relieve hand tension or writer's cramp).

PHARMACOLOGICAL OPTIONS FOR THE TREATMENT OF ANXIETY

When anxiety significantly interferes with a person's functioning or causes distress, short-term or intermittent pharmacotherapy may be indicated as an adjunct to nonpharmacological approaches. Chronic or long-term pharmacotherapy for anxiety should not be undertaken unless it has been established that the patient cannot be comfortable or function adequately with short-term or intermittent therapy. This is a judgment call which the physician should make in conjunction with the patient. Certain diagnostic groups are more likely to respond to specific therapies, but, as noted above, individualized treatment planning is essential.

Beta Blockers

Beta-adrenoreceptor blocking agents (BABAs) have the potential to play a valuable but somewhat unpredictable role in the treatment of anxiety disorders and related symptomatology. Patients with situational or performance anxiety, anxiety secondary to mitral valve prolapse, anxiety associated with stress-related unmasking of essential (familial) tremor, social phobias, mild or limited PD, or benzodiazepine-withdrawal hyperarousal may at times benefit from treatment with BABAs, alone or in combination with other agents. Since these indications are not approved by the U.S. Food and Drug Administration (FDA) for the use of BABAs, cautious use and careful documentation are indicated and essential. Although many BABAs exist, the author's clinical experience has focused on three agents for this varied group of patients. Propranolol (see Table 3-9) has had the greatest use in anxiety-related conditions and has the most extensive literature documentation. Propranolol is highly lipophilic and is a nonselective BABA with a relatively short duration of action. Thus, it frequently requires multiple dosing during the day. However, a slow-release form is available (120 mg). Atenolol, a beta-1 selective BABA, has the advantage of once-a-day dosing (see

TABLE 3-9 Some Beta-Adrenoreceptor Blocking Agents (BABAs) Useful in Anxiety Disorders

BABA	Typical Daily Dosage Schedule	Time of Peak Concentration (hours)	Elimination Half-Life (hours)	Strengths Available (mg)	Typical Daily Dosage (mg)
Propranolol	three times[a]	1–1.5	4	10, 20, 40, 60, 80, 90	10–80
Atenolol	once or twice	2–4	6–7	50, 100	25–50
Acebutolol	once or twice	2.5	2–4	200, 400	200–400
(Diacetolol[b])		3.5	8–13	—	—

[a] A slow-release (longer-acting) form is marketed (120 mg).
[b] An active metabolite of acebutolol.

Table 3-9) and is the least lipophilic (most hydrophilic) of currently marketed BABAs. Because it is not extensively metabolized by the liver, atenolol should be used with special care in patients with renal impairment or reduced renal clearance (e.g., the elderly). Acebutolol is also a beta-1 selective BABA (see Table 3-9) which can be given once daily. It is quite hydrophilic and undergoes hepatic metabolism yielding an active metabolite, diacetolol.

In addition to the three BABAs with which the author has had the most extensive experience, five other oral BABAs are currently marketed in the United States: labetalol, metoprolol, nadolol, pindolol and timolol. Like acebutolol and atenolol, nadolol has low lipid solubility and high water solubility. The other four BABAs are intermediate between these three and the highly lipid-soluble propranolol.

All BABAs may be contraindicated in some patients (the reader should consult a current package insert for up-to-date information before prescribing). My clinical experience leads me to recommend avoidance of BABAs or particular caution and monitoring when the following conditions are present in addition to the patient's anxiety symptoms: bronchial asthma (may increase asthmatic symptomatology or block effective treatment with beta agonists); sinus bradycardia (may further slow heart rate or block treatment) and second or third degree heart block; hyperthyroidism (may mask symptomatology and confuse treatment); or concomitant use of catecholamine-depleting drugs (e.g., reserpine).

The following cases capture two instances in which BABAs were particularly effective:

> *Case 1*: A 35-year-old woman sought help after a series of treatment encounters (individual psychotherapy for 2 years, relaxation therapy, biofeedback, imipramine, alprazolam, which had either been ineffective or caused unwanted side effects) for mild panic attacks, limited agoraphobia, and claustrophobia. Her panic attacks could occur up to three times a day, primarily when she was working in her small cubicle as a computer programmer. History and physical examination revealed bronchial asthma since childhood and previously undiagnosed mitral valve prolapse (subsequently confirmed by echocardiogram). Atenolol (50 mg/day each morning) produced complete symptom relief within 2 weeks, without side effects or aggravation of her asthma.

She has remained symptom-free for 4 years, although her symptoms returned during an elective interval off atenolol when she conceived and bore a child.

Case 2: A 40-year-old woman sought a consultation after unsuccessful prior treatment for essential tremor (familial) which was mostly troublesome when she was stressed by work or relationships. Barbiturates and propranolol had been ineffective or caused side effects at high doses. Alcohol (self-prescribed) helped on occasion. Alprazolam had not helped, but diazepam at 20–40 mg/day would mute the tremor; however, sedation and impaired coordination occurred as unwanted side effects. Acebutolol (200 mg/day or 200 mg twice a day when she anticipated more stress) accomplished the desired symptom relief without side effects. Of interest is that, once on acebutolol, she was intolerant of alcohol (it caused too much sedation even with limited intake), a common effect reported by patients on BABAs.

Benzodiazepines (BZDPs)

Benzodiazepines are safe and effective treatments for a variety of anxiety states. Nine BZDPs, currently marketed in the United States, are useful for the treatment of anxiety. They vary widely in milligram potency and also have qualitative differences in the speed of onset of action and duration of clinical activity after single doses. With multiple-dose (chronic) therapy, the qualitative differences among BZDPs become more subtle.

BZDP usage should involve an understanding of their pharmacokinetic and pharmacodynamic characteristics. It is beyond the scope of this chapter to discuss each of the nine BZDPs in detail, but certain global principles can be summarized. The rate of absorption and volume of distribution (determined largely by lipid solubility) after single, oral doses of BZDPs are the major determinants of the onset and duration of their clinical activity. During multiple-dose or chronic therapy, the rate and extent of accumulation for a given BZDP is determined by half-life and rate of clearance. BZDPs may be classified into three somewhat arbitrary groups according to their rates of clearance (as reflected in their elimination half-lives):

1. Ultrashort half-life BZDPs have elimination half-lives of less than 5 hours. These do not accumulate. Drugs of this cate-

gory are almost always used as hypnotics rather than as antianxiety agents; none of the nine BZDPs considered here is classified as ultrashort.

2. Short and intermediate half-life BZDPs have elimination half-lives of 5–24 hours. Limited drug accumulation occurs with this group, and accumulation of active metabolites is not significant. Patient's age has little effect on drug clearance for drugs of this group metabolized by conjugation (e.g., oxazepam); however, oxidatively metabolized agents (e.g., diazepam) have impaired clearance in the elderly, resulting in an increased potential for accumulation.

3. Long half-life (slow BZDPs) have elimination half-lives greater than 24 hours, frequently have active metabolites, and both parent drugs and metabolite(s) may accumulate during chronic therapy (clearance is not uncommonly impaired in the elderly).

As noted, half-lives of BZDPs are important determinants of their duration of clinical antianxiety activity. Since BZDPs do not "cure" anxiety, for chronically anxious patients reappearance of anxiety should be anticipated; the time of this reappearance is likely to be a function, in part, of the individual BZDP's elimination half-life. While tolerance usually develops to the sedative properties of BZDPs used in an anxiolytic dosage range (i.e., below the range for hypnotic effects), tolerance to the anxiolytic effects is less common even with extended use. Since many patients' anxiety states are intermittent rather than persistent, use of benzodiazepines should be time-limited until the responsible physician has established that chronic use is the only way to provide the patient with sufficient relief to function in relationships, work, and play. During the typical 4-week trials employed in drug studies, BZDPs demonstrate consistent efficacy for appropriately symptomatic patients with manifest anxiety.

Which patients are candidates for BZDP therapy? The efficacy of benzodiazepines is adequately established to my satisfaction for patients meeting DSM-III criteria for GAD (i.e., 1 month of persistent, mixed symptomatology). While it is likely that BZDPs will have comparable efficacy in GAD patients meeting DSM-III-R criteria (6 months' duration and prominent worries), this has not been established.

In addition to beneficial effects in GAD patients, in my clinical experience, all BZDPs are likely to be helpful for the anticipatory anxiety of PD patients. BZDPs (probably by lowering overall tension and anxiety levels) in many instances will lower the frequency of panic attacks. Although not yet FDA-approved for the treatment of PD, two BZDPs, alprazolam and clonazepam, appear to block panic attacks when given chronically. Doses vary for this latter effect (for alprazolam, 1–8 mg is common with 3–6 mg being modal and 0.5–12 mg a range encountered by many clinicians who treat large numbers of PD patients; for clonazepam, 0.5–3 mg is common with 1–2 mg being modal and 0.5–5 mg being the range). Much variability is present in the response of PD patients, depending in part on the frequency of panic attacks and on their level of concurrent background stress and anxiety.

Because sedation is more common with intermittent single dosing and memory impairment can occur with single dosing (5), BZDPs are not optimal agents for use in situational anxiety. Some patients do find these agents useful, however, so that their use for this purpose can be attempted with caution and appropriate warnings to the patient. When acute anxiety interferes with a patient's falling asleep, single nighttime dosing may be helpful, particularly with BZDPs that have either a rapid onset of action (e.g., diazepam) or, if taken slightly earlier in the evening, an intermediate duration of action (e.g., lorazepam).

Table 3–10 lists these nine BZDPs used in the treatment of anxiety and details selected properties and available dosage strengths.

Common unwanted effects of BZDPs are related to their depression of the central nervous system (CNS): drowsiness, sleepiness, impaired intellectual performance, clumsiness or impaired fine-motor coordination, and impairment of recall and memory. Most of these effects are dose-dependent in individual patients, and the threshold for their appearance is variable. BZDPs potentiate the effects of alcohol and other CNS depressants. Although the frequency of physiological addiction to BZDPs has been exaggerated in the popular press, some patients do have withdrawal states (e.g., tremulousness, sweating, hyperacusis, photophobia, insomnia, nightmares, gastrointestinal complaints, systolic hypertension). Withdrawal is more common when high dosages have been used over extended time periods, but in occasional patients withdrawal can

TABLE 3–10 Characteristics of Benzodiazepines Currently Marketed in the United States for the Treatment of Anxiety[a]

Administered Drug	Approved Indications	Rate of Appearance after Oral Dose	Active Substances in Blood	Overall Rate of Elimination	Dosage/Strength (mg) Tablets	Dosage/Strength (mg) Capsules
Alprazolam	Anxiety Anxiety-depression	Intermediate	Alprazolam	Intermediate	0.25, 0.5, 1	
Chlordiazepoxide	Anxiety Alcohol withdrawal Preoperative sedation	Intermediate	Chlordiazepoxide Desmethylchlordiazepoxide Demoxepam Desmethyldiazepam	Slow		5, 10, 25
Clonazepam[a] Clorazepate	Seizure disorders Anxiety Seizure disorders Alcohol withdrawal	Intermediate Rapid	Clonazepam Desmethyldiazepam	Intermediate Slow	0.5, 1, 2 3.75, 7.5, 15	
Diazepam[b]	Anxiety Alcohol withdrawal Muscle spasm Preoperative sedation Status epilepticus	Rapid	Diazepam Desmethyldiazepam	Slow	2, 5, 10	
Halazepam	Anxiety	Intermediate to slow	[Halazepam][c] Desmethyldiazepam	Slow	20, 40	
Lorazepam	Anxiety Anxiety-depression Preoperative sedation	Intermediate	Lorazepam	Intermediate	0.5, 1, 2	
Oxazepam	Anxiety Anxiety-depression Alcohol withdrawal	Intermediate to slow	Oxazepam	Intermediate to rapid	15	10, 15, 30
Prazepam	Anxiety	Slow	Desmethyldiazepam	Slow	10	5, 10, 20

[a]Clonazepam does not have use in anxiety as a current FDA-approved indication.
[b]A slow-release form is available in 15-mg capsules.
[c]Of minor clinical significance.

occur with discontinuation of typical therapeutic doses. Gradual tapering should be undertaken whenever possible when BZDPs are discontinued, and duration of drug exposure should be kept to the minimum time consistent with the chronicity of the patient's anxiety. BABAs are occasionally warranted to reduce withdrawal symptomatology. Some clinicians are noting that tapering of alprazolam at times needs to be particularly gradual to avoid withdrawal symptoms. On occasion, even extremely gradual tapering has not avoided alprazolam-withdrawal effects (6). Clonidine or carbamazepine has been employed successfully in some cases to treat alprazolam-withdrawal symptomatology, but these strategies have not been consistently effective.

Buspirone

A novel azaspirodecanedione, buspirone was marketed late in 1986 as an oral anxiolytic agent. Typically effective in the 15–60 mg/day range in divided dosing (usually three times a day), modal dosage appears to be 20 mg/day for typical adult and geriatric patients. Buspirone seems indicated at this point for the symptoms and course of manifest anxiety diagnosed as GAD. Its onset of action is often slow (perhaps 1–2 weeks); it probably has little value for single-dose use for situational anxiety. Given its effectiveness in treating generalized anxiety disorder symptoms, buspirone may be expected to lessen the frequency of panic attacks and reduce anticipatory anxiety in patients with panic disorder (perhaps by raising the lowered threshold for the occurrence of attacks which occurs with heightened background, interattack or anticipatory anxiety). There would be little reason to expect that it would block panic attacks per se, and this has indeed been the case in my preliminary clinical experience with buspirone.

Although its apparent activity in animal studies (increased central dopaminergic and noradrenergic activity and decreased serotonergic activity in the absence of meaningful BZDP receptor-binding or actions on gamma-amino butyric acid [GABA] binding) is becoming known, there is at this time no convincing hypothesis for buspirone's mechanism of action. Buspirone appears to lack significant anticonvulsant, hypnotic, or muscle-relaxant properties. Whether it may have proconvulsant properties in unusual circumstances (e.g., acute alcohol withdrawal) remains to be clarified. The beta-phase elimination half-life for the parent compound is 2–3 hours. After oxidative metabolism, at least one potentially active metabolite, 1-pyrimidinyl piperazine (1-PP), is formed which has a half-life of 4–5 hours.

Advantages to buspirone (when it is effective) appear to be in its pattern and the relatively small number of clinically significant side effects. Usage suggests little impairment of daytime wakefulness, motor performance (e.g., automobile driving) or cognitive functions. There seems to be minimal potential for abuse (although there are always some individuals who will misuse anything) or withdrawal reactions. Potentiation of the CNS depressant effects of alcohol and other CNS depressant agents seems negligible to date. Side effects include, but are not limited to, dizziness, faintness, nervousness, restlessness, headache, dysphoria (at higher doses), parenthesias, nausea, diarrhea, weakness, lethargy, and fatigue.

It would appear from preliminary clinical observations that buspirone is optimally used in patients who have never taken BZDPs or when a reasonably long interval has elapsed since BZDP usage. Concurrent chronic use of buspirone with BZDPs, beta blockers, or alcohol has not been well studied. Preliminary clinical experience suggests that elevated blood pressure may occur when buspirone is combined with monoamine oxidase inhibitors. Data from accidental or purposeful overdosing are extremely limited. Monitoring and supportive and symptomatic care in association with gastric lavage are the approach that can be recommended at this time. In contrast to barbiturates and BZDPs or meprobamate, buspirone is not a scheduled controlled substance at this time.

The following case illustrates the type of patient whom I have found to be responsive to buspirone:

> *Case 3*: A 57-year-old professional man who had experienced two prior episodes of major affective disorder (recurrent, unipolar) was left with residual morning dread and apprehension following recovery from his second episode some five years before. Maintenance antidepressants (amitriptyline, imipramine, desipramine, doxepin) given by prior physicians had not helped with the morning anxiety, although they had eliminated other symptoms (particularly bedtime ruminations and early morning awakening). He had also been given benzodiazepines (diazepam, lorazepam, oxazepam) which would inconsistently suppress his morning dread and apprehension (mainly in the form of worries about his business, his adult children, properties he

owned, and his own health) and were always accompanied by a sense of being sedated and disconnected which he did not like. He was started on buspirone and responded after 8 days to 5 mg twice a day. He had been started at this low dosage because of his apparent sensitivity to sedation from benzodiazepines. He has remained comfortable for 3 months (i.e., up to the time of the writing of this chapter) at that dose and has not complained of side effects.

MONOAMINE OXIDASE INHIBITORS (MAOIs) AND ANTIDEPRESSANTS

As noted earlier, many patients with generalized manifest anxiety present with accompanying symptoms of depression (e.g., low mood, discouragement, occasional tearfulness, irritability, lack of energy or vitality, difficulty having pleasure, hypochondriasis). While some of these patients may respond to supportive and clarifying interpersonal therapies and to therapies that address the patient's negative cognitive set, and some may respond to BZDPs or buspirone, others may respond to MAOIs or other antidepressants.

Monoamine oxidase inhibitors were among the earliest of the modern generation of psychopharmacological agents. Beginning with iproniazid in the early 1950s, a number of MAOIs have been studied for the treatment of depression or anxiety. Despite their early arrival in our modern pharmacopeia, MAOIs are among the least well-studied agents in terms of numbers of adequately designed, controlled, clinical trials. For a number of decades in the United States, MAOIs were seen as second-line agents to be used only when other approaches were not successful. Some of this negative set no doubt can be attributed to the hepatotoxicity of several of the early hydrazine MAOIs, their inconsistent efficacy in patients with major depression with melancholic features (a group in which they were often tried when standard antidepressants failed), and their hypotensive properties. In addition, serious problems can occur with these agents in the presence of dietary intake of foods containing tyramine-like pressor agents, certain medications (e.g., sympathomimetic amines, meperidine, L-dopa, tricyclic antidepressants, and alpha-methyldopa) and cocaine. The interested reader should consult more detailed texts and current package inserts to obtain more information on these important concerns before prescribing MAOIs.

Nevertheless, MAOIs can be helpful to certain anxious patients and are an important part of our armamentarium. Table 3-11 lists three MAOIs currently marketed in the United States for the treatment of depression. My experience indicates that tranylcypromine is often too stimulating to be useful for anxious patients. A nonhydrazine MAOI and analogue of amphetamine, tranylcypromine was actually synthesized in an effort to produce a psychostimulant. The following discussion refers to the two hydrazine MAOIs phenelzine and isocarboxazid.

Phenelzine and isocarboxazid may be helpful for those anxious–depressed patients whose anxiety involves phobic, panic attack, and hypochondriacal (e.g., illness fears and worries) elements and whose depression is more reactive than autonomous, particularly in response to rejection, criticism, or disappointment. These patients are at times called "atypical depressives" when the depressive elements predominate.

In addition to their value in patients with mixed anxiety and depression, MAOIs may also be helpful in treating patients with PD. Placebo-controlled studies have been conducted with phenelzine in PD patients that establish its efficacy. I know of no comparable studies with isocarboxazid, but my clinical experience has been positive. Many PD patients respond to a single tablet per day, but higher dosages may at times be required and must be individualized for each patient.

For most patients, dosing before 1 P.M. is indicated to avoid drug-induced insomnia. However, for an occasional patient the reverse is true and bedtime dosing is more helpful. Other common unwanted effects associated with isocarboxazid and phenelzine are listed in Table 3-12.

Perhaps the most frequent concern raised when patients or physicians seek a consultation about MAOIs is the issue of diet.

TABLE 3-11 Some MAOIs Currently Marketed in the U.S.

Generic Name	Initial Dose (mg)	Usual Dose Range (mg/day)
Isocarboxazid	10	10–50
Phenelzine	15	15–90
Tranylcypromine	10	10–50

TABLE 3-12 Some Side Effects with Isocarboxazid and Phenelzine

More Frequent (perhaps > 10%)	Less Frequent (usually < 10%)
Anorgasmia/impotence	Disorientation
Chills	Drowsiness
Falling, passing out, hypotension	Edema
	Headaches
Hypomania	Hypertensive crises
Insomnia	Myoclonic jerking
Weight gain	Paresthesias
Withdrawal nightmares	Rashes
	Urinary retention

Table 3-13 is a guideline for dietary restrictions. It is essential that the treating physician instruct the patient about to receive an MAOI about diet and the importance of compliance. In practice, however, many patients, despite careful and explicit warnings, are noncompliant. They will drink a glass or two of wine or eat a piece of slightly aged cheese and have no ill effects. They then begin to question the importance of dietary compliance. I suggest trying to anticipate this by indicating to patients that some individuals are less sensitive to the tyramine–MAOI interaction, that amounts of tyramine present in a given food or the amounts absorbed after a given ingestion may vary and that not following the diet is like playing Russian roulette.

All currently marketed antidepressants have been helpful to individual patients with mixed anxiety–depression states. Doxepin and amitriptyline in low dosages are particularly popular with family physicians and internists. In addition, antidepressants have been effective in blocking panic attacks in patients with PD. Imipramine has received the greatest attention in controlled trials, but other agents can be helpful to individual patients, and choice varies according to the patients' tolerance of a given drug's unwanted properties (e.g., sedation, dry mouth). As with MAOIs, small doses of antidepressants may be sufficient to block panic attacks. For some patients whose panic attacks are blocked by MAOIs or antidepressants, concomitant use of a BZDP may be helpful to treat the accompanying anticipatory anxiety. This use should be time-limited. In most patients, once panic attacks are blocked, anticipatory anxiety will be extinguished.

TABLE 3-13 Some Dietary Restrictions with MAOIs[a]

Foods to Avoid	Usually Safe	Unlikely to Pose Problems When Used in Moderation
Aged cheeses	Cottage cheese, cream cheese, farmer cheese	Yogurt, sour cream
Beer, red wine, sherry, liqueurs	Vodka, gin, dry white wines	Other alcoholic beverages
Fermented sausage, beef or chicken liver, smoked or pickled fish, caviar	All fresh meats and fish	
Canned or overripe figs, whole bananas, banana peel fiber	Banana pulp	Other fruit, if not overripe
Fava or broad bean pods	Shelled beans, peas	Avocado, New Zealand spinach
Yeast/protein extracts		Soy sauce
		Chocolate, caffeine-containing beverages

[a]Modified with permission from D. G. Folks, (1983). *Journal of Clinical Psychopharmacology* 3:249–252.

REFERENCES

1. Freud, S. (1926). *The Problem of Anxiety*. New York: W. W. Norton.
2. *Diagnostic and Statistical Manual of Mental Disorders*, rev. 3rd ed. (1987). Washington, DC: American Psychiatric Association.
3. Mitchell, S. W. (1904). Evolution of the rest treatment. *Journal of Nervous and Mental Disease*, 31:368–373.
4. Shader, R. I., and Greenblatt, D. J. (1986). Some practical approaches to the understanding and treatment of the symptoms of anxiety and stress. In *American Handbook of Psychiatry*, vol. 8, ed. P. A. Berger and H. K. H. Brodie, pp. 597–619. New York: Basic Books.
5. Shader, R. I., Dreyfuss, D., Gerrein, J. R., et al. (1986). Sedative effects and impaired learning and recall after single oral doses of lorazepam. *Clinical Pharmacology and Therapeutics* 39:526–529.
6. Browne, J. L., and Hauge, K. J. (1986). A review of alprazolam withdrawal. *Drug Intelligence and Clinical Pharmacology* 20:873–841.

4

Mania

David L. Dunner, M.D.

The 1970s were termed the decade of affective disorders. Indeed, at the beginning of the 1970s, the diagnostic nomenclature and treatment parameters for affective disorders were confusing and varied considerably among clinicians. However, by the end of that decade, the nomenclature was standardized (DSM-III) (1). The application of DSM-III (1) broadened the concept of affective disorders and particularly mania in this country and standardized criteria for the diagnosis of affective disorders. Furthermore, treatment of affective disorders advanced considerably with the introduction of lithium carbonate and several new antidepressants. The use of medication on a long-term basis (maintenance therapy) for both recurrent bipolar affective disorder as well as recurrent depression has become an integral part of modern clinical practice. This chapter discusses the treatment of mania, which depends on understanding its classification and course of illness. Thus, this chapter includes sections on the diagnosis of affective disorder, treatment of acute mania, and maintenance therapy for recurrent bipolar affective disorder.

DIAGNOSTIC CONSIDERATIONS

In the 1960s a U.S./U.K. study documented the diagnostic discrepancies regarding affective disorder, particularly mania, between American-trained and British-trained psychiatrists (2). Although these diagnostic discrepancies existed, they had few treatment implications since the treatment for most psychotic illnesses in the 1960s was antipsychotic drugs, particularly chlorpromazine. In the 1950s and 1960s lithium salts were introduced in Europe as a more specific treatment for acute mania and later for maintenance therapy for bipolar affective disorder. This provided an impetus for the development of a classification system in the United States that would be broader in its concept of affective disorders and narrower in its concept of schizophrenia. Furthermore, this diagnostic formulation should have greater reliability so that different clinicians would be apt to make the same diagnosis on the same patient. Whereas DSM-II was descriptive and largely intuitive, DSM-III as a classification system evolved as a triage-type diagnosis with both inclusion and exclusion criteria.

The road to development of DSM-III went from the St. Louis (Feighner) criteria (3) to the Research Diagnostic Criteria (4), and then to the current DSM-III operational criteria. One of the difficulties in applying DSM-III diagnoses to treatment considerations is that most of the treatment literature from the 1960s and 1970s used older criteria, which were often idiosyncratic to the investigator. Thus, bipolar affective disorder in DSM-III is not entirely congruent with manic depressive illness as diagnosed by previous investigators. For example, the concept of bipolar I affective disorder entailed a hospitalization specifically for mania (5), whereas severity of illness is not a consideration in diagnosing bipolar subtypes in DSM-III. Therefore, in this chapter we will at times use DSM-III criteria but attempt to correlate diagnostic considerations with the newer criteria.

The DSM-III subdivisions of affective disorders are:

1. Bipolar

   - bipolar affective disorder
   - cyclothymic disorder
   - atypical bipolar disorder

2. Depressive only
   - major depressive disorder
   - dysthymic disorder
   - atypical depression

The bipolar disorders are characterized by manic episodes. DSM-III defines a manic episode as a 1-week or longer syndrome of elevated or irritable mood associated with such symptoms as increased activity, overtalkativeness, racing thoughts, grandiosity, decreased need for sleep, distractibility, and impulsivity. Exclusion criteria are also delineated.

Those DSM-III subtypes of affective disorder that include manic episodes are bipolar disorder, cyclothymic disorder, and atypical bipolar disorder. The latter term is described as corresponding to "bipolar II," which identified cases of recurrent depression and hypomania.

One of the clinically confusing points about the DSM-III criteria relates to the presence of psychotic symptoms during affective states. About one-third of patients with mania will evidence the so-called "Schneiderian first-rank" symptoms during mania (6). Among the exclusion criteria for affective disorders are cases where the clinical condition is predominated by mood-incongruent delusions. The distinction between mood-incongruent and mood-congruent delusions may be difficult to make at the time one is treating the patient and may only be clarified by the course of illness and the relationship of these psychotic symptoms to overall symptomatology.

Schizo-affective disorder is a term that was considerably more widely used in the 1970s than currently. DSM-III lists the term but there are no specific diagnostic criteria given. Thus, the use of schizo-affective as a clinical diagnosis is quite difficult. This is probably for the betterment of diagnostic classification since the term was frequently misapplied prior to DSM-III and was used to describe patients of different clinical descriptions and idiosyncratically by physicians who employed the term at all. On the other hand, atypical psychosis has become a rather broadly used term for many patients with psychotic symptoms in whom the diagnosis cannot be clarified by initial history.

TREATMENT OF ACUTE MANIA

There are basically two conditions relating to acute mania for which treatment should be considered. One is psychotic mania and the second is hypomania. Psychotic mania essentially requires hospitalization or some form of confinement. This is to protect the patient from doing social or physical harm to himself/herself or others. The onset can be acute over a few days or subacute over a few weeks. In some cases the onset is over several weeks and the patient may develop expanding grandiosity which is on the borderline between psychosis and reality. Such patients may be very difficult to treat and may be difficult to convince to come to the hospital voluntarily. Indeed, in many instances even involuntary commitment of such patients is quite difficult. However, it should be stressed that control of the patient's behavior and treatment is paramount and this is best effected for the acute manic patient by hospitalization.

Once a patient is hospitalized, the question of which drug to use depends largely on the degree and type of symptomatology. If the patient is grandiose and excitable, if psychotic symptoms are not too severe, and if the patient is willing to take oral medication, lithium alone may be the treatment of choice. However, if the patient is paranoid, very agitated, and not willing to take oral medications, then beginning treatment with an antipsychotic medication and adding lithium carbonate may be of considerable benefit. In general, it takes 4-7 days to attain a therapeutic lithium blood level, whereas the antipsychotic drug will provide early sedation for the manic patient.

Untreated mania is described in the literature as a 6-month-to 1-year illness. In modern times it is unusual to hospitalize a patient for acute mania for more than a few weeks. This has been effected by the use of high doses of antipsychotic drugs in combination with lithium. However, several points of caution are worth noting. First, it is important to obtain blood lithium levels frequently in order to prevent neurotoxicity. Second, the patient who does not respond within a few weeks may have an underlying manic illness that is more severe than other patients and may require a few more weeks for treatment to be effective. One frequently overlooked cause of failure to respond to treatment is that patients who are psychotic frequently do not take their medication. Thus low blood lithium levels in the face of what seem to be adequate doses may simply reflect the patient not taking the medication. This can be prevented by giving lithium in a liquid form and the antipsychotic drug intramuscularly. Third, in the 1970s there were reports of neurotoxicity resulting from the combination of high doses of lithium carbonate and of neuroleptics (7). This neurotoxicity appears clinically similar to malignant neuroleptic syndrome in some instances (fever, extrapyramidal signs, stupor), whereas in other patients the syndrome appears as lithium toxicity. Higher-potency antipsychotic medications have been implicated in the malignant neuroleptic syndrome toxicity, whereas lower-potency medications (such as thioridazine) have been implicated in cases resembling pure lithium toxicity (8). Although neurotoxicity/malignant neuroleptic syndrome occur rarely, it is useful to monitor fluid intake, hydration, and clinical status in patients receiving combined treatment. Treatment of lithium toxicity involves stopping medication and maintaining fluid and electrolytes. Treatment of malignant neuroleptic syndrome is more complicated, involving stopping medication and possible use of medication such as dantrolene or bromocriptine (9).

Although there are several techniques described for determining a lithium steady-state dose by giving a test dose and obtaining a blood level some hours thereafter, I do not recommend this form of beginning lithium therapy as the doses administered this way may lead to lithium toxicity. It is suggested that the patient be begun on a dose of lithium at a relatively low level in order to prevent initial gastrointestinal side effects and that this dose be rapidly and steadily increased with frequent (every other day) monitoring of lithium levels. Patients who have underlying medical problems or elderly patients who do not tolerate lithium well should have their doses increased less frequently and blood levels monitored more frequently. Careful observation during initiating lithium treatment is clinically warranted. In general, the blood level for the medically healthy patient who is acutely manic will be from 1.0 to 1.5 mEq/L. The use of red blood cell plasma:lithium ratios is sometimes advantageous in monitoring lithium doses. Lithium is normally actively excreted from red blood cells. The activity of this "lithium pump" is dependent on lithium dose level in an inverse fashion such that with higher plasma levels lithium tends to build up increasingly in erythrocytes. Thus, a patient who may not be responding to treatment at what seem to be therapeutic lithium blood levels may be found to have a low intracellular lithium level. Further increases of the lithium dose may produce satisfactory cellular or therapeutic levels of lithium.

If antipsychotic medication is also used, the choice of this drug will vary depending on the symptoms of the patients. Thus, if the patient requires intramuscular medication, some of the more potent antipsychotic medications such as haloperidol or thiothixine may be of use. If the patient is able to take oral medication, thioridazine or chlorpromazine may be quite useful. In general, the dose of antipsychotic medication is elevated quite rapidly in order to produce sedation. Additional medication for sleep may be useful. Lithium doses are increased gradually, and when the manic symptoms begin to decrease the antipsychotic drug dose can be lowered.

It is important to realize that the usual course of mania is triphasic: premanic depression, manic excitement, and postmanic depression. One is never sure that the mania is complete until the postmanic depression sets in. Thus, it is advisable to continue treatment with lithium and a neuroleptic through the development of a postmanic depressive phase. At that time the dose of the antipsychotic drug can be tapered. Whereas sleep and grandiosity symptoms improve rapidly during the initial phase of treatment of mania, judgment and insight may take longer to change. Thus, one should be careful, for example, in sending patients out of the hospital on passes, until one is certain that the patients have sufficient insight and judgment so that their behavior will not cause untoward social effects.

Other treatments for acute mania include electroconvulsive therapy (ECT). ECT has been used successfully in some patients who are refractory with treatment of antipsychotic drugs or lithium. However, it is important that patients not be given ECT while taking lithium carbonate as neurotoxicity can develop with this combination. Similarly, patients who have difficulty taking lithium have been treated with carbamazepine. Post and colleagues have shown that the time course of treatment response of acutely manic patients was similar for treatment with carbamazepine, pimozide, or placebo (10). Lerer recently reviewed several nonlithium therapies for bipolar disorder (11). Although lithium efficacy has been established through controlled treatment of several hundred acutely manic patients, other agents have been reported to have antimanic effects in small series or case reports. Thus, medication such as sodium valproate and clonidine have been reported to have antimanic effects. Verapamil, a calcium agonist, has also been reported to have antimanic effects (12).

Other treatments for acute mania include L-tryptophan, which has been shown to be somewhat effective for some manic patients. At times, patients may have medical complications that preclude the use of antipsychotic drugs and in these patients high doses of barbiturates or benzodiazepines can be useful in temporizing manic symptoms until lithium doses can be raised to therapeutic levels. Electroconvulsive therapy is also useful in the treatment of acute mania. However, lithium therapy should be discontinued prior to initiation of ECT as neurotoxic effects have been reported with concomitant use of ECT and lithium (13).

Other treatments for acute manic excitement include exercise and psychosocial structure. Often while the patient is hospitalized it is useful to have the patient in a socially deprived area such as a seclusion room several times a day in order to decrease social stimulation.

Hypomania is a condition which is less severe than mania and is seen in patients termed bipolar II. Most patients with hypomania do not require specific treatment for their manic symptoms. Hypomanic symptoms are the same as those described by DSM-III for mania. However, psychotic features are usually absent. Usually, hypomanic patients who need treatment can be treated on an outpatient basis with small doses of antipsychotic medication, such as thioridazine, or by adjusting the lithium level alone. Patients who relapse from maintenance therapy into a hypomanic episode, and who previously had manic episodes (see maintenance therapy below), often can be successfully treated out of the hospital by adjusting the lithium dose upward slightly and by adding relatively small doses of antipsychotic medication. Exercise is frequently a useful adjunct in the treatment of the hypomanic patient.

Secondary Mania

One of the difficulties in treating the acute manic episode relates to the problem of secondary mania. Krauthammer and Klerman (14) outlined medical and other conditions that could present with manic-like syndromes. These include illnesses such as lupus psychosis, Cushing's disease, drug intoxication, epilepsy, caffeinism, and thyrotoxicosis. To this list we add the problem of patients who have extensively abused hallucinogenic drugs in the past and who have continued to have a psychiatric syndrome which persists often for many years after these drugs have not been used. This syndrome has been called the post-LSD syndrome. Its DSM-III classification is problematic, although the term *organic affective* or *organic delusional syndrome* may be appropriate. This syndrome in general consists of mood shifts from affective highs to depressions, impulsive behavior, and hallucinations, delusions, and difficulty in thinking. Although tryptophan has been suggested as a possible treatment for this condition, at times patients with this condition will be misdiagnosed as having acute mania. The response of such patients to conventional treatment may be different since their illness is not typical mania. The issue of secondary mania is a critical one for treatment of the acute manic syndrome since a "nonendogenous" manic syndrome may have a different innate course and not have the characteristic treatment responses of the typical manic syndrome.

MAINTENANCE THERAPY

Acutely manic patients used to be quite frequently seen in psychiatric hospitals. However, this seems to be no longer the case in many psychiatric centers. It is our belief that this change in inpatient characteristics is a reflection of good psychopharmacology practice by clinicians in preventing recurrent attacks of what ordinarily is a disabling illness. Thus, the episode frequency of bipolar affective disorder prior to maintenance therapy was about four episodes in 10 years, and approximately 80% of these episodes involved a rehospitalization for mania (15). With lithium carbonate maintenance therapy, these attacks are either nonexistent or considerably attenuated in such a way that they are treated more frequently on an outpatient than inpatient basis. Thus, a major effect of maintenance therapy has been to reduce the number of true manic cases one sees in the hospital who are relapsing after their first episode.

The early studies by Baastrup and Schou (16) suggested that the continuation of lithium salts in patients who had recurrent manic depressive illness was useful in reducing the subsequent frequency of such attacks. These open clinical studies were severely questioned, and the need for placebo-controlled data resulted in a series of double-blind, controlled, lithium-maintenance studies being performed in the late 1960s and early 1970s. The results of these research trials clearly show that lithium is an effective treatment in the prevention of recurrent attacks of both mania and depression in bipolar patients (17). Indeed, for bipolar I patients the frequency of mania was reduced to about one-eighth, and the severity of relapses was also considerably reduced. Similarly, for bipolar II patients (most of whom do not ordinarily require treatment for hypomania) there were no cases of treated hypomania when lithium was applied as compared to placebo (18).

The use of lithium salts for maintenance can begin during the manic episode when lithium is continued through what is usually a postmanic depressive episode, and then to maintenance levels. In general, maintenance levels are somewhat lower than therapeutic levels for acute mania, and are of the range of 0.7–1.0 mEq/L. It is important to obtain lithium blood tests, and our recommendation is that patients be seen at least monthly for the first 6 months of maintenance treatment (since a higher relapse rate has been noted during this interval) and then at least every other month for several years thereafter. If a patient has been stable for several years, the interval between visits can be decreased to every 3 months or so. However, manic relapses on lithium can occur even after several years of stabilization. The patient should be made aware of this fact and advised to seek help should typical symptoms recur.

In the selection of patients for lithium maintenance treatment, one should consider that patients with a first cycle of bipolar affective disorder may not relapse at all or may take several years to have their second cycle. Thus, the concept of episode frequency is relevant for determining who should be treated with lithium maintenance. Our guidelines have been that patients who show two episodes within a 5- to 7-year period merit lithium maintenance therapy. Certainly, the age and medical condition of the patient should be considered along with episode frequency when the decision is made regarding lithium maintenance.

Some patients have an interim cyclothymia between episodes which they find is benefited by lithium maintenance therapy. Thus, the patient with a low episode frequency may decide that the cyclothymia benefits from lithium maintenance and opt for lithium maintenance even though the frequency of the attacks does not in itself warrant maintenance therapy. This is not an unimportant consideration since lithium has a number of side effects, and the risk of long-term lithium effects on the kidney, heart, and thyroid in particular should be weighed against the potential benefit regarding reduction of frequency and severity of attacks.

Rapid Cyclers

Rapid cyclers have been defined as patients who have two cycles (four episodes or more of affective disturbance) in a 1-year period. Such patients are relatively rare but have comprised approximately 15% of lithium research centers where such refractory patients are often referred. The patient with rapid cycling illness should be studied for the possibility of underlying thyroiditis by obtaining antithyroid antibodies. That is, high thyroid antibody titers have been reported in some patients with rapid cycling disorder, and such patients when treated with lithium frequently develop a hypothyroid state. The addition of thyroid hormone to patients who have high thyroid titers may be advisable. Furthermore, rapid cyclers may benefit from a combination of lithium and antipsychotic medications. Antidepressants should be avoided in rapid cycling patients because these drugs appear to increase the cycle frequency.

Another drug that has been proposed for maintenance is carbamazepine. It has been found to be beneficial in maintenance therapy as well as in acute mania (10,19,20). Rapid cycling bipolars as well as bipolars with mild electroencephalographic (EEG) abnormalities may particularly benefit from treatment with carbamazepine. Lithium should be used cautiously with carbamazepine as this combination has been reported to produce neurotoxicity, even at therapeutic blood lithium concentrations (21). Carbamazepine has a series of side effects relating to blood dyscrasias, and white blood cell counts should be obtained as well as serum carbamazepine levels during treatment. More recently it has been suggested that the new antidepressant drug, bupropion, may have maintenance effects for bipolar patients. Further research regarding this compound would be important prior to its widespread use as a maintenance drug. Studies of maintenance therapy in patients with bipolar and unipolar recurrent depression have recently been reviewed at a "consensus development panel (22)." The conclusions of this panel include lithium being the drug of choice for maintenance therapy of bipolar disorder. Lithium or tricyclic antidepressants are effective in recurrent unipolar depression. However, choice of medication may be determined by such factors as age, intercurrent medical problems, and concomitant medication as well as diagnosis.

Baseline medical workups for patients undergoing lithium therapy should include a physical exam and medical history, complete blood count, thyroid function tests, kidney function test (at least blood urea nitrogen and creatinine), electrocardiogram for patients over 40, and urinalysis. Lithium has antithyroid effects, and myxedema occurring early in the course of treatment has been reported. If this condition is suspected, an elevated thyroid-stimulating hormone (TSH) level should be correlated with the appropriate diagnosis. Such patients can be successfully treated by adding a thyroid hormone to the lithium regimen.

The side effects (particularly renal side effects) of lithium were controversial for a while, but more recent studies have suggested that long-term clinically serious renal side effects are limited to a small percentage of patients. A slight polyuria occurs in most patients who are undergoing lithium maintenance therapy. This is related to an antidiuretic hormone effect of lithium and an inability to concentrate urine, with resulting increased thirst, polydipsia and polyuria. A small percentage of patients will develop a severe nephrogenic diabetes insipidus and will urinate more than 3 L/day. Treatment of this condition should be considered, although the condition itself may be episodic and aggravated during manic relapses. Various treatments have been proposed including treatment with diuretics or lowering the lithium dose. Lithium has effects in older patients in producing sinus node dysfunction and this should be part of the differential diagnosis if syncopal episodes occur in an elderly patient taking lithium.

Maintenance effects of lithium include decreased frequency of both manic and depressive episodes in bipolar I patients (those who have recurrent cycles of bipolar affective disorder involving hospitalization for mania). In bipolar II patients, lithium maintenance results in a diminution of future attacks of both hypomania and depression. Rapid cyclers also show a positive response to lithium pharmacotherapy, although such patients often continue to have affective episodes in spite of lithium treatment. Patients who seem to have a poor response to lithium should be considered for treatment with carbamazepine. As newer medications are developed for affective disorder, their use in maintenance therapy of bipolar affective disorders will need to be assessed.

REFERENCES

1. *Diagnostic and Statistical Manual of Mental Disorders*, (3rd ed.). (1980). Washington, DC: American Psychiatric Association.
2. Cooper, J. E., Kendell, R. E., Gurland, B. J., et al. (1972). *Psychiatric Diagnosis in New York and London.* London: Oxford University Press.
3. Feighner, J. P., Robins, E., Guze, S. B., et al. (1972). Diagnostic criteria for use in psychiatric research. *Archives of General Psychiatry* 26:57–63.
4. Spitzer, R. L., Endicott, J., and Robins, E. (1978). Research diagnostic criteria: rationale and reliability. *Archives of General Psychiatry* 35:773–782.
5. Dunner, D. L., Gershon, E. S., and Goodwin, F. K. (1976). Heritable factors in the severity of affective illness. *Biological Psychiatry* 11:31–42.
6. Rosenthal, N. E., Rosenthal, L. N., Stallone, F., et al. (1980). Toward the validation of RDC schizoaffective disorder. *Archives of General Psychiatry* 37:804–810.
7. Cohen, W. J., and Cohen, N. H. (1974). Lithium carbonate, haloperidol, and irreversible brain damage. *Journal of the American Medical Association* 230:1383–1387.
8. Spring, G., and Frankel, M. (1981). New data on lithium and haloperidol incompatibility. *American Journal of Psychiatry* 138:818–821.
9. Levenson, J. L. (1985). Neuroleptic malignant syndrome. *American Journal of Psychiatry* 142:1137–1145.
10. Post, R. M., Ballenger, J. C., Uhde, T. W., and Bunney, W. E., Jr. (1984). Efficacy of carbamazepine in manic-depressive illness: implication for underlying mechanisms. In *Neurobiology of Mood Disorders*, ed. R. M. Post, and J. C. Ballenger, pp. 777–816. Baltimore, MD: Williams & Wilkins.
11. Lerer, B. (1985). Alternate therapies for bipolar disorder. *Journal of Clinical Psychiatry* 46:309–316.
12. Dubovsky, S. L., Franks, R. D., and Schrier, D. (1985). Phenelzine-induced hypomania: effect of verapamil. *Biological Psychiatry* 20:1009–1014.
13. Small, J. G., Kellams, J. J., Milstein, V., et al. (1980). Complications of electroconvulsive treatment combined with lithium. *Biological Psychiatry* 15:103–112.
14. Krauthammer, C., and Klerman, G. (1978). Secondary mania: manic symptoms associated with antecedent physical illness. *Archives of General Psychiatry* 35:1333–1339.
15. Dunner, D. L., Murphy, D., Stallone, F., and Fieve, R. R. (1979). Episode frequency prior to lithium treatment in bipolar manic depressive patients. *Comprehensive Psychiatry* 20:511–515.
16. Baastrup, P. C., and Schou, J. (1967). Lithium as a prophylactic agent: its effects against recurrent depression and manic-depressive psychoses. *Archives of General Psychiatry* 16:162–172.
17. Fieve, R. R., Kumbaraci, T., and Dunner, D. L. (1976). Lithium prophylaxis of depression in bipolar I, bipolar II and unipolar patients. *American Journal of Psychiatry* 133:925–929.
18. Dunner, D. L., Stallone, F., and Fieve, R. R. (1982). Prophylaxis with lithium carbonate: an update. *Archives of General Psychiatry* 39:1344–1345.

References

19. Ballenger, J. C., and Post, R. M. (1980). Carbamazepine in manic-depressive illness: a new treatment. *American Journal of Psychiatry* 137:782-790.
20. Okuma, T., Kishimoto, A., Inoue, K., et al. (1973). Anti-manic and prophylactic effects of carbamazepine on manic-depressive psychosis. *Folia Psychiatrica et Neurologica Japonica* 27:283-297.
21. Shukla, S., Goodwin, C. D., Long, L. E. B., and Miller, M. G. (1984). Lithium-carbamazepine neurotoxicity and risk factors. *American Journal of Psychiatry* 141:1604-1606.
22. Consensus Development Panel. (1985). Mood disorders: pharmacologic prevention of recurrences. *American Journal of Psychiatry* 142:469-476.

5

Violence

Joe P. Tupin, M.D.

Violence by individuals usually results from an interaction of various factors. These have been described in detail in other sources, and the literature continues to evolve. Even a brief listing would include cultural, social, demographic, psychological, developmental, physical, psychiatric, and substance-abuse elements (1). Although these are often identified in retrospective studies and thus are mostly correlative and descriptive rather than experimentally proven, they nonetheless are often clinically useful. These putative causes of violence often coexist, suggesting interaction. Occasionally, single factors seem adequate to explain violent behavior. For example, amphetamine abuse or specific types of brain disease may be independent of any pre-existing or continuing factors; thus, when removed, violence disappears. This is rare. Conversely, not all individuals exhibiting a high-risk profile, for example paranoid psychosis, develop actual violence. Thus, careful examination of the patient's history, physical and neurological status, psychiatric diagnosis, and other factors is mandatory in organizing and implementing a rational treatment program.

This chapter focuses exclusively on the psychopharmacology as it relates to the origin and treatment of violence by individuals. Psychotherapy (2), behavior therapy (3), education (4), and other intervention strategies (4) are not reviewed.

PSYCHOPHARMACOLOGY OF THE ORIGINS OF VIOLENCE

This area has had little systematic study. Most observations arise from case reports, brief surveys, or retrospective analysis of individual violent acts. Drugs may elicit violence, either on the basis of their direct effect or at the time of withdrawal. A variety of direct effect that is poorly understood but familiar to clinicians is disinhibition or paradoxical excitement. The best example of the direct effect of drugs leading to an increased risk for violence includes the central nervous system stimulants (5) such as amphetamines, phencyclidine, and cocaine. These drugs may produce hyperactivity, irritability, lability, delusions, or hallucinations, which may be the direct antecedent of the violent behavior. Delirium may be present. Drugs such as atropine, meperidine, and hallucinogens may increase the risk for violence by creating a delirium, perceptual distortion, lability delusions and altered sensorium (5). Disinhibition or paradoxical excitement (5) has been associated with alcohol, benzodiazepines, barbiturates, and other sedative hypnotics.

Drug withdrawal states that produce delirium may also lead to violent behavior. Typically these are sedative–hypnotic drugs where tolerance has developed. Multiple drug abuse may be a component of this syndrome. Likewise, these will occur occasionally in general hospitals when inadvertent "cold-turkey" withdrawal occurs. Typically, violence associated with delirium is impulsive, "purposeless," poorly organized, and reactive.

Certain benzodiazepines have been associated with increased incidence of hostility and occasionally violence. These include alprazolam, clonazepam, diazepam, and chlordiazepoxide (6).

TREATMENT OF SYNDROMES

Treatment can be divided into two broad strategies, short term and long term. Philosophy, goals, setting, and drug selection will differ dramatically.

Short-Term Treatment

Short-term treatment usually occurs in an urgent or emergency situation. The patient may be unknown and is often brought to the emergency treatment setting by police or ambulance. Also, short-term control of agitation, increased psychotic symptoms, or violence will occur when the patient is well known to the institution and already hospitalized.

Goals of short-term treatment. The desired outcome is the safety of the staff and patient, and if the patient is unknown to the institution, to obtain opportunity for evaluation. Adjunctive treatment often includes seclusion and restraints, quiet rooms, supportive psychotherapy, and careful institution of environmental precautions. Since short-term control of behavior is the goal, the result can be rather nonspecific; that is, sedation or tranquilization may be all that is desired, whereas other specific serious symptomatology may continue, for example, delusions. Treatment may occur prior to establishment of a diagnosis or even prior to any definitive evaluation.

Medications for short-term treatment. Three types of medication can be prescribed in this situation: barbiturates, benzodiazepines, or anti-psychotics. Historically, barbiturates have been used to produce sedation (7); however, because of the risk of depressing cardiorespiratory function with serious consequences, including death, they are rarely used (although they are occasionally a welcome alternative). An anti-psychotic given either orally, intramuscularly, or intravenously in doses of 100–300 mg often is adequate to produce general sedation. Intravenous administration should be slow, e.g., 50 mg every 1–2 minutes with careful monitoring of respiration, blood pressure, and pulse. In addition to respiratory depression, disinhibition can occur.

Benzodiazepines currently play an increasingly important role (8). They are relatively safe and generally do not depress respiration significantly unless there is prior physical disease (e.g., chronic lung disease) or if other central nervous system depressant drugs have been ingested. Most of the benzodiazepines are reasonably well absorbed and active orally; however, the prodrugs (8), prazepam and clorazepate, require an acid milieu in the stomach for conversion to an active form. None of the drugs is available as a liquid. Generally, shorter-acting medications such as oxazepam or lorazepam may be preferable because they do not require liver metabolism. The emergency-room patient may have a coexisting liver disease. Likewise, longer-acting drugs will interfere with an adequate evaluation for a longer period of time. Another important consideration with this group of drugs is the dose form. Diazepam can be given intravenously as can lorazepam. Diazepam can be given effectively intramuscularly if given in the deltoid area (8), and lorazepam is well absorbed from any site intramuscularly. Chloradiazepoxide is not advised to be given parenterally.

Benzodiazepines may be given alone and have been reported favorably in small, uncontrolled studies for the control of manic excitement and other forms of agitation (9). Often, they are also given as an adjunct to antipsychotics. Antipsychotic drugs are usually given to patients who are agitated and combative. High-potency drugs are usually chosen because of their lack of sedation and significant effect on blood pressure (10). Double-blind control studies have indicated that this characteristic of high-potency drugs is a significant clinical advantage (see Chapter 1). Fluphenazine, haloperidol, and thiothixene are all available in oral and intramuscular forms. There has been a great deal of experience of haloperidol given intravenously in its present parenteral formulation, although no explicit approval exists for that use (dose 5–10 mg, I.V. slowly) (11).

Droperidol (12) (Inapsine), structurally similar to haloperidol, is widely used in Europe for treating acute and chronic psychosis. However, in this country, it is approved for anesthesia-related I.V. uses but is used for emergencies such as combativeness and severe agitation at a dose of 1–50 mg, I.V. One recent paper (12), in which doses of 5 mg intramuscularly were studied has indicated it is comparable to more accepted antipsychotics, but the authors conclude that it afforded more rapid relief of acute psychiatric symptoms and is somewhat shorter acting (12). Doses of 1.5–5 mg are adequate and can be repeated in 30 minutes.

A recent review (13,14) of rapid neuroleptization suggested that there may be relatively little clinical benefit in using extremely high doses of high-potency antipsychotics but there may be increased side effects which may masquerade or aggravate the underlying psychosis. Consequently, doses equivalent to 300–1,000 mg of chlorpromazine are adequate for most patients. Little is gained with higher doses, except side effects. Fluphenazine hydrochloride (5–30 mg), thiothixene (15–60 mg), and haloperidol (5–30 mg) is generally adequate for most patients. The dosages are usually divided: for example, haloperidol is given in 5- to 10-mg doses every 30–60 minutes until the patient is controlled or the above dose limits are achieved. If the upper limit is achieved without adequate control of combative, agitated behavior, then the addition of a benzodiazepine, for example, lorazepam given intramuscularly 1–2 mg every 30–60 minutes (maximum dose, 10 mg), will be useful for most patients who have not responded to the antipsychotic alone. Occasionally, barbiturates may be used in this same manner in low doses.

Monitoring vital signs is particularly important, especially since these patients may not be well known to the institutions and may have other drugs, either legal or illegal, on board. Occasional cases of sudden death have been reported with antipsychotic medications.

As soon as possible, even before giving medication, a brief mental status should be obtained to assess any evidence of organic brain disease and to gather any other psychiatric information. As soon as safety is assured, neurological evaluation should be completed and toxicological screens begun (15,16). Dementias, delirium, substance abuse, personality disorders, major psychoses, and neurological conditions should all be considered.

Phencyclidine psychosis is probably best treated at this time by a high-potency antipsychotic with a predominantly dopamine receptor-site blockade characteristic (17). Haloperidol is typical of this group.

Long-Term Treatment

Violence tends to be repeated. The known violent or potentially violent individual needs an effective prophylactic treatment program which begins after an adequate evaluation. The medication choice is a direct result of a complete evaluation. Most often, there has been previous violent behavior. However, occasionally there are patients where there is no history but whose threats, fantasies, delusions, hallucinations, results of psychological testing, or other data suggest the potential for violence.

Goals of long-term treatment. Prevention is the goal, and the clinician must implement a program that may include medication, psychotherapy, behavior modification, or education. Diagnostic evaluation should pay particular attention to brain injury in repetitively violent individuals. A recent study of death-row inmates emphasized the presence of nonspecific neuropsychological abnormalities (18).

Psychotically depressed individuals may also be violent. My clinical experience is that they usually exhibit early developmental characteristics of deprivation, and the like, that differentiate them from nonviolent, psychotically depressed patients. The usual diagnosis associated with violence, for example, paranoid schizophrenia, is treated in the usual way with antipsychotics. Occasionally these individuals may also have other factors that contribute to violence and must not be overlooked. For example, substance abuse or brain injury may be independent of their paranoid schizophrenia and may require special attention.

Medications for long-term treatment

Antipsychotics. These medications are traditionally used for the treatment of various types of schizophrenia, schizo-affective disorders, agitated and/or delusionally demented individuals, and for short-term control of delirium. They also have recently been identified as an important part of the treatment of the delusionally depressed patient. Generally, the medication is given orally, but intramuscular, long-acting dosage is also indicated. Doses and selection of medication are thoroughly discussed in Chapter 1 ("Psychosis") and Chapter 2 ("Depressive Disorders"). Violence not directly related to psychotic features may not remit with antipsychotics.

Antidepressants. These medications are part of the treatment for the delusionally depressed individual who may carry out a murder and suicide act. Antipsychotics have already been mentioned as an important part of the pharmacological treatment of these individuals, but antidepressants are also critical. Electroconvulsive therapy may be of importance. Poor responders to pharmacological interventions are particularly dangerous. Less severe forms of depression may also be associated with irritability, anger, and assault.

Attention-deficit disorder has been linked to impulsivity in adults and there is some evidence to suggest that these individuals may be violent. The usual treatment of stimulants is indicated for the child or adolescent. This is less-well studied in the adult and is reviewed in Chapter 12.

To the extent that panic disorders can be associated with inadvertent violence, antidepressants, which are often quite effective for this condition, can be very helpful.

Antimanic Medications. Usually these medications are used for the initial control of manic symptomatology and also for the long-term prevention of recurrent bipolar illness. These are well reviewed in Chapter 4. Lithium is the oldest of this group of drugs. Carbamazepine (19) has recently been widely studied and is considered to be effective in the initial control of manic symptoms as well as for prophylaxis of bipolar symptoms.

Benzodiazepines, particularly lorazepam and diazepam (20), have been used as part of the initial control of manic symptomatology. Also, clonidine (21) has been used in doses of 0.4–1.2 mg/day for control of acute manic symptomatology, and it has been suggested that it may be a useful addition to other antimanic agents to control difficult cases. Violence can occur in manic episodes. Both lithium and carbamazepine have been identified as occasionally being useful adjuncts in the treatment of schizophrenia and schizoaffective illness.

There is a group of poorly understood patients often with a diagnosis of personality disorder and repeated explosive violence that may respond to lithium (22) and possibly carbamazepine. Patients studied have been both adult and children, brain injured and nonbrain injured, and may carry a variety of other psychiatric diagnoses, including mental retardation. The identifying characteristics of the lithium responders have been suggested (23) to be: (a) easy provocation (minimal stimuli may produce a significant angry, hostile, or assaultive outburst); (b) poor control (once provoked, their anger is inappropriate, persistent, and the assaultiveness grossly inappropriate to the stimulus); and (c) cognition (these individuals report that between the stimulus and the assaultive outburst they have no reflective assessment of the social situation or the nature of the stimulus, whether it was accidental or whether there was personal risk of harm or arrest). Lithium dose and blood levels are maintained at the same level as for prophylaxis of manic-depressive illness.

Carbamazepine has also been studied in patients having rage outbursts with apparent favorable activity specifically for hyperactivity, perhaps representing adults with attention-deficit disorder (24). Other experimental treatments for bipolar illness are discussed in Chapter 4.

Antianxiety Drugs. To the extent that anxiety is a preliminary state to violent outbursts, for example, homosexual panic, this type of medication may be useful for long-term control. In addition, antianxiety agents may be a useful adjunct in the control of agitation associated with schizophrenia, schizo-affective disorder, or bipolar illness. Alprazolam has been reported to provoke hostility (25).

Miscellaneous Medications. There is a keen interest in studies involving a variety of medications often not used for psychiatric purposes but perhaps useful in the control of episodic violence. These include beta-adrenergic blockers (26), anticonvulsants, calcium channel blockers (27), and antiandrogen hormones (28). The beta blockers are the most carefully studied; however, carefully done placebo control studies have yet to be completed in large numbers. Propranolol and nadolol, both beta-1 and beta-2 blockers, have been reported to be effective (26). Propranolol is lipophilic while nadolol is hydrophilic. There is also one brief mention of metropolol, a beta-1 blocker, as being effective (24). Trazadone is being used for violent, brain-damaged, and elderly patients. Undoubtedly, additional reports will be forthcoming.

Anticonvulsants. Carbamazepine has been previously mentioned. Literature also refers to diphenylhydantoin, valproic acid, and clonazepam. None of these has been carefully or exhaustively studied; however, the most work has been done with carbamazepine. In those patients with demonstrable brain injury, even without epileptogenic abnormalities on the electroencephalogram or clinical history of seizures, anticonvulsants may be an appropriate choice.

Calcium channel blockers (27) remain even more speculative. Although there are few case reports, these drugs may be useful.

Hormonal treatment for sexually associated aggression has been the subject of a great deal of study (28). Two compounds, both of which block androgens, have been fairly widely used. They are medroxyprogesterone and cyproterone acetate. The former inhibits the release of androgens by suppressing luteinizing hormone release. The latter blocks androgen receptor sites. Only medroxyprogesterone is available in the United States. Doses are 100–800 mg given intramuscularly every 7 days. The average dose is about 500 mg. Reports indicate that these drugs reduce drive, arousal, fantasy, and ejaculation while increasing control. They have been used in a variety of sexually deviant aggressive individuals including rapists, pedophiles, and exhibitionists.

Initial control for short-term purposes only serves the purpose of providing a safe environment for patients and staff and allows for thorough evaluation for continuing with any specific treatment. Long-term treatment is a complex issue demanding careful diagnostic assessment where numerous factors may interact to produce violent behavior. Specific pharmacological interventions must be chosen on the basis of the findings (29).

REFERENCES

1. Daniels, D. N., Gilula, M. F., and Ochberg, F. M., eds. (1970). *Violence and the Struggle for Existence.* Boston: Little, Brown.
2. Madden, E. J. (1976). Psychological approaches to violence. In *Rage, Hate, Assault, and Other Forms of Violence,* ed. E. J. Madden and J. R. Lion, pp. 135-151. New York: Spectrum.
3. Wong, S. E., Slaman, K., and Lieberman, R. P. (1985). Behavioral analysis and therapy for aggressive psychiatrically and developmentally disabled patients. In *Clinical Treatment of the Violent Person,* ed. L. H. Roth. Washington, DC: U.S. Department of Health and Human Services, Public Health Service.
4. Lion, J. R., and Reid, W. A., eds. (1983). *Assaults within Psychiatric Facilities.* New York: Grune & Stratton.
5. Tinklenberg, J. R., Woodrow, K. M., and Frazier, S. H., eds. (1973). Drug use among assaultive and sexual offenders. In *Human Aggression: Proceedings of the 1972 Annual Meeting for the Association for Research in Nervous and Mental Disease.* Baltimore, MD: Williams & Wilkins.
6. Kochansky, G. E., Salzman, C., Shader, R. I., et al. (1975). The differential effects of oxazepam and chlordiazepoxide upon hostility in a small group setting. *American Journal of Psychiatry* 132:861-863.
7. Sheard, M. H. (1984). Clinical pharmacology of aggressive behavior. *Clinical Neuropharmacology* 7:173-183.
8. Shader, R. I., Greenblatt, D. J., and Abernathy, D. (1983). Current status of benzodiazepines. *New England Journal of Medicine* 309:410-416.
9. Salzman, C., Green, A. I., Rodriguez-Villa, F., and Jaskow, G. I. (1986). Benzodiazepines combined with neuroleptics for management of severe disruptive behavior. *Psychosomatics* 27:17-23.
10. Donlon, P. T., Hopkin, J., and Tupin, J. P. (1979). Overview: efficacy and safety of the rapid neurolepticization method with injectable haloperidol. *American Journal of Psychiatry* 136:273-278.
11. Tesar, G. E., Murray, J. B., and Cassem, N. H. (1985). Use of high-dose intravenous haloperidol in the treatment of agitated cardiac patients. *Journal of Clinical Psychopharmacology* 5:344-347.
12. Resnick, M., and Burton, B. T. (1984). Droperidol versus haloperidol in the initial management of acutely agitated patients. *Journal of Clinical Psychiatry* 45:298-299.

13. Tupin, J. P. (1985). Focal neuroleptization: an approach to optimal dosing for initial and continuing therapy. *Journal of Clinical Psychopharmacology* 5:15s-21s.
14. Cole, J. O. (1982). Antipsychotic drugs: is more better? *McLean Hospital Journal* 7:61-87.
15. Ellinwood, E. H. (1976). Amphetamine psychosis: description of the individuals and process. *Journal of Nervous and Mental Diseases* 144:273-283.
16. Pitts, F. N., Allen, R. E., Aniline, O., and Burgoyne, R. W. (1982). The dilemma of the toxic psychosis: differential diagnosis and the PCP psychosis. *Psychiatric Annals* 12:762-768.
17. Giannini, A. J., Nageotte, C., Loiselle, R. H., et al. (1984-1985). Comparison of chlorpromazine, haloperidol, and pimozide in the treatment of phencyclidine psychosis: DA-2 receptor specificity. *Clinical Toxicology* 22:573-579.
18. Lewis, D. O. (1986). Psychiatric, neurological and psychoeducational characteristics of 15 death row inmates in the United States. *American Journal of Psychiatry* 143:838-845.
19. Post, R. M., Rubinow, D. R., and Uhde, T. W. (1984). Biochemical mechanisms of action of carbamazepine in affective illness and epilepsy. *Psychopharmacology Bulletin* 20:585-590.
20. Arana, G. W., Ornsten, L., Canter, F., et al. (1986). The use of benzodiazepines for psychotic disorders: a literature review and preliminary clinical findings. *Psychopharmacology Bulletin* 22:77-87.
21. Bond, W. S. (1986). Psychiatric indications for clonidine: the neuropharmacologic and clinical basis. *Journal of Clinical Psychopharmacology* 6:81-88.
22. Tupin, J. P., Smith, D. G., Clanon, T. L., et al. (1973). The long-term use of lithium in aggressive prisoners. *Comprehensive Psychiatry* 14:311-317.
23. Tupin, J. P. (1977). Letter to the editor: usefulness of lithium for aggressiveness. *American Journal of Psychiatry* 135(9):1118.
24. Roy-Byrne, P. P., Uhde, T. W., and Post, R. M. (1984). Carbamazepine for hyperactivity, anxiety, and withdrawal syndromes. *International Drug Therapy Newsletter*, September, p. 19.
25. Rosenbaum, J. F., Woods, S. W., Groves, J. E., and Klerman, G. L. (1984). Emergence of hostility during alprazolam treatment. *American Journal of Psychiatry* 141:792-794.
26. Silver, J. M., and Yudofsky, S. (1988). Propranolol for aggression: literature review and clinical guidelines. *International Drug Therapy Newsletter*, March, p. 20.
27. Montgomery, P. T., and Mueller, M. E. (1985). Treatment of PCP intoxication with verapamil. *American Journal of Psychiatry* 142:882.
28. Gagne, P. (1981). Treatment of sex offenders with medroxyprogesterone acetate. *American Journal of Psychiatry* 138(5):644-646.
29. Dubin, W. R., Weiss, K. J., and Dorn, J. M. (1986). Pharmacotherapy of psychiatric emergencies. *Journal of Clinical Psychopharmacology* 6:210-223.

6

Substance Abuse

Domenic A. Ciraulo, M.D.
Ann Marie Ciraulo, R.N.

While recruiting at a Boston Alcoholics Anonymous (AA) meeting, one of our research associates was asked about the interests of our laboratory. Quite innocently she replied that we were interested in which medications used in psychiatry could be helpful to alcoholics and other substance abusers. The AA member quipped, "Well you sure are in luck. Just listen to the people here tonight, and you'll have your answer." After a suitable dramatic pause he added, "None. Lady, these people need to be *off* of those drugs." The prepossessions of some recovering substance abusers lead them to regard the use of psychotropic agents in this population as flagitious. Clinical and research data, however, reveal this to be a biased position.

There are at least five areas in which drug treatment of substance abusers has immediate clinical relevance. Psychotropics are used to (a) treat abstinence syndromes; (b) block the subjective or euphoric effects of abused drugs; (c) produce adverse consequences if an abused substance is ingested; (d) block craving; and (e) treat anxiety, depression, and other psychiatric disturbances in alcoholics and addicts. This chapter reviews the clinically relevant data regarding the use of psychoactive drugs in substance abusers.

ALCOHOL WITHDRAWAL SYNDROME

Signs and Symptoms

Chronic ingestion of ethanol leads to tolerance and an abstinence syndrome upon abrupt discontinuation or significant reduction of alcohol intake. The severity and duration of the syndrome depend on numerous factors, such as the amount and duration of heavy drinking, the overall medical condition of the individual, concomitant use of other drugs, and the severity of an individual's previous withdrawal symptoms.

The characteristic symptoms of alcohol withdrawal generally begin within hours after ingestion of the last drink (1). Symptoms peak at 24–48 hours and gradually subside within 5–7 days. Mild alcohol withdrawal symptoms may include anxiety, tremulousness, sleep disturbance, and mild gastrointestinal upset. The severe symptoms are nausea, vomiting, tachycardia, elevated blood pressure, sweating, fever, irritability, and agitation. The individual may become confused, disoriented, and delusional and experience vivid hallucinations (delirium tremens). Over the past 20 years, the mortality rate for delirium tremens has declined from 20% to 1%. Grand mal seizures ("rum fits"), occur between 7 and 48 hours after the cessation of drinking with the highest incidence at 24 hours. Some experts believe the maximum risk of seizures is later, between 31 and 48 hours after stopping drinking (2). Seizures that occur after 48 hours are most likely due to other causes (e.g., dependence on other drugs, cranial injury, or metabolic disturbances) and diagnostic evaluations are required.

Treatment

General procedures. Effective nursing care, accurate diagnosis and management of medical and surgical complications, and the judicious use of medications are the major factors responsible for reducing morbidity and mortality from alcohol withdrawal. The importance of nursing care is demonstrated by programs that successfully treat mild withdrawal without medication (3,4). With this approach patients with mild dependence, no serious medical or psychiatric problems, and a history of uncomplicated withdrawal are detoxified from alcohol in 2–7 days in a nonmedical inpatient setting which relies on intensive staff contact with patients. Counselors are trained to use interpersonal techniques such as reassurance and reality orientation to reduce the anxiety associated with withdrawal.

Nutritional supplementation, fluids, and electrolytes. Nutritional deficiencies commonly occur in the chronic alcoholic. Wernicke's encephalopathy, Korsakoff's syndrome (alcohol amnestic disorder resulting from thiamine deficiency), megaloblastic anemia (due to folate deficiency), peripheral neuropathy, and prolonged prothrombin time (as a result of vitamin K deficiency) are the result of vitamin deficiencies. It has become standard procedure to administer thiamine, 50–100 mg intramuscularly (IM) or intravenously (I.V.) daily, for the first 3 days, usually with daily multivitamins. If prothrombin time is prolonged, vitamin K is administered (5–10 mg IM). Patients with megaloblastic anemia or peripheral neuropathy should receive 1–5 mg folic acid orally or IM. Most alcoholics are magnesium-depleted regardless of serum concentrations, and this may result in lethargy, arrhythmias, weakness, and decreased seizure threshold. Although the apparent depletion may be a distributional phenomenon, some clinicians recommend replacement therapy. Magnesium sulfate, however, does not appear to be an effective prophylactic agent against alcohol withdrawal seizures (5). Potassium deficiency is also quite common and causes weakness, fatigue, and cardiac arrhythmias. Supplemental potassium is administered either orally or I.V. The usual daily replacement dose is 100–140 mEq. Renal function should be carefully monitored during potassium replacement. Hypophosphatemia is also common in alcoholics. Serum phosphate levels below 1 mg% are accompanied by anorexia, weakness, lethargy, bone pain, tremor, cardiomyopathy, hemolysis, and respiratory failure. Dietary intake in the hospital is usually sufficient to replace phosphate; however, if a patient is not eating, supplementation may be required. Hypoglycemia can occur as the result of liver disease or accompanying medical illnesses. If glucose administration is required, it may further deplete thiamine and can precipitate the onset of Wernicke's encephalopathy. Although many alcoholics appear to be dehydrated, tissue water levels are higher than normal in most alcoholics (6,7). The routine use of parenteral fluid replacement is not justified. On the other hand, some patients in severe withdrawal may be volume depleted. Determining daily weights, urine specific gravity, and urinary sodium concentration will assist in monitoring hydration (8).

Benzodiazepines. The benzodiazepines are the drugs of choice in treatment of the alcohol withdrawal syndrome because of their anxiolytic, anticonvulsant, sedative, and muscle-relaxing properties which provide effective and safe control of most withdrawal symptoms (see Table 6-1). For patients who are hallucinating or have a previous history of seizures, neuroleptics or anticonvulsants may be necessary. If the delirium is well established, higher doses of benzodiazepines are generally required.

The pharmacokinetic properties that distinguish the various benzodiazepines are important in planning rational drug therapy (9). Diazepam and chlordiazepoxide are long-acting benzodiazepines that are metabolized via demethylation to the active metabolite desmethyldiazepam (DMDZ) which has an elimination half-life of 50-100 hours in normal adults. Similarly, halazepam (Paxipam) and prazepam (Centrax) are also converted to DMDZ by the liver, while clorazepate is a prodrug that is hydrolyzed to DMDZ in the stomach.

The longer-acting drugs have the advantage of being self-tapering due to the cumulative effects of active metabolites. An initial loading dose can thus be administered with the onset of withdrawal symptoms, and quickly or even abruptly discontinued without adverse effects. Longer-acting drugs have the disadvantage of occasionally leading to drug and metabolite accumulation which may result in confusion, sedation, and ataxia. Diazepam and chlordiazepoxide are erratically and incompletely absorbed from IM injection in the gluteal area, therefore the oral or I.V. route of administration is preferable. Diazepam may be more reliably absorbed from IM injection in-to the deltoid. Oxazepam (Serax) and lorazepam (Ativan) are short-acting benzodiazepines that are metabolized by glucuronidation. The glucuronide is inactive, highly water soluble, and rapidly eliminated by the kidney. This can be advantageous in the elderly or cirrhotic alcoholics.

In controlling alcohol withdrawal symptoms with benzodiazepines, one approach is to use an initial loading dose to achieve sedation. Using this technique, an initial 50- to 100-mg oral dose of chlordiazepoxide is administered. Additional doses of 50-100 mg of chlordiazepoxide may then be given hourly until symptom suppression is achieved; total dosage for a 24-hour period should rarely exceed 600 mg (8). Due to the self-tapering action of the long-acting benzodiazepines, once the withdrawal symptoms are suppressed, further medication is not necessary. A similar strategy has been pro-

TABLE 6-1 Benzodiazepine Protocols for Moderate-to-Severe Alcohol Withdrawal

Drug	Initial Dose	Advantages	Disadvantages
Lorazepam (Ativan)	2-4 mg orally every 2 hours until patient is sedated. Taper drug over 5-7 days.	Less likely to accumulate and cause excessive sedation Duration of action after single dose is actually longer than diazepam Intramuscular preparation reliably absorbed Disposition not altered by cirrhosis or aging	Tapering required because of short elimination half-life Must be given on a thrice daily regimen
Diazepam (Valium)	20 mg orally every 1-2 hours until sedated	Active metabolites allow for self-tapering permitting a shorter prescribing period and less fluctuation of plasma levels between doses Less conflict with patient over drug doses	Multiple doses can accumulate causing unwanted sedation, confusion, and ataxia Intramuscular preparation is not reliably absorbed (diazepam may be better absorbed from the deltoid rather than gluteal region) Disposition impaired in cirrhosis and aging
Chlordiazepoxide (Librium and others)	50-100 mg every 1-2 hours until patient is sedated; drugs may either be discontinued abruptly after sedation is achieved or preferably quickly tapered over the next 1-2 days		

posed by Sellers and colleagues (10). In their protocol they administer 20 mg of oral diazepam every 1-2 hours, titrated to symptom improvement. After the loading dose, additional drug is not required.

Alternatively, a short-acting benzodiazepine can be used. With this method we prefer lorazepam because, if needed, an IM formulation is available that is rapidly and reliably absorbed. Lorazepam, 2-4 mg, is administered orally every 1-2 hours until sedation is achieved. Over the next 24 hours, the patient is stabilized on a four-times-daily basis, total dosage depending on the clinical situation. The dosage is then tapered over 5-7 days or 25% per day. The drug should be tapered by lowering each dose rather than by omitting one of the four daily doses. Oxazepam in an initial dose of 30-60 mg can also be used; however, an IM formulation is not available.

Beta blockers. Propranolol may reduce tremor, tachycardia, blood pressure, and diaphoresis during withdrawal (i.e., the hyperadrenergic symptoms of withdrawal) (11,12). Some clinicians suggest it is useful in mild abstinence syndromes or for patients in whom a hyperadrenergic state would seriously impair cardiovascular functioning. Propranolol will not prevent seizures, nor is it effective in delirium. Furthermore, it may mask those withdrawal symptoms that the clinician uses to assess severity. It should not be given to patients with a history of asthma, congestive heart failure, or insulin-dependent diabetes. Atenolol has also been used to treat mild-to-moderate alcohol withdrawal (13).

Lithium. Lithium carbonate (300 mg, three times a day) was found to improve subjective ratings of anxiety and sleep quality during alcohol withdrawal, being most effective when given 3 days prior to cessation of drinking (14). It was not effective in the treatment of tachycardia, elevated blood pressure, or tremors. Animal studies have shown that high doses of lithium actually potentiate withdrawal symptoms in alcohol-dependent rats (15). Given that there are efficacious and safe pharmacological therapies for the alcohol abstinence syndrome, the clinical use of lithium for this purpose is not indicated.

Chlormethiazole. Chlormethiazole is a sedative-hypnotic with anticonvulsant activity. It has a rapid onset of action, but a shorter duration of action than the long-acting benzodiazepines.

Cases of abuse and overdose have been reported. Although widely used in Great Britain and Europe, it is not currently available in the United States.

Chloral hydrate. Chloral hydrate is rarely used in the treatment of alcohol withdrawal. Its use is limited by lack of a parenteral form and its short elimination half-life (6-8 hours).

Alpha-adrenergic agonists. Clonidine, a centrally active imidazolene derivative used to treat hypertension, has also been used in opiate and alcohol abstinence syndromes. In an open trial comparing clonidine to carbamazepine plus a neuroleptic in the alcohol withdrawal syndrome, both drug regimens were effective (16). The lack of a placebo control limits these findings. Clonidine has also been shown to block alcohol withdrawal symptoms in laboratory animals (17).

Presumably clonidine acts by virtue of its alpha-2 receptor mediated inhibition of brain noradrenergic activity. Common side effects are hypotension, dry mouth, and light-headedness. One disadvantage of clonidine is its potential to mask the signs and symptoms of sedative-hypnotic withdrawal delaying appropriate pharmacological treatment.

Lofexidine is an alpha-adrenergic agonist with less sedative and hypotensive effects than clonidine. Recent studies suggest that it too may be effective in the treatment of alcohol withdrawal (18). At present there is no evidence to suggest that alpha-adrenergic agonists offer any advantages over benzodiazepines; they may have dangerous side effects (e.g., hypotension) and disadvantages in combined sedative-hypnotic-alcohol dependence.

Barbiturates. The barbiturates (pentobarbital, phenobarbital, and secobarbital) are effective in management of the alcohol withdrawal syndrome and have excellent antiseizure properties. They are still used in Europe and occasionally in the United States. The barbiturates are more likely to produce respiratory depression than benzodiazepines and therefore have limited clinical applicability.

Neuroleptics. In some cases of severe alcohol withdrawal, it may be necessary to control psychotic symptoms associated with delirium. Haloperidol has been useful in control of hallucinations and may be given 0.5–2.0 mg IM every 2 hours until the symptoms clear or to a total of five doses given in 24 hours (19). The antipsychotics are not as effective or safe as the benzodiazepines and have the added disadvantage of producing hypotension and lowering seizure threshold. They have limited usefulness in the treatment of withdrawal symptoms.

Paraldehyde. Historically, paraldehyde played an important role in the treatment of alcohol withdrawal syndrome. However, due to numerous problems it should be considered obsolete (19). Paraldehyde is more toxic and less effective than the benzodiazepines. It is available only as a liquid and has a somewhat noxious, unpleasant odor. When administered orally, it causes gastric irritation; intramuscularly, it is painful and causes sterile abcesses; intravenously, there is a risk of fat embolization; rectally, it causes proctitis, and is slowly and erratically absorbed. Paraldehyde is hepatotoxic and may cause respiratory depression, apnea, and death.

Anticonvulsants. Seizures during withdrawal are most often nonfocal, grand mal, and one or two in number (2). Phenytoin does not suppress alcohol withdrawal seizures in animal models (20) and its use in prophylaxis or treatment of such seizures in humans is of uncertain value. Patients with a pre-existing seizure disorder on the other hand, may benefit. Phenytoin (300 mg/day) in combination with chlordiazepoxide (up to 400 mg/day) is more effective than placebo in such patients (21). In patients with a known history of seizure disorder, who have stopped phenytoin maintenance for at least 5 days, phenytoin is most effective when a loading dose of 10 mg/kg in 250–500 ml of 5% dextrose in water is infused I.V. over a period of 1–4 hours. Maintenance doses of 300–400 mg daily should be started the next day (22). For patients without an underlying seizure disorder, the benzodiazepines have adequate anticonvulsant activity. Other anticonvulsants may be more rational choices than phenytoin in the treatment of alcohol withdrawal seizures. Mephenytoin, phenacemide, paramethadione, valproic acid, and carbamazepine all suppress withdrawal seizures in animal models (20,23). Clinical experience in this country using these agents in alcohol withdrawal is limited.

Carbamazepine has been studied by a number of investigators (24–30). It appears to be as effective as chlormethiazole and tiapride and superior to placebo in the treatment of alcohol withdrawal syndrome (27–29). Clinicians experienced in its use suggest that it is effective, well-tolerated, and especially useful for the dysphoric symptoms of withdrawal. It is also said to be effective in the treatment of delirium tremens. It is typically administered in a 600- to 800-mg divided daily dose during the first 48 hours of withdrawal and then tapered by 200 mg daily. Post and colleagues have suggested that repeated episodes of alcohol withdrawal are associated with increased neuronal excitability in cortical and subcortical tissues and lead to a progressive increase in severity of symptoms due to a kindling-like process (30). Carbamazepine, which inhibits limbic kindling, may thus be of benefit in acute and chronic withdrawal syndromes.

Ethanol. The administration of ethanol is not recommended for the treatment of the abstinence syndrome. Although a clinical trial in a small number of burn patients has shown that ethanol given intravenously may prevent withdrawal (31), routine administration is not recommended. Administration of ethanol intravenously to control withdrawal symptoms requires excessive fluid administration, is associated with toxicity, and is of questionable efficacy in severe withdrawal.

ALCOHOL HALLUCINOSIS

Alcohol hallucinosis is a condition associated with cessation or reduction of alcohol ingestion, and is characterized by vivid auditory hallucinations and delusions. The auditory hallucinations may be hissing or buzzing sounds, or voices talking about the individual in the third person (32). Often in response to the content of hallucination, which may be threatening or accusatory, the patient will act out by defending himself or herself, running away, or calling the police for protection. The age of onset is generally around 40–45 years, and follows 10 or more years of heavy drinking.

The onset of the syndrome occurs during the first 48 hours after the cessation of drinking following an extended period of intoxication. Some authorities suggest that this syndrome may also appear during a drinking bout, several weeks to a month after the drinking stopped, or during withdrawal (8, 33). The duration of the syndrome is from several hours to weeks or months and in a small percentage the syndrome advances to a chronic state.

The differential diagnosis of alcohol hallucinosis may be difficult due to the blurring of symptoms with other disorders, such as paranoid schizophrenia, amphetamine- or other stimulant-induced psychosis, or alcohol withdrawal delirium. Differential diagnosis is made by obtaining a careful history of the present illness, family history of affective disorder or schizophrenia, blood and urine alcohol and drug screening, and by the absence of signs and symptoms of withdrawal delirium. These patients may require hospitalization because there is a higher rate of depressive symptomology and suicide attempts in alcoholics with psychotic symptoms (33). Alcohol hallucinosis is best treated with low doses of a neuroleptic, although on occasion we have seen the symptoms respond to benzodiazepines.

DRUG TREATMENT OF ALCOHOLICS AFTER DETOXIFICATION

Psychiatric Symptoms after Detoxification

The use of psychotropic drugs after completion of alcohol withdrawal is a highly controversial issue. On the one hand, medication use may merely substitute drug dependence for alcohol, lead to combined dependency, or provide the tools for suicide. On the other hand, some evidence suggests that anxious and dysphoric states persist after the acute withdrawal phase. We have found that approximately 15% of alcoholics entering an inpatient psychiatric facility will continue to show elevated scores on a variety of self-rating scales of depression 4-6 weeks after alcohol intake (34). Furthermore mean scores on the Beck Depression Inventory after a 4- to 6-week period of detoxification remain higher than scores of a control population. Despite the persistence of high scores on self-rating scales of depression, major depression is less common. On our psychiatric inpatient unit at the Boston Veterans Administration Medical Center, major depression was present in only 10 of 88 patients with a DMS-III diagnosis of alcoholism (see Table 6-2). Of these, only six stayed in the hospital long enough for adequate drug trial. Three received tricyclic antidepressants, one alprazolam (after an unsuccessful trial of two tricyclic antidepressants), one electroconvulsive treatment

TABLE 6-2 DSM-III Axis I Diagnoses of Alcoholics
Requiring Psychiatric Admission[a]

Diagnosis	N	Percent of Total ($N = 88$)
Bipolar disorder (total)	20	23
With mood-congruent psychotic features	12	14
With mood-incongruent psychotic features[b]	8	9
Mixed substance abuse or dependence	14	16
Post-traumatic stress disorder	12	14
Major depression	10	11
Schizophrenia (all types)	8	9
Dysthymic disorder	5	6
Agoraphobia and/or panic	4	5
Paranoid disorder	2	2
Dementia associated with alcoholism	2	2
Alcohol hallucinosis	2	2

[a]Some patients had more than one Axis I diagnosis; others had none. Borderline personality disorder ($N = 12$) was the most common Axis II diagnosis. These patients usually presented intoxicated with suicidal ideation or after an attempt.
[b]Clinicians diagnosed all of these patients as schizo-affective.

followed by lithium prophylaxis, and one who had previously used antidepressants in a suicide attempt refused drug therapy. Despite only an 11% incidence of major depression in our hospitalized alcoholics, milder dysphoria is commonplace. The efficacy of drug treatment in mild depressive symptoms in alcoholics has not been studied.

Similarly, anxiety disorders are frequent in alcoholics. Mullaney and Trippett found that one-third of 102 inpatient alcoholics had disabling phobias and another third had less severe phobias (35). Those with severe phobias developed alcohol problems at an earlier age than mild phobics and phobic alcoholics reported that alcohol problems occurred after the anxiety symptoms first appeared. A somewhat lower percentage of alcoholics with phobia (18%) was reported by Smail and colleagues, who suggest that even though phobias antedate alcoholism, chronic ethanol consumption exacerbates agoraphobia and social phobia (36). Substantial improvement in phobic anxiety occurs with abstinence (37). Quitkin and colleagues suggest that high rates of alcoholism occur in panic disorder patients (38). In an unpublished study of drug treatment of panic disorder, we found fourteen of twenty (70%) reported the use of alcohol to relieve symptoms. Another study of 48 inpatient alcoholics using structured interviews found that one-fourth suffered from symptoms of agoraphobia, social phobia, or mixed phobias (39). The mean ages of onset of alcoholism and phobias were 25.3 years and 16.3 years, respectively. Given that effective pharmacological treatments exist for anxiety and panic disorder, the role of these agents requires further investigation.

Antidepressants

Antidepressants are commonly prescribed in outpatient alcoholics (40). Yet the literature on antidepressants in alcoholism does not provide a definitive answer on efficacy. We have recently reviewed the literature and found that most studies failed to differentiate major depression from sadness or withdrawal symptoms, to measure plasma levels to ensure adequate dosage and compliance, or to assess changes in mood as well as drinking patterns (41). In addition most studies began treatment immediately after withdrawal, when any spontaneous improvement would obscure drug-induced improvement. We have shown that alcoholics have lower steady-state levels of imipramine and metabolites than nonalcoholic depressed controls and 2.5 times greater intrinsic clearance (42), presumably due to induction of the hepatic drug-oxidizing enzymes. Furthermore, protein-binding changes during withdrawal (due to higher levels of alpha-1 acid glycoprotein) alter the free fraction of antidepressants (43). Desipramine clearance is also enhanced (43) as is that of amitriptyline (44). All of these findings suggest that higher doses are required in alcoholic depressed patients.

Although there is little doubt that most sad moods observed early in withdrawal improve spontaneously, approximately 8–15% of patients who are hospitalized will have persistent severe depressed moods (45). For such patients, antidepressants may be indicated. They should be used with the awareness that most alcoholics without cirrhosis will have lower plasma levels than nonalcoholic depressed patients given the same dose. The clinician should be aware of the potential for adverse effects of antidepressants and alcohol when taken in combination, and should carefully limit the amount of antidepressant given at any one time. Antidepressants may also be of value in panic disorder and agoraphobic patients with alcoholism.

Antidepressants that affect serotonergic function may decrease alcohol consumption in laboratory animals and problem drinkers (46). The decrease is a modest one and at present is of more theoretical than clinical importance.

Monoamine oxidase inhibitors may be of value in some patients with atypical depression and alcohol dependence. An open pilot study (Jaffe and Ciraulo, unpublished data) showed that patients with elevated phobic anxiety and depression scores on the Hopkins Symptom Check List-90 were more likely to have a positive response to tranylcypromine than those with depression in the absence of anxiety. Limitations of the monoamine oxidase inhibitors are the need for careful dietary restrictions, a possible disulfiram-like reaction if taken with ethanol, and liver toxicity with the hydrazine derivatives (phenelzine).

Benzodiazepines

Even more controversial than the antidepressant treatment is the use of antianxiety agents in alcoholics after acute withdrawal has subsided. Most nonmedical treatment personnel have a particular antipathy toward the use of drugs that may induce dependence. Even though alcoholics appear to be at greater risk to develop benzodiazepine dependence, the probability of abuse is lower than generally believed. In the largest sample (over 14,000 patients) surveyed, the prevalence of combined alcohol and benzodiazepine was 3.4% (47). A report of seventeen New York alcoholism treatment centers indicated 12.7% of alcoholics also used "tranquilizers" prior to entering treatment (48). Another study suggested that 5% of 750 patients entering treatment were alcohol and benzodiazepine dependent (49). Only 4% of 413 alcoholics developed problems with benzodiazepines in still another study (50). Other studies and clinical reports suggest that concurrent use may range from 2 to 80%, although the majority of studies and those studying the largest number of patients support lower percentages (51–55).

There are several problems with many of the aforementioned studies, including failure to (a) distinguish *use* of benzodiazepines from *abuse*, (b) use standardized diagnoses of anxiety and/or phobia, (c) report data on plasma or urine levels of drugs, or (d) distinguish use of barbiturates or other sedative hypnotics from benzodiazepines. There is substantial evidence that barbiturates are more reinforcing (i.e., lead to continuous self-administration of high doses) than benzodiazepines (56). There is even evidence to suggest that, among the benzodiazepines, there is a spectrum of abuse potential. Clinical lore has taught that chlordiazepoxide and oxazepam have relatively low abuse potential (57,58), and the lower abuse potential of oxazepam has recently been documented (59). We have found that halazepam produced minimal euphoria even at supratherapeutic doses, whereas diazepam increases euphoria in alcoholics (60).

The dropout rate from treatment after acute withdrawal may be as high as 90%, often as a result of return to alcohol use. To the degree that early relapse is a result of protracted withdrawal expressed as anxiety, depression, and insomnia, low doses of benzodiazepines may enhance retention in treatment (61,62). Some alcoholics find benzodiazepines helpful in stopping alcohol use without abusing them, while others may substitute benzodiazepines for alcohol. If dosage is maintained within a therapeutic range, long-term benzodiazepine therapy is safer than continued alcohol use.

We believe that there is an important but limited place for benzodiazepines in the treatment of alcoholics. When there is a diagnosable anxiety disorder that persists for 2–3 weeks after detoxification, benzodiazepines may be used. Chlordiazepoxide, oxazepam, and halazepam may have less potential for abuse than other drugs in this class. No greater than a 1-week supply of medication should be given at any one time. Pill counts, urine drug screens, and periodic benzodiazepine plasma levels should be obtained to ensure that dosage is not being escalated and that other drugs are not being taken surreptitiously. Using this protocol, we estimate that abuse (defined as escalation of dose, patient or family reports of drug intoxification, "lost" prescriptions) to be about 1% for patients who stay in treatment 3 months or longer. With people who are diagnosed as having alcohol abuse rather than dependence ("problem drinkers") with good premorbid adjustment, the abuse rate is lower.

As with any medical treatment, benefits must be weighed against risks. If patients combine alcohol with benzodiazepines, there is additive or synergistic sedation and psychomotor impairment. Such a combination can lead to serious overdose or automobile accidents. If a combined dependence on alcohol and benzodiazepines occurs, some evidence suggests that prognosis is poor (48) and withdrawal more complex (63).

Buspirone is a nonbenzodiazepine antianxiety agent with efficacy comparable to diazepam in neurotic outpatients. Its sedative properties in normal volunteers were not accentuated by combination with alcohol (64). Drug abusers do not find its acute affects reinforcing, and its abuse potential should be lower than that of diazepam (65).

Lithium

The published clinical trials of lithium treatment in alcoholics have not yielded definitive results. The promise of studies that showed that lithium reduced alcohol intake in laboratory animals (66) and blocked some of the subjective and psychomotor effects of ethanol (67–69) has not been fulfilled in clinical trials. Published studies suffer from high dropout rates (percentage of subjects completing trial ranges from 17–53).

Kline and colleagues were the first to study the effects of lithium in chronic alcoholics (70). They studied seventy-three male veterans with elevated Zung depression scale scores. At the end of the 48-week double-blind phase of the study, only sixteen lithium and fourteen placebo patients remained in the study. Although Zung scores of placebo and lithium patients were comparable, lithium patients had significantly fewer days of pathological drinking and hospitalization for alcoholism.

Merry and associates (71) studied seventy-one alcoholics (sixty men, eleven women), 48% of whom had Beck depression inventory scores above 15 which is indicative of clinically significant depression. After an average of 41 weeks of treatment, Beck scores declined in both groups, with the lithium group showing greater improvement. Depressed patients on lithium ($N = 9$) had significantly fewer days drinking and fewer days of incapacitating drinking compared to depressed patients on placebo ($N = 7$).

Pond and colleagues studied forty-seven alcoholics using a 3-month crossover design in which the maximum period on lithium was 3 months (72). Nineteen subjects completed the study. No significant difference in Minnesota Multiphasic Personality Inventory (MMPI) scores or drinking patterns were found between drug and placebo conditions.

Fawcett and associates investigated the efficacy of lithium in eighty-four alcoholic subjects admitted to two different alcoholism treatment programs (73). Subjects were randomly assigned to either lithium or placebo for a period of 18 months. The dropout rate was 17% at 6 months, 32% at 12 months and 43% at 18 months. Both medication compliance and therapeutic serum lithium levels (defined by the investigators as greater or equal to 0.4 mEq/L) were associated with abstinence. Compliance was defined as at least 15 days compliance per month to the prescribed regimen for at least 4 months of the first 6-month period. The therapeutic lithium level/compliant group showed 87%, 62%, and 50% abstinence rates at 6-, 12-, and 18-month follow-ups, respectively. The subtherapeutic lithium level/compliant group showed abstinence rates of 38%, 25%, and 0% for the same follow-up periods. The placebo/compliant group showed rates of 52%, 36%, and 38%, while noncompliant groups showed 0% for all three periods. These findings suggest that patients who comply with their medication regimen relapse less frequently than noncompliers, but also that lithium in serum levels of 0.4 mEq/L or greater improves the chances of abstinence. A somewhat higher than expected rate of depressive illness (two-thirds met Research Diagnostic Criteria [RDC] for major depression, 88% met criteria for depression in their lifetime) was present in this population, although this is probably an artifact of assessment too early in the detoxification period or failure to differentiate primary depressive symptoms from those secondary to alcohol intake.

Establishing the efficacy of lithium in alcoholics has been difficult. High dropout rates, compliance issues, and concurrent psychosocial treatments all affect the quality and interpretation of the lithium studies. Although it appears that lithium may reduce drinking in some alcoholics, the characteristics of this subgroup remain to be identified. Furthermore, substantial risk of overdose and toxicity accompanies lithium treatment of the alcoholic. Even if lithium proves to be an effective agent in reducing alcohol consumption in alcoholics, there is the possibility that other drugs may be as or more effective and less toxic. All in all, the results of clinical trials of lithium in alcoholics are encouraging though inconclusive.

Alcohol Sensitizing Agents

Although many drugs alter the physiological response to alcohol, only two, disulfiram and calcium carbimide, are used in alcoholism treatment. If alcohol is consumed in the presence of these drugs, acetaldehyde oxidation is impaired resulting in a toxic reaction that varies in intensity from mildly unpleasant to fatal (the severity depending on drug, dose, and the amount of alcohol consumed). The signs and symptoms of the disulfiram–ethanol reaction (DER) are:

- facial flushing,
- warm, hot, or itching sensations,
- tachycardia,
- palpitations,
- nausea,
- vomiting,
- hypotension,
- generalized flushing,
- seizures,
- loss of consciousness,
- cardiovascular collapse, infarction,
- death.

The pharmacokinetics of disulfiram have recently been reviewed (74). The drug is rapidly absorbed following oral administration and reduced to diethyldithiocarbamate (DDC), which in turn is metabolized to diethylamine, carbon disulfide (CS_2), DDC methylester, DDC glucuronide, and DDC sulfate. In humans, 90% of orally administered disulfiram is eliminated within 3 days and principal metabolites in urine are DDC and DDC glucuronide and, to a lesser extent, DDC sulfate. CS_2 is eliminated in the breath and is responsible for an unpleasant odor. Breath CS_2 is sometimes used as a measure of compliance. Although usually administered orally, disulfiram can also be surgically implanted. The usual procedure is the subcutaneous implantation of ten 100-mg disulfiram implants into the abdominal wall. Blood levels of DDC and CS_2 are lower with the implant procedure and may be insufficient to exert an alcohol sensitizing effect (75)

Adverse effects from disulfiram are common. In addition to acetaldehyde dehydrogenase, disulfiram inhibits a variety of other enzymes including dopamine beta-hydroxylase, xanthine oxidase, hexokinase, 3-phosphoglyceraldehyde oxidase. It also inhibits hepatic microsomal drug-metabolizing enzymes, such as the mixed function oxidase system (76,77). Thus, in addition to the toxicity of the disulfiram-ethanol reaction caused by the accumulation of acetaldehyde, adverse effects can occur as a result of multiple drug interactions, alterations in levels of normal body constituents and neurotransmitters, as well as from other toxic effects of disulfiram or its metabolites.

The DER can sometimes be quite severe. Although severe reactions are usually associated with high-dosage disulfiram (500 mg/day) and more than 2 ounces of alcohol, deaths have occurred with lower dosage and after a single drink (78–80). Most DERs are self-limited, and conservative measures to handle hypotension (modified Trendelenburg position) are usually adequate. Vagal-induced bradycardia may require cholinergic blockers. No demonstrably effective treatments for the DER are available. Although vitamins and antihistamines are often used, there is no evidence for their efficacy. In volunteers pretreated with disulfiram or carbimide, the drug 4-methylpyrazol, which inhibits the metabolism of alcohol to acetaldehyde, produced a prompt fall in blood acetaldehyde levels and an associated decrease in symptoms. Penicillamine reportedly binds to acetaldehyde and has lowered blood levels in rats (78).

In addition to the risks of the DER, the use of disulfiram is associated with numerous side effects and toxicities including drowsiness, lethargy, peripheral neuropathy, hepatotoxicity, and hypertension. Disulfiram and DDC inhibit dopamine beta-hydroxylase resulting in decreased brain norepinephrine levels and increased dopamine levels. The exacerbation of schizophrenic symptoms in schizophrenics and occasionally their appearance in nonschizophrenics, as well as the development of depression, may be linked to these actions. Alcoholics with low cerebrospinal fluid dopamine beta-hydroxylase activity are more likely to develop dysphoric or psychotic symptoms (80,81).

The efficacy of disulfiram has been difficult to establish. Disulfiram therapy provides a unique problem in drug study design because the effect of disulfiram depends on the expectation that harm will come if alcohol is consumed. Early studies that suggested that disulfiram was an effective treatment for alcoholism suffered from serious methodological flaws including failure to (a) randomly assign patients, (b) adequately match controls (or even have controls), (c) use double-blind procedures, (d) define outcome criteria, (e) corroborate outcome with family members, (f) measure compliance, or (g) follow patients long enough (82).

There are three published studies using a placebo-controlled design. The first of these found no differences between drug and placebo groups after 3 years of treatment (83). The second study compared disulfiram implantation to a sham operation and found no differences between groups initially, but after 2 years, improvement was greater for the implant group (84). Improvement was seen primarily in those alcoholics who experienced a DER. In a third study, patients were given disulfiram (1 mg or 250 mg daily) or placebo (50 mg riboflavin) (85,86). The patients were told whether they were taking placebo or disulfiram, but did not know the dose. No significant differences were found in drinking or social stability after 1 year; however life-table analysis found that, at 1 month, 77% of the 250-mg group, and 63% of the 1-mg group were abstinent, compared to only 48% of the placebo group. At 6 months, 42% and 35% of the two disulfiram groups were abstinent but only 17% of the placebo group was. By the end of 1 year, however, the percentages of abstinence between groups was not statistically significant. There was almost no difference between the two groups, suggesting that the therapeutic effects of disulfiram were due more to psychological rather than pharmacological factors. A Veterans Administration Cooperative Study (as yet unpublished) has shown that abstinence rates at 1 year do not differ between groups on disulfiram 250 mg, 1 mg, or placebo; however, number of days drinking is lower in the disulfiram 250 mg group.

The efficacy of disulfiram remains unestablished, although it may be useful for some patients, especially early in abstinence. Daily dosage is usually 250 mg; however, a number of patients report they can drink safely with this dose. Although 500 mg will more reliably produce a DER, side effects are common. Sellers and co-workers set fairly stringent exclusionary criteria for using disulfiram, as well as rules for monitoring its safety, and for discontinuing its use in the event of noncompliance (80). Contraindications include myocardial disease; severe pulmonary insufficiency; severe liver dysfunction; chronic renal failure; organic mental disturbances; neuropathy; psychosis; difficulties in impulse control or recurrent suicidal ideation; the need for treatment with vasodilators, beta-adrenergic antagonists, monamine oxidase inhibitors, tricyclic antidepressants or antipsychotic agents; pregnancy; and unwillingness to attend monthly meetings for medical and psychosocial assessment. They also recommend an initial complete mental and physical exam, including a laboratory screen and electrocardiogram as well as psychosocial assessment. This is followed by a monthly repeat of mental and physical exams, a quarterly repeat of selected laboratory work, and semiannual repeat of all initial exams. Some clinicians believe that such stringent criteria and routine exams may largely preclude the use of disulfiram in most alcoholics, or raise the cost of its use to prohibitive levels (87). We find no contradiction to combining disulfiram with tricyclic antidepressants, provided that allowances are made for alterations in metabolism of the latter (88).

Calcium carbimide (citrated calcium carbimide, Temposil, Abstem) is another drug that inhibits aldehyde dehydrogenase and is used as an alcohol sensitizing agent, although it is not currently available in the United States. It is hydrolyzed in the gut to carbimide (cyanamide) which is rapidly absorbed. Whereas aldehyde dehydrogenase is irreversibly inhibited with disulfiram, there is reversible inhibition with carbimide: 80% of enzyme activity is restored within 24 hours and complete recovery occurs in 6 days (89). The usual dosage is 50 mg given twice daily.

The intensity of the alcohol reaction depends on the dose of calcium carbimide, length of treatment prior to ethanol exposure, and amount of alcohol consumed. There is great variability in the intensity of the reaction in different individuals or even in the same individual during different drinking episodes. Repeated drinks after an initial reaction will tend to produce progressively less severe reactions, a phenomenon sometimes referred to as "burning off the drug" (74,80).

Calcium carbimide produces less side effects than disulfiram, although neuropathy and hepatotoxicity have been reported (90,91). Because calcium carbimide does not inhibit the wide range of enzymes affected by disulfiram, there is less likelihood of adverse drug interactions or behavioral toxicity. The efficacy of calcium carbimide is not established.

Other drugs may also cause altered sensitivity and adverse responses to ethanol. Among them are some monoamine oxidase inhibitors (pargyline and perhaps phenelzine and tranylcypromine), antibiotics (the beta-lactam cephalosporins, moxalactam, cefamandol, cefoperazone) and metronidazole (Flagyl) (92). The latter was tried but found ineffective in treatment of alcoholism. In certain susceptible individuals taking oral hypoglycemic agents, chlorpropamide and tolbutamide, alcohol ingestion can produce a flushing reaction associated with modest rises in blood acetaldehyde levels (93,94). Other sensitizing substances include hydrogen sulfide, tetraethyl lead, pyrogallol, 4-bromopyrazole, and coprine (1-aminocyclopropranol), the active ingredient in the inky-cap mushroom (*Coprinus atramentarius*) (19,76,80). The ethanol–chemical interaction appears to be due to the increase of acetaldehyde in the blood following aldehyde dehydrogenase inhibition (95).

BARBITURATE DETOXIFICATION

Tolerance to the clinical effects of barbiturates and an abstinence syndrome occurring upon abrupt discontinuation of administration was first described in the 1950s (96–99). Wikler classified the symptoms of withdrawal as major and minor (99). Table 6–3 describes the signs and symptoms of the barbiturate abstinence syndrome occurring after the abrupt withdrawal of secobarbital or pentobarbital following chronic intoxication at oral doses of 0.8–2.2g/day for 6 weeks or more. Minor symptoms (apprehension, muscular weakness, tremors, postural hypotension, twitches, insomnia, diaphoresis, paroxymal discharges in the electroencephalogram [EEG], and an-

TABLE 6–3 Signs and Symptoms of Barbiturate Withdrawal (modified from reference 95)

Signs and Symptoms	Day of Onset	Duration (days)
Apprehension and uneasiness	1	3–14
Muscular weakness	1	3–14
Coarse tremors	1	3–14
Postural faintness, orthostatic hypotension	1	3–14
Anorexia and vomiting	1	3–14
Twitches, myoclonic jerks	1	3–14
Grand mal seizures	2–3	8
Delirium	3–8	3–14

orexia) occur within 24 hours of the last barbiturate dose and continue up to 2 weeks. Major abstinence phenomena include clonic-tonic seizures and delirium. The interictal EEG shows recurrent 4/second spike wave discharges. The delirium may be accompanied by hyperthermia, which can be fatal. Chronic intoxication with pentobarbital at daily doses of 0.6–0.8 g for periods of 35–57 days produces a clinically significant withdrawal syndrome, while daily doses of 0.2–0.4 g for 90 days or more rarely leads to withdrawal symptoms (99).

Treatment of the barbiturate withdrawal syndrome is by gradual discontinuation of the drug to prevent the occurrence of major symptoms and to avoid the development of intolerable minor symptoms. The current procedure is based on protocols described by several authors (96,99,100). The first step is to determine the severity of tolerance. If the patient is intoxicated, no additional barbiturate should be given until these symptoms have resolved. If there is substantial evidence or strong suspicion of chronic barbiturate use, it is not necessary or desirable to wait until withdrawal symptoms appear prior to the first dose. A 200-mg oral dose of pentobarbital is given on an empty stomach to a sober patient (that is, one who is not exhibiting signs of barbiturate intoxication), and the effects are observed at 1 hour. The patient's condition 1 hour after the test is done is used to determine the daily dose for stabilization (see Table 6–4).

TABLE 6–4 Estimation of Pentobarbital Requirement for Detoxification

Patient's Condition 1 Hr after 200 mg oral Pentobarbital	Degree of Tolerance Indicated	Estimated 24-Hr Pentobarbital Requirement, mg
Asleep but arousable	None	None
Drowsy, slurred speech, coarse nystagmus, Rombergism	Definite tolerance	500–600
Comfortable, fine lateral nystagmus is only sign of intoxication	Marked tolerance	800
No sign of drug effect; perhaps signs of abstinence persisting	Extreme tolerance	1000–1200 or more

Courtesy of J. A. Ewing and W. E. Bakewell: Diagnosis and management of depressant drug dependence. *American Journal of Psychiatry* 123: 909–917, 1967. Copyright 1967 by the American Psychiatric Association. Reprinted by permission.

If no physical changes are observed after 1 hour, the test is repeated 3 hours later using 300 mg. If there is no response to the 300-mg dose, the probable 24-hour requirement is above 1600 mg/day. The daily dose is given every 4–6 hours for a 2- to 3-day stabilization period. Withdrawal regimens must be individualized, but the initial reduction is usually 10% of the daily stabilization dose. Some clinicians recommend the use of phenobarbital for stabilization and withdrawal since it is longer acting and may provide a smoother course of withdrawal (101). Phenobarbital doses are one-third those suggested for pentobarbital. The barbiturate withdrawal protocol can also be used for other sedative-hypnotic abstinence syndromes (e.g., chloral hydrate, glutethimide, meprobamate).

OPIATE WITHDRAWAL

Signs and Symptoms

The signs and symptoms of opiate withdrawal are listed in Table 6–5 (102). With short-acting opiates such as heroin, morphine, and oxycodone, early signs occur 8–12 hours after the last dose, peak at 48–72 hours and subside over 7–10 days. With long-acting opiates, such as methadone, the first symptoms are seen 24–48 hours after the last dose, peak at 3 days or later, and may last as long as several

TABLE 6–5 Signs and Symptoms of Opiate Withdrawal

Early	Middle	Late
Lacrimation	Restless sleep	Increased severity of earlier symptoms
Yawning	Dilated pupils	Nausea
Rhinorrhea	Anorexia	Vomiting
Sweating	Gooseflesh	Diarrhea
	Restlessness	Abdominal cramps
	Irritability	Tachycardia
	Tremor	Increased blood pressure
		Mood lability
		Depression
		Muscle spasms
		Weakness
		Bone pain

weeks. Deep bone pain is reported to be more severe in methadone withdrawal as compared to the shorter-acting drugs. A protracted opiate abstinence syndrome characterized by physiological disturbances (blood pressure, temperature, sleep) and subjective changes (mood lability, irritability, drug craving) may persist for many months (103). Either methadone or clonidine is used for detoxification from opiates. This can be done on an inpatient or outpatient basis, although we prefer the former. Inpatient withdrawal allows for close monitoring of patients, reduces the likelihood of illicit drug use, and permits drug education and counseling to begin on an intensive basis.

Methadone Detoxification

The protocol we use is a modification of that of Green and associates (104). The patient is observed for signs of withdrawal (see Table 6-5), and is given 10-20 mg of methadone orally, after appearance of these symptoms. Clinical effects are seen 1-2 hours after the oral dose and peak effect is seen at about 4 hours (103). There is a moderate decline in subjective effects over the next 12 hours (with the exception of "liking" scores, which increase). After the initial dose, incremental doses of 5-10 mg may be given every 3 hours. Patients rarely require more than 40 mg/day; however, patients with a documented history of tolerance to this dose, or addicted health professionals who may have been using very large amounts, may require higher methadone doses. Objective signs of withdrawal such as pupil size, pulse, blood pressure, and respiratory rate, should guide the dosage adjustment. Somnolence is an indication of methadone intoxication. The total dose given over the first 24 hours is given on each of the second and third days in two divided doses (morning and evening). After stabilization over the first 3 days, reductions are made either of 5 mg/day or as a 15% to 20% dose reduction each day. Most patients are detoxified in 1-2 weeks. Patients being withdrawn from methadone maintenance may require longer periods to complete detoxification.

Clonidine Detoxification

The alpha-2 adrenergic agonist clonidine, introduced as an antihypertensive, has also been used as a withdrawal agent in opiate addicts (105-107). A widely used clinical protocol is that of Kleber and Kosten (Table 6-6) (108). After the patient's daily dose of methadone is reduced to 25 mg (or equivalent if the patient is addicted to another opiate; see Table 6-7), a single, 0.1-mg dose of clonidine is administered, and the patient is observed for adverse effects over the next hour. Adverse reactions include hypotension, sedation, dizziness, dry mouth, and facial pain. Blood pressure should be checked prior to each dose and the dosage should be held if blood pressure is less than 85/55. The next dose should not be given until the pressure rises. Tolazine, a clonidine antagonist, should be available, although it is rarely required. Average starting doses are between 0.3 and 0.5 mg/day for the first day. Daily doses should be divided and administered every 6-8 hours.

Withdrawal from narcotics with short elimination half-lives (e.g., heroin, oxycodone) requires that a higher dose of clonidine is reached sooner because peak withdrawal symptoms occur earlier. Likewise the duration of clonidine therapy is shorter. Amelioration of withdrawal symptoms begins within 30 minutes and reaches maximum at 2-3 hours. Some withdrawal symptoms that are not relieved

TABLE 6-6 Suggested Protocol for Administration of Clonidine

Time	Methadone, mg/day	Short-Acting Opiate mg/day[a]
Day 0	Usual dose of narcotic	Usual dose of narcotic
Day 1	0.3-0.6	0.3-0.6
Day 2	0.4-0.6	0.4-0.8
Day 3	0.5-0.8	0.6-1.2
Day 4	0.6-1.2	0.6-1.2
Day 5	0.6-1.2	0.6-1.2
Day 6	0.6-1.2	Cut dose in half, but not more than 0.4 mg
Day 7	0.6-1.2	Cut dose in half
Day 8	0.6-1.2	Cut dose in half
Day 9	0.6-1.2	
Day 10	0.6-1.2	
Day 11	Cut dose in half, but not more than 0.4 mg	
Day 12	Same as day 11	
Day 13	Same as day 11	
Day 14	Same as day 11	

[a] Heroin, oxycodone, etc.
Reprinted courtesy of H. D. Kleber and T. R. Kosten, Naltrexone induction: psychotic and pharmacologic strategies. *Journal Clinical Psychiatry* 45: 31, 1984.

TABLE 6-7 Relative Potencies of Opioids
(modified from reference 98)

Generic Name	Proprietary Name	Approx. Equiv. Anal. Dose (mg)
Methadone	Dolophine	7–10
Morphine		10
Hydromorphone	Dilaudid	1.5
Codeine		120
Oxycodone	Percodan	10–15
Meperidine	Demerol	80–100
Heroin		3
Levorphanol	Levo-Dromoran	2–3
Fentanyl	Sublimaze	0.1

Note: Equivalent doses are for subcutaneous and/or intravenous administration. When patients are taking opioids orally, equivalencies may differ due to absorption factors and first-pass metabolism in the liver.

by clonidine are insomnia, irritability, and muscle aches. One advantage of clonidine withdrawal is that naltrexone can be started sooner than when methadone detoxification is used.

Methadone Maintenance

Methadone maintenance therapy provides daily doses of methadone (40–120 mg/day) to opiate addicts. It was developed because of the recognition that addicts rarely achieved total abstinence, perhaps due to a protracted withdrawal syndrome and resultant craving for opiates (109). High doses of methadone not only reduce the craving, but also block the acute effects of heroin. The U.S. Food and Drug Administration has stringent regulations regarding program approval, patient eligibility for maintenance, and maximum dosages for maintenance. Methadone programs have higher retention rates compared to other programs for opiate addicts. Heroin use decreases in treated patients, although there is frequent use of other illicit drugs. Criminal behavior also declines. L-alpha-acetyl methadol is an experimental long-acting opiate, similar to methadone which is given three times a week and has the potential for reducing patient visits. It is not yet available for general clinical use.

Naltrexone

Since the 1940s, addiction specialists have written about the need for a long-acting narcotic antagonist to block the euphoric effects of opiates (110). Cyclazocine, nalorphine, naloxone, and naltrexone have been studied (111-115). The dysphoric symptoms induced by cyclazocine and nalorphine have limited their clinical usefulness. Naloxone has a short half-life and requires parenteral administration making it unsuitable for chronic administration to addicts. Naltrexone on the other hand is long-acting, can be administered orally and produces little (116) or no dysphoria (115).

The half-life of naltrexone ranges from 3.7 to 4.8 hours and the half-life of its major metabolite, naltrexol, ranges from 7.7 to 13.9 hours (117-119). The ability to antagonize opioids, however, has a duration of 48-72 hours after an oral dose, suggesting that plasma levels may not reflect pharmacodynamic activity.

Prior to starting naltrexone, the patient should be narcotic-free, 5 or more days for short-acting opiates, such as heroin, 10 or more days for long-acting drugs, such as methadone, to avoid acutely precipitating withdrawal. We feel inpatient withdrawal and induction is preferable to outpatient because there is less likelihood for abuse of street drugs, and the inpatient staff has the ability to closely monitor and treat subtle persistent withdrawal symptoms such as anxiety and insomnia. Obvious disadvantages of hospitalization are expense and disruption of the patient's employment and family life. Most studies support the greater success of inpatient induction (108).

Detoxification with clonidine or lofexidine rather than methadone is recommended, because this allows for a shorter waiting period prior to institution of naltrexone. Before starting naltrexone, naloxone (0.8 mg) is administered intramuscularly to establish that the patient is opiate-free. If withdrawal symptoms develop after naloxone is given, the patient should be treated with clonidine and the test readministered either 24 or 48 hours after. Protocols for naltrexone induction vary among centers. A typical initial dose is 25 mg daily and this is gradually increased to 150 mg over a 6-day period; a common maintenance dose is 100 mg on Monday and Wednesday, and 150 mg on Friday. Most authorities suggest that outpatients should be observed by clinic staff or family to ensure compliance (120). Benzodiazepines may be judiciously used to treat anxiety and insomnia in naltrexone-maintained patients. Naltrexone appears to be relatively free of clinically important adverse effects, but has been shown to stimulate the secretion of luteinizing and follicle-stimulating hormones (LH and FSH) by enhancing the secretion of luteinizing hormone-releasing hormone (LHRH), and in large doses to stimulate the secretion of ACTH, cortisol and catecholamines (121). It has little or no effect on prolactin, the pituitary-thyroid axis, growth hormones, insulin, glucagon, vasopressin, or gut hormones (121). Clinical implications of these findings are unknown. Some studies have reported that naltrexone reduces food intake and causes weight loss in humans (121).

The efficacy of naltrexone is not established, because of the same problems as encountered with disulfiram. As pointed out by O'Brien, the placebo-controlled paradigm may not be valid, because after a subject reads a consent form, the placebo takes on the qualities of the drug (as long as the opiate blockade is not tested) (120). Dropout rates from naltrexone programs are quite high. In one study only 16.9% of patients remained more than 90 days (122). Patients reported to do best are addicted middle-class businessmen, physicians, and other health professionals (123).

PSYCHOSTIMULANTS

Prolonged high doses of amphetamine, its derivatives, methylphenidate, and cocaine can induce psychotic symptoms in nonschizophrenic individuals. The most common form of psychosis is paranoid in nature and characterized by delusions of persecution, ideas of reference, auditory, visual, tactile, and olfactory hallucinations, agitation, panic, stereotyped behavior (termed "punding"), hypersexuality, and labile affect. With prolonged intake of gradually increasing doses, a fairly typical pattern of behavioral changes results (124). Initially there is behavioral activation, talkativeness, euphoria, hypersexuality, insomnia, and concern with minutiae and philosophical concepts. Later there is stereotyped behavior such as repetitive grooming or compulsive performance of meaningless tasks. Some experts believe that such stereotypes occur most often in prepsychotic addicts who eventually become paranoid (125). The last symptoms to develop are paranoid delusions, visual illusions, and finally hallucinations. Such patients may become violent.

Psychosis most commonly develops only after high oral doses are taken for prolonged periods or after several months of intravenous use. Once psychotic symptoms have developed, they occur more easily with subsequent drug ingestion. Treatment of the psychosis consists of discontinuation of the stimulant and administration of a neuroleptic. Benzodiazepines may be used to sedate agitated patients. Abrupt discontinuation of amphetamines results in an abstinence syndrome characterized by fatigue, lethargy, and dysphoria ("crashing") which is self-limited. Some have suggested tricyclic antidepressants may hasten mood normalization in nonpsychotic patients in withdrawal.

Recent open trials have suggested that antidepressants may be of some value in reducing craving and dysphoria in chronic cocaine abusers (126,127). Such a treatment strategy is consistent with what is known about neurotransmitter and receptor changes occurring during chronic cocaine administration. Animals administered cocaine develop increased beta-adrenergic and dopaminergic receptor binding (128,129). Similar receptor changes are thought to occur in depression and perhaps also may account for the mood changes seen with chronic cocaine use. Antidepressants produce the opposite receptor changes which may explain their usefulness in decreasing dysphoria and craving in cocaine abusers. Although preliminary studies are encouraging, larger blinded studies are needed.

Bromocriptine, a dopamine agonist, may also be useful in cocaine withdrawal states. Two female cocaine abusers reported decreased drug craving after receiving 0.625 mg orally (130). Although acute cocaine ingestion increases dopamine transmission, chronic administration probably depletes brain dopamine and may be a neuromechanism of craving.

Although some investigators have found that lithium blocks cocaine-induced euphoria (131,132), the only published clinical trial found it useful only for cyclothymic patients (127). Anecdotal reports suggest that methylphenidate may be of some value in the treatment of cocaine abusers, especially those with attention deficit disorder, residual type (127,133). Given its potential for abuse, the usefulness of this drug is clinically limited but of theoretical importance.

REFERENCES

1. Mendelson, J. H., and Mello, N. K. (1985). Diagnostic criteria for alcoholism and alcohol abuse. In *The Diagnosis and Treatment of Alcoholism*, ed. J. H. Mendelson and N. K. Mello. New York: McGraw-Hill.
2. Sellers, E. M., and Kalant, H. (1976). Alcohol intoxication and withdrawal. *New England Journal of Medicine* 294:757-762.
3. Whitfield, E. L., Thompson, G., Lamb, A., et al. (1978). Detoxification of 1,024 alcoholic patients without psychoactive drugs. *Journal of the American Medical Association* 293:1409-1410.
4. Whitfield, C. (1980). Nondrug detoxification. In *Phenomenology and Treatment of Alcoholism*, W. E. Fann, I. Karacan, A. D. Pokorny, and R. Williams, pp. 305-320. New York: Spectrum.
5. Wilson, A., and Vulcano, B. A. (1984). A double-blind placebo-controlled trial of magnesium sulfate in the ethanol withdrawal syndrome. *Alcoholism: Clinical and Experimental Research* 8:542-545.
6. Besson, J. A., Glen, A. I. M., Foreman, E. I., et al. (1981). Nuclear magnetic resonance observations in alcoholic cerebral disorder and the role of vasopressin. *Lancet* 2:923-924.
7. Eisenhofer, G., Whiteside, E., Lambie, D., and Johnson, R. (1982). Brain water during alcohol withdrawal. *Lancet* 1:50.
8. Holloway, H. C., Hales, R. E., and Watanabe, H. K. (1984). Recognition and treatment of acute alcohol withdrawal syndromes. *Psychiatric Clinics of North America* 7:729-743.
9. Greenblatt, D. J., Shader, R. I., and Abernathy, D. R. (1983). Drug therapy: current status of benzodiazepines. *New England Journal of Medicine* 309(6):354-358, 410-416.
10. Sellers, E. M., Naranjo, C. A., Harrison, M., et al. (1983). Diazepam loading: simplified treatment of alcohol withdrawal. *Clinical Pharmacology and Therapeutics* 34:822-826.
11. Gross, G. A. (1982). The use of propranolol as a method to manage acute alcohol detoxification. *Journal of the American Osteopathic Association* 82:206-207.
12. Zilm, D. H., Sellers, E. H., MacLeod, S. M., and Degani, N. C. (1975). Propanolol effect on tremor in alcohol withdrawal. *Annals of Internal Medicine* 83:234-236.
13. Kraus, M. L., Gottlieb, L. D., Horwitz, R. I., and Anscher, M. (1985). Randomized clinical trial of atenolol in patients with alcohol withdrawal. *New England Journal of Medicine* 313:905-909.
14. Sellers, E. M., Cooper, S. D., Zilm, D. H., and Shanks, C. (1976). Lithium treatment during alcohol withdrawal. *Clinical Pharmacology and Therapeutics* 20:199-206.
15. Ho, A. K. S., and Tsai, C. S. (1976). Effects of lithium on alcohol preference and withdrawal. *Annals of the New York Academy of Sciences* 273:371-377.
16. Walinder, J., Balldin, J., Bokstrom, K., et al. (1981). Clonidine suppression of the alcohol withdrawal syndrome. *Drug and Alcohol Dependence* 8:345-348.

17. Kostowski, W., and Trzaskowska, E. (1980). Effects of lesion of the locus coeruleus and clonidine treatment on ethanol withdrawal syndrome in rats. *Polish Journal of Pharmacology and Pharmacy* 32:617.
18. Cushman, P., Forbes, R., Lerner, W., and Stewart, M. (1985). Alcohol withdrawal syndromes: clinical management with lofexidine. *Alcoholism: Clinical and Experimental Research* 9:103–108.
19. Jaffe, J. H., and Ciraulo, D. A. (1985). Drugs used in the treatment of alcoholism. In *Diagnosis and Treatment of Alcoholism*, ed. J. H. Mendelson and N. K. Mello, pp. 355–389. New York: McGraw-Hill.
20. Gessner, P. K. (1979). Drug therapy of the alcohol withdrawal syndrome. In *The Biochemistry and Pharmacology of Ethanol*, ed. E. Majchrowicz and E. Noble, pp. 375–434. New York: Plenum.
21. Sampliner, R., and Iber, F. L. (1974). Diphenylhydantoin control of alcohol withdrawal seizures: results of a controlled study. *Journal of the American Medical Association* 230:1430–1432.
22. Greenblatt, D. J., and Shader, R. I. (1975). Treatment of the alcohol withdrawal syndrome. In *Manual of Psychiatric Therapeutics*, ed. R. I. Shader, pp. 211–236. Boston: Little, Brown.
23. Shaw, G. K. (1982). Alcohol dependence and withdrawal. *British Medical Bulletin* 38:99–102.
24. Chu, N. S. (1979). Carbamazepine: prevention of alcohol withdrawal seizures. *Neurology* 29:1397–1401.
25. Brune, F., and Busch, H. (1971). Anticonvulsive-sedative treatment of delirium alcoholicum. *Quarterly Journal of Studies on Alcohol* 32:334–342.
26. Bjorkqvist, S. E., Isohanni, M., Makela, R., and Malinen, L. (1976). Ambulant treatment of alcohol withdrawal symptoms with carbamazepine: a formal multicentre double-blind comparison with placebo. *Acta Psychiatrica Scandinavica* 53:333–342.
27. Ritola, E., and Malinen, L. (1981). A double-blind comparison of carbamazepine and clomethiazole in the treatment of alcohol withdrawal syndrome. *Acta Psychiatrica Scandinavica* 64:254–259.
28. Poutanen, P. (1979). Experience with carbamazepine in the treatment of withdrawal symptoms in alcohol abusers. *British Journal of Addiction* 74:201–204.
29. Agricola, R. (1982). Treatment of acute alcohol withdrawal syndrome with carbamazepine: a double-blind comparison with tiapride. *Journal of International Medical Research* 10:160–165.
30. Post, R. M., Ballenger, J. C., Putnam, F., and Bunney, W. E. (1983). Carbamazepine in alcohol withdrawal syndromes: relationship to the kindling model. *Journal of Clinical Psychopharmacology* 3:204–205.
31. Hansbrough, J. F., Zapata-Sirvent, R. L., Carroll, W. J., et al. (1984). Administration of intravenous alcohol for prevention of withdrawal in alcohol burn patients. *American Journal of Surgery* 148:266–269.
32. (1980). *Diagnostic and Statistical Manual of Mental Disorders*, 3rd ed. American Psychiatric Association, Washington, DC.
33. Schuckit, M. A. (1982). The history of psychotic symptoms in alcoholics. *Journal of Clinical Psychiatry* 43:53–57.
34. Jaffe, J. H., and Ciraulo, D. A. (1986). Depression and alcoholism. In *Psycho-

pathology and Addictive Disorders, ed. R. E. Meyer, pp. 293–320. New York: Guilford Press.
35. Mullaney, J. A., and Trippett, J. A. (1979). Alcohol dependence and phobias: clinical description and relevance. *British Journal of Psychiatry* 135:565–573.
36. Smail, P., Stockwell, T., Canter, S., and Hodgson, R. (1984). Alcohol dependence and phobic states: I. a prevalence study. *British Journal of Psychiatry* 144:53–57.
37. Stockwell, T., Smail, P., Hodgson, R., and Canter, S. (1984). Alcohol dependence and phobic anxiety states: II. a retrospective study. *British Journal of Psychiatry* 144:58–63.
38. Quitkin, F. M., Rifkin, A., Kaplan, J., and Klein, D. F. (1972). Phobic anxiety syndrome complicated by drug dependence and addiction. *Archives of General Psychiatry* 27:159–162.
39. Bowen, R. C., Cipywnyk, D., D'Arcy, C., and Keegan, D. (1984). Alcoholism, anxiety disorders and agoraphobia. *Alcoholism: Clinical and Experimental Research* 8:48–50.
40. Gee, S. (1980). *Part II. Mental Hygiene Clinic Survey, Day Treatment Center Survey, Day Hospital Survey*, Vol. 7, pp. 29–49. Washington, DC: Reports and Statistics Service, Office of Controller, Veterans Administration.
41. Ciraulo, D. A., and Jaffe, J. H. (1981). Tricyclic antidepressants in the treatment of depression associated with alcoholism. *Journal of Clinical Psychopharmacology* 1:146–150.
42. Ciraulo, D. A., Alderson, L. M., Chapron, D. J., et al. (1982). Imipramine disposition in alcoholics. *Journal of Clinical Psychopharmacology* 2:2–7.
43. Ciraulo, D. A., and Barnhill, J. (1986). Pharmacokinetic mechanisms of ethanol-psychotropic drug interactions. In *Strategies for Research on the Interactions of Drugs of Abuse*, pp. 73–88. Washington, D.C. NIDA Monograph Series, #68.
44. Sandoz, M., Vandel, S., Vandel, B., et al. (1983). Biotransformation of amitriptyline in alcoholic depressive patients. *European Journal of Pharmacology* 24:615–621.
45. Jaffe, J. H., and Ciraulo, D. A. (1986). Depression and alcoholism. In *Psychopathology and Addictive Disorders*, ed. R. E. Meyer, pp. 293–320. New York: Guilford Press.
46. Naranjo, C. A., Sellers, E. M., and Lawrin, M. O. (1986). Modulation of ethanol intake by serotonin uptake inhibitors. *Journal of Clinical Psychiatry* (Suppl.):47(4):16–22.
47. Tuchfield, B. S., McLeroy, K. R., and Waterhouse, G. J. (1975). *Multiple Drug Use Among Persons with Alcohol-Related Problems.* Research Triangle Park, NC: Research Triangle Institute.
48. Sokolow, L., Welte, T., Hynes, G., and Lyons, J. (1981). Multiple substance use by alcoholics. *British Journal of Addiction* 76:147–158.
49. Cushman, P., and Benzer, D. (1980). Benzodiazepines and drug abuse: clinical observations in chemically dependent persons before and during abstinence. *Drug and Alcohol Dependence* 6:365–371.
50. Krypsin-Exner, K. (1967). Misuse of benzodiazepine derivatives by alcoholics. *Quarterly Journal of Studies on Alcohol* 28:768.

51. Rothstein, E., Cobble, J. C., and Sampson, H. (1976). Chlordiazepoxide: long-term use in alcoholism. *Annals of the New York Academy of Sciences* 273:381-384.
52. Carroll, J. F., Malloy, T. E., and Kenrick, F. M. (1977). Drug abuse by alcoholics and problem drinkers: a literature review and evaluation. *American Journal of Drug and Alcohol Abuse* 4:317-341.
53. Freed, E. X. (1973). Drug abuse by alcoholics: a review. *International Journal of the Addictions* 8:451-473.
54. Schuckit, M. A., and Morrissey, E. R. (1979). Drug abuse among alcoholic women. *American Journal of Psychiatry* 136:607-611.
55. Busto, U., Simpkins, J., Sellers, E. M., et al. (1983). Objective determination of benzodiazepine use and abuse in alcoholics. *British Journal of Addiction* 78:429-435.
56. Griffiths, R. R., Bigelow, G. F., and Liebson, I. (1978). Experimental drug self-administration: generality across species and type of drug. In *Self-Administration of Abused Substances: Methods for Study*, Vol. 20, ed. N. A. Krasnegor, pp. 24-43. Washington, DC: National Institute on Drug Abuse Research Monograph.
57. Bliding, A. (1978). The abuse potential of benzodiazepines with special reference to oxazepam. *Acta Psychiatrica Scandinavica* (Suppl.) 24:111-116.
58. Kissin, B. (1977). Medical management of the alcoholic patient. In *The Biology of Alcoholism*, vol. 5: *Treatment and Rehabilitation of the Chronic Alcoholic*, ed. B. Kissin and H. Begleiter, pp. 55-103. New York: Plenum.
59. Griffiths, R. R., McLeod, D. R., Bigelow, G. E., et al. (1984). Comparison of diazepam and oxazepam: preference, liking and extent of abuse. *Journal of Pharmacology and Experimental Therapeutics* 229:501-508.
60. Jaffe, J., Ciraulo, D., Nies, A., Dixon, R., and Monroe, L. (1983). Abuse potential of halazepam and diazepam in patients treated for acute alcohol withdrawal. *Clinical Pharmacology and Therapeutics* 34:623-630.
61. Kissin, B., and Gross, M. M. (1970). Drug therapy in alcoholism. *Current Psychiatric Therapies*, pp. 135-144.
62. Rosenberg, C. M. (1974). Drug maintenance in the outpatient treatment of chronic alcoholism. *Archives of General Psychiatry* 30:373-377.
63. Schuster, C. L., and Humphries, R. H. (1981). Benzodiazepine dependency in alcoholics. *Connecticut Medicine* 45:11-13.
64. Seppala, T., Aranko, K., Mattila, M. J., and Shrotriya, R. C. (1982). Effects of alcohol on buspirone and lorazepam actions. *Clinical Pharmacology and Therapeutics* 32:201-204.
65. Cole, J. O., Orzack, M., Beake, B., et al. (1982). Assessment of the abuse liability of busprione in recreational sedative users. *Journal of Clinical Psychiatry* 43:69-74.
66. Ho, A. K. S., and Tsai, C. S. (1975). Lithium and ethanol preference. *Journal of Pharmacy and Pharmacology* 27:58.
67. Linnoila, M., Mattila, M. J., and Kitchell, B. S. (1979). Drug interactions with alcohol. *Drugs* 18:299-311.
68. Judd, L., Hubbard, B., Janowsky, D., et al. (1978). Ethanol-lithium interactions in alcoholics. In *Alcoholism and Affective Disorders*, ed. D. Goodwin and C. Erickson. New York: Spectrum.

69. Judd, L., and Huey, L. (1984). Lithium antagonizes ethanol intoxication in alcoholics. *American Journal of Psychiatry* 141:1517–1521.
70. Kline, N. S., Wren, J. C., Cooper, T. B., et al. (1974). Evaluations of lithium therapy in chronic and periodic alcoholism. *American Journal of the Medical Sciences* 268:15–22.
71. Merry, J., Reynolds, C. M., Bailey, J., and Copper, A. (1976). Prophylactic treatment of alcoholism by lithium carbonate. *Lancet* 2:481–482.
72. Pond, S. M., Becker, C. E., Vandervoort, R., et al. (1981). Evaluation of the effects of lithium in the treatment of chronic alcoholism. *Alcoholism: Clinical and Experimental Research* 5:247–251.
73. Fawcett, J., Clark, D. C., Gibbons, R. D., et al. (1984). Evaluation of lithium therapy for alcoholism. *Journal of Clinical Psychiatry* 45:494–499.
74. Peachey, J. E. (1981). A review of the clinical use of disulfiram and calcium carbimide in alcoholism treatment. *Journal of Clinical Psychopharmacology* 1:368–375.
75. Wilson, A., Davidson, W. J., and Blanchard, R. (1980). Disulfiram implantation: a trial using placebo implants and two types of controls. *Journal of Studies on Alcohol* 41:429–436.
76. Fried, R. (1980). Biochemical actions of anti-alcoholic agents. *Substance and Alcohol Actions/Misuse* 1:5–27.
77. Marchner, H. (1984). The pharmacology of alcohol-sensitising drugs. In *Pharmacological Treatments for Alcoholism*, ed. G. Edwards and J. Littleton. New York: Metheun.
78. Lindros, K. O., Stowell, A., Pikkarainen, P., and Salaspuro, M. (1981). The disulfiram (Antabuse)-alcohol reaction in male alcoholics: its efficient management by 4-methylpyrazole. *Alcoholism: Clinical and Experimental Research* 5:528–530.
79. Peachey, J. E., and Annis, H. (1984). Pharmacologic treatment of chronic alcoholism. *Psychiatric Clinics of North America* 7:745–756.
80. Sellers, E. M., Naranjo, C. A., and Peachey, J. E. (1981). Drugs to decrease alcohol consumption. *New England Journal of Medicine* 305:1255–1262.
81. Major, L. F., Lerner, P., Ballenger, J. K., et al. (1979). Dopamine beta-hydroxylase in the cerebrospinal fluid: relationship to disulfiram induced psychosis. *Biological Psychiatry* 14:337–344.
82. Fuller, R. K. (1984). A critical analysis of the efficacy and toxicity of the alcohol sensitizing drugs. In *Pharmacologic Treatment for Alcoholism*, ed. G. Edwards and J. Littleton. New York: Methuen.
83. Yalovoi, A. Y. (1978). Substitution of the antabuse-alcohol test in the treatment of alcoholism by placebo. In *Disulfiram in the Treatment of Alcoholism*, ed. S. Busse, C. T. Malloy, and C. E. Weise. Toronto: Addiction Research Foundation.
84. Wilson, A., Davidson, W. J., Blanchard, R., and White, J. (1978). Disulfiram implantation: a placebo-controlled trial with two-year follow-up. *Journal of Studies on Alcohol* 39:809–819.
85. Fuller, R. F., and Roth, H. P. (1979). Disulfiram for the treatment of alcoholism: an evaluation in 128 men. *Annals of Internal Medicine* 90:901–904.
86. Fuller, R. K., and Williford, W. O. (1980). Life-table analysis of abstinence in a

study evaluating the efficacy of disulfiram. *Alcoholism: Clinical and Experimental Research* 4:298–301.
87. Graff, D. M. (1982). Drugs to decrease alcohol consumption. *New England Journal of Medicine* 306:747.
88. Ciraulo, D. A., Barnhill, J., and Boxenbaum, H. (1985). Pharmacokinetic interaction of disulfiram and antidepressants. *American Journal of Psychiatry* 142:1373–1374.
89. Marchner, H., and Tottmar, O. (1978). A comparative study on the effects of disulfiram, cyanamide and aminocyclopropanol on the acetaldehyde metabolism in rats. *Acta Pharmacologica et Toxicologica (Copenhagen)* 43:219–232.
90. Vazquez, J. J., and Cervera, S. (1980). Cyanamide-induced liver injury in alcoholics. *Lancet* 1:361–362.
91. Reilly, T. M. (1976). Peripheral neuropathy associated with citrated calcium carbimide. *Lancet* 1:911–912.
92. Elenbaas, R. M., Ryan, J. L., Robinson, W. A., et al. (1982). On the disulfiram-like activity of moxalactam. *Clinical Pharmacology and Therapeutics* 32:347–355.
93. Barnett, A. H., Gonzalez-Auvert, C., Pyke, D. A., et al (1981). Blood concentrations of acetaldehyde during chlorpropamide-alcohol flush. *British Medical Journal* 283:939–941.
94. Capretti, L., Speroni, C., Girone, M., et al. (1981). Chlorpropamide- and tolbutamide-alcohol flushing in non-insulin dependent diabetics. *British Medical Journal* 283:1361–1362.
95. Marchner, H., and Tottmar, O. (1978). A comparative study of the effects of disulfiram, cyanamide and l-aminocyclopropanol on the acetaldehyde metabolism in rats. *Acta Pharmacologica et Toxicologica (Copenhagen)* 43:219–232.
96. Isbell, H. (1950). Manifestations and treatment of addiction to narcotic drugs and barbiturates. *Medical Clinics of North America* 34:425–438.
97. Wikler, A., Fraser, H. F., Isbell, H., and Pescor, F. T. (1955). Electroencephalograms during cycles of addiction to barbiturates in man. *Electroencephalography and Clinical Neurophysiology* 7:1–13.
98. Fraser, H. F. (1954). Use of miotic effect in evaluating analgesic drugs in man. *Archives Internationales de Pharmacodynamie et de Therapie* 98:443–451.
99. Wikler, A. (1968). Diagnosis and treatment of drug dependence of the barbiturate type. *American Journal of Psychiatry* 125:758–765.
100. Ewing, J. A., and Bakewell, W. E. (1967). Diagnosis and management of depressant drug dependence. *American Journal of Psychiatry* 123:909–917.
101. Shader, R. I., Caine, E. D., and Meyer, R. E. (1975). Treatment of dependence on barbiturate and sedative-hypnotics. In *Manual of Psychiatric Therapeutics*, ed. R. I. Shader. Boston: Little, Brown.
102. Jaffe, J. H., and Martin, W. R. (1980). Opioid analgesics and antagonists. In *The Pharmacological Basis of Therapeutics*, ed. A. G. Gilman, L. S. Goodman, and A. Gilman. New York: Macmillan.
103. Martin, W. R., Jasinski, D. R., and Mansky, P. A. (1973). Naltrexone, an antagonist for the treatment of heroin dependence. *Archives of General Psychiatry* 28:784–791.
104. Green, A. I., Meyer, R. E., and Shader, R. I. (1975). Heroin and methadone

abuse: acute and chronic management. In *Manual of Psychiatric Therapeutics*, ed. R. I. Shader. Boston: Little, Brown.
105. Gold, M. S., Redmond, D. E., Jr., and Kleber, H. D. (1978). Clonidine blocks acute opiate withdrawal symptoms. *Lancet* 2:599–602.
106. Gold, M. S., Pottash, A. L. C., Sweeney, D. R., and Kleber, H. D. (1980). Opiate withdrawal using clonidine. *Journal of the American Medical Association* 243:343–346.
107. Gold, M. S., Pottash, A. L. C., Sweeney, D. R., and Kleber, H. D. (1980). Effect of methadone dosage on clonidine detoxification efficacy. *American Journal of Psychiatry* 137:375–376.
108. Kleber, H. D., and Kosten, T. R. (1984). Naltrexone induction: psychologic and pharmacologic strategies. *Journal of Clinical Psychiatry* 45:29–38.
109. Dole, V. P., Nyswander, M. E., and Warner, A. (1968). Successful treatment of 750 addicts. *Journal of the American Medical Association* 206:2708–2714.
110. Wikler, A. (1948). Recent progress in research on the neurophysiologic basis of morphine addiction. *American Journal of Psychiatry* 105:329–338.
111. Resnick, R. B., Washton, A. M., Stone-Washton, N., and Rawson, R. A. (1981). Psychotherapy and naltrexone in opioid dependence. In *Problems of Drug Dependence, 1980*, ed. L. S. Harris. Washington, DC: National Institute on Drug Abuse Research Monograph 34.
112. Martin, W. R. (1966). Assessment of the dependence producing potentiality of narcotic analgesics. In *International Encyclopedia of Pharmacology and Therapeutics*, vol. 1, ed. C. Radouca-Thomas and L. Lasagna, pp. 155–180. Glasgow: Pergamon Press.
113. Freedman, A. M., Fink, M., Sharoff, R., and Saks, A. (1968). Clinical studies of cyclazocine in the treatment of narcotic addiction. *American Journal of Psychiatry* 124:1499–1505.
114. Zaks, A., Jones, T., Fink, M., and Freedman, A. M. (1971). Naloxone treatment of opiate dependence. *Journal of the American Medical Association* 215:2108–2110.
115. Ginzburg, H. M., and Glass, W. J. (1984). The role of the National Institute on Drug Abuse in the development of naltrexone. *Journal of Clinical Psychiatry* 45:4–6.
116. Crowley, T. J., Wagner, J. E., Zerbe, G., and MacDonald, M. (1985). Naltrexone-induced dysphoria in former opioid addicts. *American Journal of Psychiatry* 142:1081–1084.
117. Meyer, M. C., Straughn, A. B., Man-Wai, L., et al. (1984). Bioequivalence, dose proportionality, and pharmacokinetics of naltrexone after oral administration. *Journal of Clinical Psychiatry* 45(9):15–19.
118. Vereby, K., and Mule, S. J. (1975). Naltrexone pharmacology, pharmacokinetics and metabolism: current status. *American Journal of Drug and Alcohol Abuse* 2:357–363.
119. Wall, M. E., Brine, D. R., and Perez-Reyes, M. (1981). Metabolism and disposition of naltrexone in man after oral and intravenous administration. *Drug Metabolism and Disposition: The Biological Fate of Chemicals* 9:369–375.
120. O'Brien, C. P. (1984). Summary. *Journal of Clinical Psychiatry* 45:57–58.

References

121. Atkinson, R. L. (1984). Endocrine and metabolic effects of opiate antagonists. *Journal of Clinical Psychiatry* 45(9):20–24.
122. Tennant, F. S., Rawson, R. A., Cohen, A. J., and Mann, A. (1984). Clinical experience with naltrexone in suburban opioid addicts. *Journal of Clinical Psychiatry* 45:42–45.
123. Washton, A. M., Pottash, A. C., and Gold, M. S. (1984). Naltrexone in addicted business executives and physicians. *Journal of Clinical Psychiatry* 45:39–41.
124. Griffiths, R. R., Brady, J. V., and Bradford, L. D. (1978). Predicting the abuse liability of drugs with animal drug self-administration procedures: psychomotor stimulants and hallucinogens. In *Advances in Behavioral Pharmacology*, ed. T. Thompson and P. Dens. New York: Academic Press.
125. Ellinwood, E. H. (1969). Amphetamine psychosis: a multi-dimensional process. *Seminars in Psychiatry* 1:208–226.
126. Tennant, F. S., and Rawson, R. A. (1983). Cocaine and amphetamine dependence treated with desipramine. In *Problems of Drug Dependence, 1982*, Vol. 43, ed. L. S. Harris, pp. 351–355. Washington, DC: National Institute on Drug Abuse Research Monograph.
127. Gawin, F. H., and Kleber, H. D. (1984). Cocaine abuse treatment. *Archives of General Psychiatry* 41:903–909.
128. Banerjee, S. P., Sharma, V. K., King-Cheung, L. S.,et al. (1979). Cocaine and d-amphetamine induce changes in central beta-adrenoceptor sensitivity: effects of acute and chronic drug treatment. *Brain Research* 175:119–130.
129. Chanda, S. K., Sharma, V. K., and Banerjee, S. P. (1979). B-adrenoceptor sensitivity following psychotropic drug treatment. In *Catecholamines: Basic and Clinical Frontiers*, ed. E. Usdin. New York: Pergamon.
130. Dackis, C. A., and Gold, M. S. (1985). Bromocriptine as treatment of cocaine abuse. *Lancet* 1:1151–1152.
131. Cronsen, A. J., and Flemenbaum, A. (1978). Antagonism of cocaine highs by lithium. *American Journal of Psychiatry* 135:856–857.
132. Mandell, A. J., and Knapp, S. (1976). Neurobiological antagonism of cocaine by lithium. In *Cocaine and Other Stimulants*, ed. E. H. Ellinwood and M. M. Kilby, pp. 187–200. New York: Plenum.
133. Khantzian, E. J., Gawin, F. H., Riordan, C. R., and Kleber, H. D. (1984). Methylphenidate treatment of cocaine dependence: a preliminary report. *Journal of Substance Abuse Treatment* 1:107–112.

7

Memory Disturbance and Cognitive Impairment in the Elderly

Patricia I. Rosebush, M.D.
Carl Salzman, M.D.

MEMORY LOSS AND THE AGING PROCESS

Disturbances in the capacity to remember can have profound and far-reaching effects on intellect, behavior, and mood. Memory loss may simply accompany the aging process, delivering the powerful message that time is passing and that one is in a relative state of decline. Memory loss may also signal illness: at best it is a symptom of a transient, treatable, medical or psychiatric disorder; at worst it marks the beginning of an untreatable dementia. A growing geriatric population (1) and an attendant increase in the prevalence of dementia (2) and psychopathology (3,4) mean the psychiatrist must be increasingly sophisticated in both the diagnosis of age-associated memory impairment as well as familiar with efforts to treat memory decline. This chapter reviews the diagnosis and treatment of cognitive impairment of normal aging, delirium, amnestic syndrome, dementia, and pseudodementia.

History

In the evaluation of memory loss, a history should be obtained from both the patient and family or friends, whenever possible. Inquiry should be made about the following:

1. family history of neurological or psychiatric illness;
2. personal history of psychiatric illness;
3. history of neurological events, such as traumas, seizures, limb weakness, gait abnormalities or involuntary movements;
4. the nature of the onset, duration, and course of the memory impairment;
5. the use of prescribed medications, alcohol, or illicit substances;
6. concurrent medical illness;
7. difficulties in the performance of usual activities and daily tasks;
8. changes in grooming, self-care, and social behavior and the presence of incontinence;
9. episodes of confusion or disorientation, such as getting lost in familiar surroundings;
10. problems with language;
11. the patient's and family's awareness of memory impairment;
12. changes in mood, interest, and interpersonal relatedness;
13. the occurrence of major life events such as losses through death or retirement.

Evaluating Memory Loss

The clinical examination of the elderly patient who presents with a complaint of memory loss should be guided by the following series of questions (Figure 7–1).

1. Does the patient have a memory loss objectively?
2. If so, is the patient's sensorium clouded or clear? If the sensorium is clouded, the patient is suffering, most acutely, from a delirium.

Memory Loss and the Aging Process

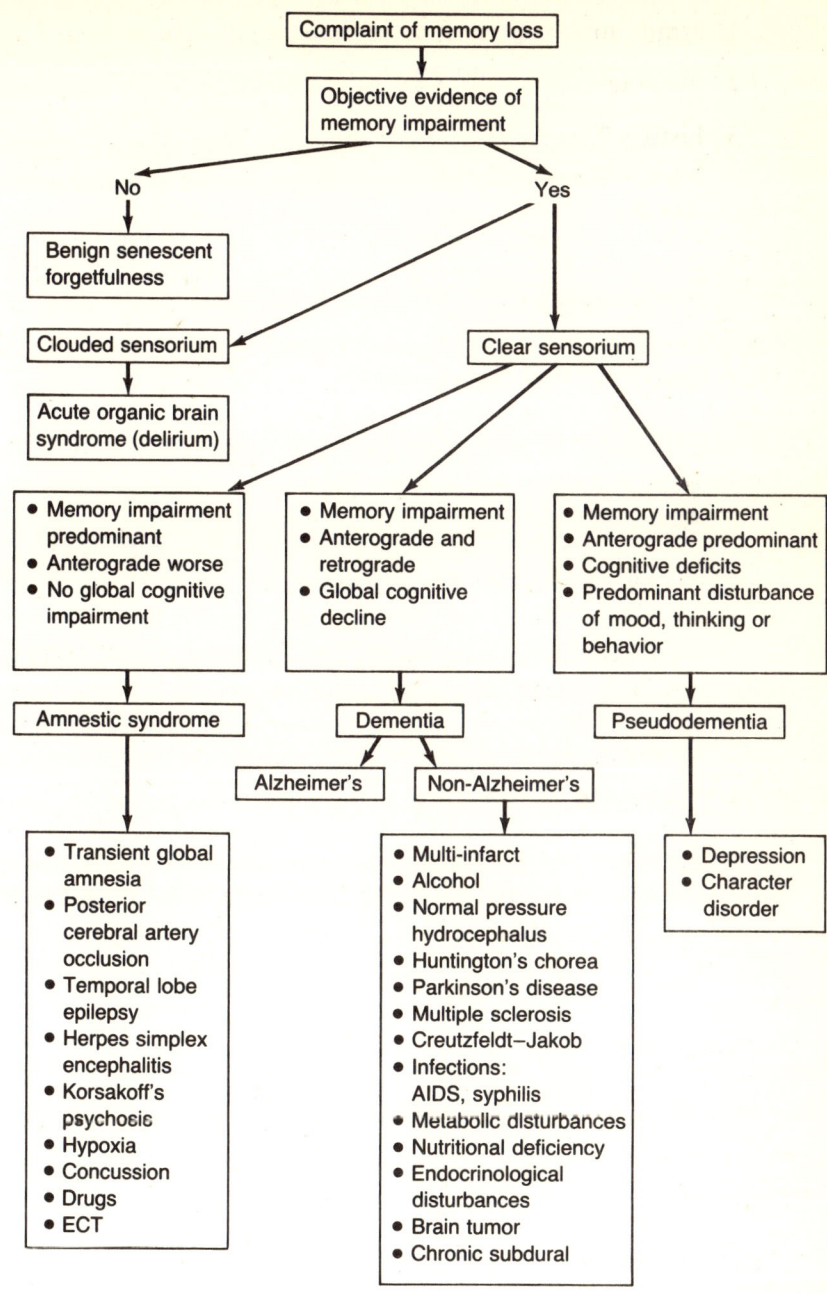

FIGURE 7-1.

3. If the patient's sensorium is clear, is the memory loss an isolated finding, as in amnestic syndrome, or is there evidence of global cognitive decline, as in dementia?

4. If global cognitive impairment is apparent, does the patient have a medical or psychiatric condition that is treatable?

5. Is there a predominant disturbance of affect or interpersonal behavior accompanying the complaint of cognitive impairment that might suggest pseudodementia?

The Mental Status Examination

A careful mental status examination is an essential tool in the evaluation of any patient with memory loss and should include the following assessments.

Sensorium or level of consciousness. This is usually described on a continuum which includes the terms alert, lethargic, drowsy, sleepy, stuporous, and comatose. Both the actual state of consciousness and the presence of fluctuations of consciousness should be noted. If the patient is anything but alert, delirium should be suspected. A patient with delirium will be unable to perform many of the tasks described below.

Orientation. Ask the patient his name, date of birth, where he is, the season and exact date. Brain dysfunction, as in delirium and dementia, usually produces a more marked and all-encompassing disorientation although this will vary with the severity of the illness. While a patient with depressive pseudodementia may not know the exact day of the week or even the month, it would be unusual for such a patient to forget the year, let alone his name or date of birth.

Attention. Valid testing of memory requires that attention be relatively unimpaired. Have the patient repeat digits forward and backward. A normal elderly individual should be able to repeat six numbers forward and five backward. Another test of attention is to read out a series of letters or numbers and ask the patient to indicate, by tapping the desk, every time a particular letter or number is repeated. The terms attention and immediate recall are often used interchangeably as are the tests of each. Both are markedly impaired in delirium; less so in dementia and pseudodementia. Attention should be normal in amnestic syndromes.

Memory

Short-term memory. Short-term memory is tested by having the patient call three or four objects after 10 minutes. If the patient is unable to recall the words, the examiner can provide categorical, phonemic, or contextual clues. Short-term or recent memory is impaired in delirium, amnesia, dementia, and depressive pseudodementia. It is often not testable in delirium because of severe inattention.

Long-term memory. This is tested by asking the patient about verifiable past events, both personal and impersonal, such as the date of marriage, place of birth, details of work history, the names of past presidents, and dates of the world wars. Like short-term memory, long-term memory is often not testable in delirium because of inattention. Long-term memory becomes impaired in the middle and late phases or stages of dementia. In amnestic syndrome, long-term memory is less severely affected than short-term memory. It is usually intact in depressive pseudodementia.

Appearance. The patient's hygiene, grooming, and appropriateness of dress should be noted, since deterioration can be seen in various psychopathological states. In delirium and in moderate to severe dementia, patients are often disheveled but show little awareness or concern. On the other hand, patients with mild-to-moderate dementia are often able to maintain their standards of personal hygiene and grooming. Patients who are cognitively impaired secondary to depression will usually show deterioration in self-care of which they are aware but unmotivated to change. Dressing errors such as socks of different colors, articles of clothing put on backward, and buttons fastened incorrectly are usually reliable signs of organic disease. Patients suffering from an amnestic syndrome would not typically show deterioration in their appearance and hygiene.

Behavior. The examiner should observe the patient's manner of greeting and his or her general attitude toward the interview.

Bewilderment, suspiciousness, or denial of the need to see a doctor are often noted in delirious and demented individuals. Gait disturbances, abnormal involuntary movements, and fluctuations in behavior are indications of brain disease and should be noted. Anxious or agitated pleading for help is usually more typical of a patient with pseudodementia.

Affect and mood. The patient's affect and mood state are important to assess. Does the patient appear depressed? How bothered is the patient by the memory impairment? A disturbance of affect and mood as well as complaints about memory disturbance are usually more prominent in patients with pseudodementia than in patients with delirium, amnestic syndrome and dementia who do not have a secondary psychiatric disturbance. However, in early dementia, patients who have insight into their impairment may be depressed, anxious, or irritable.

Thought content. The examiner should inquire about the presence of self-critical, nihilistic and guilty thoughts, suicidal ideation, suspiciousness or paranoia, and perceptual abnormalities such as illusions or hallucinations. None of these symptoms are typically present or predominant in amnestic syndrome. Paranoid thinking is a common finding in individuals with dementia regardless of etiology. Marked depressive thought content and active suicidal ideation suggest pseudodementia but may also be present in early dementia where insight is intact. Predominant perceptual abnormalities, particularly visual, tactile, or olfactory hallucinations, are characteristic of delirium.

Language. Disturbances of language are an important manifestation of brain disease, and the examiner should pay careful attention to each patient's spontaneous speech, noting errors and difficulties with fluency, grammar, vocabulary, and comprehension. Formal assessment should include the following aspects.

Comprehension. This can be tested by having the patient point to objects named or written on a piece of paper by the examiner. Simple questions that require a yes/no response can also be used to test comprehension. The examiner must be certain that visual acuity and hearing are unimpaired.

Repetition. While any words or sentences can be used, the phrase "no ifs, ands, or buts" is simple and commonly used to test repetition. Difficulties with repetition indicate organic pathology.

Naming. Patients should be asked to name common and uncommon objects. Problems in naming objects is called anomia, a common finding in dementia. Demented patients may also engage in elaborate circumlocutions in an effort to compensate and find the word they want.

Reading. Patients should be asked to read aloud a paragraph from a book appropriate to their educational level. In patients with brain disease, omissions and word substitution errors may occur.

Writing. Having a patient write a spontaneous or a dictated sentence is an excellent screen for language disturbance caused by brain dysfunction. The examiner should check for omissions, additions, perseveration, and grammatical and spelling errors. When an individual with pseudodementia is asked to write a sentence of choice, highly personalized, affectively laden material will often be expressed.

Construction. Disturbances of visual-spatial competence is an early and sensitive indicator of dementia (4,5). In the office, the physician can have the patient copy several designs such as a horizontal diamond, a two-dimensional cross, a three-dimensional cube and a three-dimensional pipe. Patients can also be asked to draw a house or clock. Pathognomonic errors in construction include (a) more than 45 degrees rotation of the figure, (b) perseveration or repetition of a part, (c) fragmentation, (d) ommission, and (e) integrative difficulty.

Praxis. The inability to carry out purposeful movements on command, in the absence of problems of comprehension, muscular strength, or coordination is a motor apraxia and indicates brain dysfunction (6). The examiner can ask the patient to whistle, fold a piece of paper and place it on the desk, or pretend to light a cigarette. Apraxias are common in Alzheimer's disease and usually appear in the middle phase of the disease (4).

Abstraction. Abstraction is a higher cortical function that can be tested by similarities, differences, and proverbs. The patient's level of intelligence and education must be taken into consideration when findings are interpreted. The examiner should proceed from simple questions to more difficult ones. Examples of similarity and difference questions are: How are an apple and an orange alike? How are a tree and a fly alike? How are a midget and a child different? Generally speaking, patients with brain dysfunction will give concrete answers and may have difficulty switching from similarities to differences. Patients with pseudodementia may give abstract but personalized responses. Highly idiosyncratic or bizarre responses are not typical of patients with pseudodementia but rather suggest a psychotic illness.

Calculations. The ability to calculate is considered to be a higher intellectual function which is compromised by brain disease such as dementia. Calculations can be tested by serial sevens and by simple addition (e.g., 4 + 5) and multiplication questions (e.g., 4 × 3). Patients with amnestic syndrome should be able to perform calculations accurately. Valid testing depends on intact attention which is impaired in delirium and often disturbed in depressive pseudodementia. Interpretation of results must take educational level into consideration.

General information. Questions of general information, like those testing abstract ability, should be asked in order of increasing difficulty. A hierarchy of six to ten questions, moving from the number of weeks in the year to more difficult inquiries about geography, politics, and literature may be constructed by the examiner and used with each patient. Interpretation will require judgment about the adequacy of responses in relationship to the patient's intelligence and level of education. Deficiencies in general information out of keeping with one's background and education suggest dementia. The performance of patients with pseudodementia may be adversely affected by inattention, psychomotor retardation, anxiety, or a lack of effort. However, with persistence and encouragement, knowledge and general information are found to be intact. Inattention and sensorial impairment make such testing difficult if not impossible in patients with delirium.

Insight. Insight can usually be tested by asking patients whether they think they have a problem, and if so, how they understand it. Insight will be severely impaired in delirium. Patients with dementia often state that they do not notice a problem with their memory even in the face of obvious impairment. It is not always clear whether this represents an organically or psychologically based form of denial. Patients suffering from pseudodementia usually acknowledge that something is wrong but do not always understand the reason.

Diagnostic Tests

All patients with a complaint of memory impairment should have a complete physical and neurological examination. While the presentation, history, and clinical examination usually reveal the diagnosis and likely etiology of the memory disturbance, certain tests are required for confirmation.

All patients should routinely have a complete blood cell count (CBC) and differential, erythrocyte sedimentation rate (ESR), electrolytes, glucose, calcium, and phosphorous, blood urea nitrogen (BUN), creatinine, liver function tests, thyroid function tests, venereal disease research laboratories (VDRL), urinalysis, vitamin B_{12}, and folate levels. In addition to laboratory tests, patients should have computed tomography (CT) scan of the head if dementia is present. Nonroutine tests that may be helpful in clarifying the diagnosis include an immunological screen, electrocardiogram (EKG), blood gases, chest x-ray, toxic and heavy metal screen, electroencephalogram (EEG), and more extensive endocrinological tests. Positron CT and nuclear magnetic resonance (NMR) are both newer diagnostic methods that are used at the research rather than at the clinical level.

The clinician who is frequently involved in the assessment of memory loss and dementia should become familiar with several simple, well-established neuropsychological tests that can easily be administered in an office setting. The Hachinski ischemia score (7) is useful in determining the presence of multi-infarct dementia (MID). It consists of a scale in which the distinguishing features of MID are each given a value of one if present. A score of 7 or more out of a possible 18 points indicates the likelihood of the cerebrovascular disease. A patient with Alzheimer's disease should have a score of less than 4. Autopsy verification of the diagnosis in a series of patients with scores of 7 or more has supported the value of the scale (8).

The Blessed Dementia Scale (9) is an easily administered instrument in which a series of questions related to the patient's daily activities and self-care (the left side of the scale) is asked of a relative or friend and another series of questions related to cognitive functions (the right side of the scale) is directed to the patient. Positive findings on each side are scored and a total dementia score is obtained, such that the higher the score the more severe the dementia. Normal elderly patients should receive a score of 3 or less. The test can be used both for screening purposes as well as over time with the same patient to demonstrate progress of the disease.

The Mini-Mental Status (10) is a short, standardized form that scores questions related to orientation, registration, attention, calculations, recall, and language. The higher the score the better. A score of 23 or less is found in patients with dementia, delirium, schizophrenia, and affective disorders but not in normal elderly people.

TYPES OF MEMORY LOSS IN THE ELDERLY

Memory loss in older people may occur as a result of benign senile forgetfulness, delirium, amnestic syndrome, dementia, or pseudodementia.

Benign Senile Forgetfulness

If an elderly patient complains of memory loss or forgetfulness, yet no impairment is found on clinical examination, the problem may be termed "benign senescent forgetfulness," a normal age-related decrease in memory function that is frightening for the individual but does not indicate a disease state. However, it is a symptom that is to be taken seriously and evaluated carefully. Patients with benign senescent forgetfulness have a clear sensorium, are usually acutely aware of their forgetfulness and often comment upon it and apologize for it. They describe frequent misplacement of objects and problems remembering names. However, episodes of disorientation and confusion have not occurred, and there is little interference with work or daily life. Global intellectual function is not compromised, and progression to more severe impairment is only minimal (11,12). Family and friends do not notice any impairment. This normal memory loss that occurs with aging is most pronounced when recall of logically disconnected material is required (13). Mild problems in naming, reduced speed in mental processing, and decreased psychomotor agility, necessitating greater time for task completion, have been described (13,14). These expectable, normal changes may be misinterpreted by the elderly patient as evidence of impending dementia.

Objectively, the patient with benign senescent forgetfulness should perform normally on tests of short- and long-term memory, have no language impairment and execute constructions accurately. The Blessed Dementia Scale and the Mini-Mental Status examination are excellent screening tests. Routine tests to rule out organic disease are appropriate. Patients with benign senescent forgetfulness often respond well to supportive intervention in the form of reassurance and education.

Delirium

Delirium is an organic brain syndrome of acute or subacute onset in which immediate recall as well as both short- and long-term memory are impaired and accompanied by a disturbance of consciousness. Inattention, distractability, disorientation, and marked disruption of the sleep–wake cycle occur. The latter is often characterized by wakefulness at night and drowsiness during the day. However, even daytime somnolence is usually interrupted by periods of restlessness and agitation. Mood lability, incoherent speech, disorganized thinking, and perceptual disturbances, such as illusions and hallucinations, are common. The clinical course is characteristically a fluctuating one changing from hour to hour or day to day. In addition to alterations in mental status and behavior, tremor, dysarthria, ataxia, asterixis, multifocal myoclonus, and autonomic dysfunction including fever, tachycardia, and hypertension can be seen (14–17). If detected early, the course is usually short and the outcome favorable. Mortality increases with the duration of the episode and the age of the patient.

The causes of delirium encompass the spectrum of most medical conditions including postoperative states, drug intoxication, and drug withdrawal. Important predisposing factors are advanced age, organic brain disease, and addiction to alcohol or drugs (14,15,17,18). The use of numerous medications by the elderly combined with impaired mechanisms of drug metabolism make them extremely susceptible to drug-induced delirium (15,19–21). Drugs commonly used by the elderly and frequently implicated in the genesis of delirium are cardiac glycosides, cimetidine, antiparkinsonian agents, benzodiazepines, psychotropic medications, steroids, antibiotics, propranolol, and other antihypertensive medications. Drugs with anticholinergic properties, such as narcotics, tricyclic antidepressants, neuroleptics, antihistamines, and substances containing atropine, frequently cause anticholinergic delirium (22). The anticholinergic syndrome is characterized by those features described above for delirium as well as tachycardia; fever; dry, flushed skin; dry mouth; mydriasis; constipation; paralytic ileus; and urinary retention.

Treatment of delirium will depend upon the underlying cause. A diagnosis of amnestic syndrome, dementia, or pseudodementia cannot be made in the presence of delirium, and evaluation of these conditions must await its complete clearing.

Amnestic Syndrome (Amnesia)

If the patient's sensorium is clear, the clinician should determine whether or not the memory disturbance is accompanied by compromise of other cognitive functions. Memory impairment in the setting of a clear sensorium and unaccompanied by general intellectual decline suggests an amnestic syndrome for which a specific organic cause can usually be discerned (16). These are listed in Figure 7-1. The amnestic syndrome is characterized by preservation of immediate recall and memory impairment that is both anterograde, as reflected in an ability to learn new material, and retrograde, as reflected in difficulty recalling past events. Recent memory is more affected than remote.

Certain psychiatric conditions included in DSM-III under dissociative disorders need to be distinguished from organically caused amnestic syndromes. Psychogenic amnesia, psychogenic fugue, and multiple personality disorder are all characterized by stress-induced periods of amnesia for which there is no underlying organic pathology. While these conditions are rarely seen for the first time in the elderly, they will be described briefly.

Psychogenic amnesia (16) is characterized by the sudden inability to recall important personal information. This failure of memory can take several forms: (a) generalized amnesia, which spans all previous life experiences; (b) continuous amnesia, which encompasses the time period following a particular event up to and including the present; (c) localized amnesia, in which there is a failure to recall all events that took place during a particular period of time; (d) selective amnesia, characterized by patchy memory failure for some events but not others within a circumscribed period of time. In all types, the patient's sensorium is clear, although there may be perplexity and disorientation. Onset and recovery are abrupt and recovery is usually complete.

In psychogenic fugue (16) the amnesia covers a period of time during which the individual travels or wanders to a new setting and assumes a new identity. During the fugue itself, a person cannot remember his or her past life and, following the episode, the events that took place cannot be recalled. There is no disturbance of consciousness and behavior is usually rational and purposeful, although there may be some disorientation and confusion.

In multiple personality disorder, an individual has two or more distinct personalities that can each be dominant at different times. The original personality has amnesia for the existence and activities of the other subpersonalities although there is some awareness of periods of lost time.

Dementia

Memory loss accompanied by global cognitive decline in a setting of clear consciousness is defined as dementia. Dementia can be divided into dementia of the Alzheimer's type (DAT) or non-Alzheimer's type (see Figure 7-1). Other terms used to refer to Alzheimer's disease include senile dementia of the Alzheimer's type (SDAT) and progressive degenerative dementia (PDD). Alzheimer's disease, a progressive, untreatable disorder, is the most common cause of dementia in the elderly, accounting for approximately 60% of all cases of global cognitive decline (4,23,24). However, the accuracy of this high prevalence has been questioned. At least 20% of all cases of Alzheimer's disease diagnosed in patients' lifetimes are found at autopsy (25,26) not to have had the disease, and several studies have found that a significant number of individuals diagnosed with Alzheimer's disease either have other treatable disorders (27) or do not follow the deteriorating course implicit in the diagnosis (28, 29). Non-Alzheimer's dementias include both treatable and untreatable illnesses as listed in Figure 7-1. Several of these conditions are briefly described before Alzheimer's disease is considered in more detail.

Multi-infarct dementia (MID) is the second most common cause of dementia, accounting for approximately 10% of patients with global cognitive decline (30). The dementia results from the cumulative effect of multiple isolated cerebral infarctions, caused by thromboembolic events within the brain. Hypertension and cardiac disease are frequent clinical findings. The history of patients with MID, usually obtained from family or friends, often reveals a stepwise deterioration characterized by abrupt, discrete episodes of neurological impairment, from which there may be full or partial recovery. The nature of the acute event will depend upon the location and size of the occluded vessel. Infarctions leading to dementia can be clinically silent at the time of the occlusion (30,31), and in these cases the history will not be helpful. On examination, asymmetric focal signs, including rigidity, hyperreflexia, muscle weakness, extensor plantar responses, as well as pathological laughing and crying are common. The Hachinski ischemia scale (7) may be helpful in distinguishing MID from other causes of dementia. Although a CT scan usually reveals findings consistent with infarctions, the lesions may be too small to be visualized (31). While NMR holds promise as a method of distinguishing Alzheimer's disease from MID, this has not been successfully demonstrated to date. NMR measures (T1 and proton density) appear to permit differentiation of either dementia (DAT or MID) from nondementia (32,33).

Alcohol may account for 5–10% of dementias (4,26,32,34). It is usually diagnosed when intellectual decline occurs in an individual with a history of alcoholism. The impairment is described as milder, more slowly progressive, and partially reversible if alcohol intake is curtailed. Constructional impairments and behavioral disturbances have been emphasized (35). However, "alcoholic dementia" is a poorly defined entity, and there is disagreement about whether it is a valid and distinct diagnosis either clinically or pathologically (18,35–37). It has been suggested that cognitive decline in alcoholics may represent chronic Wernike-Korsakoff psychosis, the additive effects of the many central nervous system (CNS) insults incurred by these individuals or the coincidental presence of another type of dementia such as Alzheimer's (18). Despite these uncertainties about whether alcohol produces a distinct and separate dementia, it is clear that alcoholics are often found to have ventricular enlargement and cortical atrophy on CT scan (18,38). The cortical atrophy is reversible if the individual remains abstinent (38).

Normal pressure hydrocephalus (NPH) accounts for approximately 6% of all dementias in the elderly (39). A prominent gait disturbance characterized by imbalance, urinary urgency, and incontinence, and impaired mental functioning constitute the classic triad of the disease (39). The cause of NPH is unknown. Diagnosis is made by the presence of the clinical triad: cerebral ventricular dilation without prominent atrophy on the CT scan, an opening lumbar puncture pressure of less than 180 mm H_2O, and abnormal isotope cisternography that shows reduced cerebrospinal fluid (CSF) reabsorption. Ventriculo-atrial shunting is effective treatment in carefully selected cases.

Huntington's disease, accounting for 3% of all dementias (34), is an autosomal dominant disorder with 100% penetrance in which there is progressive neurological deterioration characterized by involuntary choreiform movements and dementia. Memory is affected early and may be a sensitive predictor of the illness in individuals who are genetically at risk (40). Psychological disturbances, especially depression and suicide, are common. While family history and physical examination usually reveal the diagnosis, personality change, emotional disturbances, and cognitive decline can precede the motor abnormalities which may begin as late as the sixth to eight decade (18,41). Such a late-onset course can make diagnosis in the elderly difficult, especially when the family history may be obscured by ancestors who have died of other causes before the clinical expression of the disease is apparent (41).

While the cause of Huntington's disease remains unknown, various neurotransmitter changes have been confirmed. Gamma-aminobutyric acid, acetylcholine, substance P, cholecystokinin, and metenkephalin are reduced, while somatostatin, thyrotropin releasing hormone (TRH), and neurotensin are increased (41). The most striking finding on neuropathological examination is striatal cell loss and atrophy, although other parts of the brain, including the cortex, thalamus, brain stem and spinal cord, also show neuronal loss (41). A CT scan may reveal wasting of the head of the caudate nucleus and putamen bilaterally as well as cerebral atrophy.

Parkinson's disease is a degenerative neurological disorder that affects 1% of the population over age 50. Clinically, it is characterized by flat facies, decreased blinking, stooped posture, shuffling gait, slowness and paucity of movement, a resting pin-rolling tremor, and cog-wheel rigidity. Dementia is common with the estimated prevalence ranging from 20-80% (42-44). There is a positive correlation between the intellectual deficits and the severity of the neurological impairment, even on tasks that do not depend on speed or manual dexterity. It is unclear whether the dementia of Parkinson's disease (PD) represents the coexistence of two common illnesses (PD and DAT) or whether Parkinson's disease itself includes dementia. Neuropathologically there is significant neuronal loss in the pars compacta of the substantia nigra which contains dopamine cell bodies that project to the basal ganglia. This results in a reduction of dopamine in the nigrostriatal pathway.

Pick's disease deserves mention in a discussion of dementia. It is a relatively rare dementing disorder of unknown cause characterized by atrophic degeneration of the frontal and temporal lobes, hence the term lobar atrophy. Senile plaques, neurofibrillary tangles, and granulovacuolar degeneration—the characteristic histopathological changes of Alzheimer's disease—are present but to a lesser degree. Occurrence is sporadic for the most part although in 20% of cases there is autosomal dominant transmission. Whether Pick's disease is clinically distinguishable from Alzheimer's disease is controversial (18). Those who believe it is (4,45) point to the early prominence of affective and personality changes, marked language impairments, frontal lobe pathology and the frequency of the Klüver-Bucy syndrome coupled with the relatively late onset of memory and visual-spatial disturbances.

Alzheimer's disease is a progressive degenerative disorder of insidious onset characterized by memory loss and cognitive impairment. The disease may begin as early as age 40 but most often occurs after the age of 60. Clinically, Alzheimer's disease is diagnosed by exclusion, when all other known causes of dementia have been ruled out. A definite diagnosis can be made only when a particular clinical course is confirmed by specific histopathological findings on postmortem examination of the brain. Whether the dementia of Alzheimer's disease is a variant of normal aging, representing an acceleration of a natural process, or a distinct disease entity is still controversial (46,47). The distinction is particularly difficult in cases of Alzheimer's disease occurring after the age of 80. There are, as yet, no consistent established guidelines for the normal memory loss and cognitive impairment of old age, nor is there a clear understanding of the neurology, neurochemistry, or anatomical changes of age (47). In 1984, the National Institute of Neurological and Communicative

Disorders and Stroke, and the Alzheimer's Disease Related Disorders Association (NINCDS-ADRDA) work group proposed criteria to serve as a guide for the diagnosis of possible, probable, and definite Alzheimer's disease (25). These more detailed and specific criteria are compatible with present DSM-III definitions (16):

1. an insidious onset with uniformly progressive deteriorating course;

2. a loss of intellectual abilities of sufficient severity to interfere with social or occupational functioning;

3. memory impairment;

4. at least one of the following:

    - impairment of abstract thinking, as manifested by concrete interpretation of proverbs, inability to find similarities and differences between related words, difficulty in defining words and concepts, and other similar tasks;

    - impaired judgment;

    - other disturbances of higher critical function, such as aphasia (disorder of language due to brain dysfunction), apraxia (inability to carry out motor activities despite intact comprehension and motor function), agnosia (failure to recognize or identify objects despite intact sensory function), "constructional difficulty" (e.g., inability to copy three-dimensional figures, assemble blocks, or arrange sticks in specific designs);

    - state of consciousness not clouded (i.e., does not meet the criteria for delirium or intoxication, although these may be superimposed);

5. either of the following:

    - evidence from the history, physical examination, or laboratory tests, of a specific organic factor that is judged to be etiologically related to the disturbance;

    - in the absence of such evidence, an organic factor necessary for the development of the syndrome can be presumed if conditions other than organic mental disorders have been reasonably excluded and if the behavioral change represents cognitive impairment in a variety of areas;

6. Exclusion of all other specific causes of dementia by the history, physical examination, and laboratory tests.

It is unclear whether Alzheimer's disease comprises a number of biological disorders or whether different clinical types represent variations and degrees of severity of the same illness. Through careful longitudinal study and autopsy investigations, attempts are being made to determine whether, in fact, there are unique clinical subgroups that remain distinct over time and that are further distinguishable by pathological findings at autopsy. In some studies, age of onset is being used to divide patients into two groups. Patients younger than 65 are defined as having presenile Alzheimer's dementia and are thought to have a stronger family history and to differ (in terms of severity of the dementia, language impairment, and pathological and neurological findings) from patients 65 years of age or older (48,49). Presenile Alzheimer's dementia is also associated with earlier and more prominent aphasia, independent of the duration of the illness (50–53). Noradrenergic deficits, reflected in a loss of cells from the locus ceruleus appear to be more severe in female patients with presenile dementia (54).

The parkinsonian signs of akinesia, rigidity, decreased movements, and primitive reflexes are common in Alzheimer's disease (55,56) and have been associated with severity of dementia (53). In a recent study, Alzheimer's patients with psychotic symptoms were found to have significantly higher scores on the Blessed Dementia Scale and to have worse performance on neuropsychiatric testing (57). Measurements of impairment were found to be even greater in those patients with psychotic symptoms who were receiving psychotropic medication.

Etiology of Alzheimer's disease. The histological abnormalities, neurochemical pathology, and diagnostic tests in Alzheimer's disease are summarized in Tables 7–1 through 7–3. Although the cause of Alzheimer's disease remains unknown, different etiological theories or hypotheses have been proposed and recently reviewed (79).

TABLE 7-1 Histologic Findings in Normal Aging and Alzheimer's Disease

	Normal Aging	Alzheimer's Disease	References
Neuronal population	Uncertain changes	Decreased in cortex, nucleus basalis of Meynert, locus ceruleus, raphe nucleus	58–62
Neuronal plaques	Predominately in hippocampus	Widespread in cortex, hippocampus, amygdala. Suggested necessary findings, per high-powered field (HPF): 50 years: 2–5 50–65: 8 66–75: 10 75: 15	47,63
Neurofibrillary tangles	Rare	Widespread, especially in cortex, hippocampus, nucleus basalis of Meynert, raphe nucleus	60,61,64
Lipofuscin "aging pigment"	Consistently present in aged brain	More than in age-matched controls	46
Granulovacuolar organelles	Present in hippocampus after age 60	No significant difference from age-matched controls	65

TABLE 7-2 Neurochemistry of Alzheimer's Disease

Neurotransmitter	Change in Alzheimer Cortex	Pathological Finding	References
Acetylcholine	Marked decrease in synthetic enzyme choline acetyltransferase (CAT)	Cell loss from nucleus basalis of Meynert	66,67
Noradrenalin	Usually decreased	Loss of neurons from locus ceruleus	45,59,60,68,69
Serotonin	Decreased in temporal and limbic areas	Loss of neurons from raphe nucleus	48,62,63,68
Somatostatin	Levels consistently decreased	Somatostatin in plaques; degeneration and tangles in somatostatin neurons	70–73
Cholecystokinin (CCK), vasointestinal peptide (VIP), vasopressin, metenkephalin TRH, oxytocin	No reported change to date		74

TABLE 7-3 Diagnostic Test Results in Normal Aging and Alzheimer's Disease

Test	Normal Aging	Alzheimer's Disease	References
EEG	Slowing of alpha frequencies	May be normal; increase in slow-wave frequencies	4,46,75
CT scan	Atrophy and sulcal widening	Greater brain atrophy than age-matched controls but considerable overlap. Sulcal widening and gyral narrowing. Usually progressive atrophy as disease advances clinically although no clear correlation with pathological or cognitive change. Increased ventricular size	4,25,76
Visual evoked potentials	Increased latency of response	Greater latency response (50–80%) than in age-matched controls	4,25,46
Cerebral blood flow and positron-emission tomography (PET)	Blood flow decrease of approximately 23% between ages of 33 and 61. Compensation by increased extraction of O_2 and glucose	Profound reduction in blood flow, O_2 and glucose extraction, especially in frontal and parietal lobes. Changes correlate with disease severity and may be correlated with neuropsychological test performance. Changes usually have to be severe to be detected	25,47,77,78
Neuropsychological testing[a]	Reduced speed of response. Decline in nonverbal measures of WAIS. Little or no change in verbal performance	Decline in both verbal and nonverbal measures on Weschsler Adult Intelligence Scale (WAIS). Block design severely impaired	5,13,14

[a]With neuropsychological testing there is little information relating findings to pathological verification of diagnosis.

Cholinergic abnormalities. The most consistent neurochemical abnormality found postmortem in the cortex of brains of Alzheimer's disease patients is decreased concentration of choline acetyltransferase (CAT), an enzyme essential for the synthesis of acetycholine. CAT is essentially a measure of the ability of cells to produce acetylcholine and is believed to be present only in cholinergic neurons. At least 70% of CAT in the cerebral cortex is present in presynaptic terminals of axons that originate from outside the cortex in the magnocellular neurons of the nucleus basalis of Meynert in the basal forebrain. The cholinergic cells in this system (which is extrinsic to the cortex but projects into it) have been found to be severely reduced in number and/or size in patients dying with Alzheimer's disease. Muscarinic acetylcholine receptors in the cortex are essentially normal and present in normal numbers.

Genetic disposition. Family studies of Alzheimer's disease suggest that in some cases the disease may be inherited through an autosomal dominant pattern of transmission (51,80). It is not clear whether there is more than one faulty gene or whether the abnormality produces an inborn error of metabolism, causing a deficiency in the production of an essential protein that is only apparent when the individual ages. Further support for the importance of genetic factors in DAT is provided by the finding of an increased incidence of Down's syndrome (trisomy 21) in the families of afflicted individuals (49,81,82). Also, all Down's syndrome patients develop neuropathological changes consistent with Alzheimer's disease by 40 years of age and at least 30% develop the clinical signs and symptoms of the illness (47,83).

Abnormal protein accumulation. Amyloid is an abnormal protein found surrounding blood vessels and within neuritic plaques in the brains of patients with Alzheimer's disease. The number of neuritic plaques is significantly related to the severity of the dementia. To date, it is unknown whether these abnormal proteins are infectious, toxic, or an expression of altered genetic processes.

Infections. Kuru and Creutzfeldt-Jakob disease are degenerative neurological disorders associated with dementia and caused by transmissible agents. The clinical expression of these infections becomes apparent only after a long dormant period. While the term "slow virus" has been used to describe the agent of transmission, it is actually not a virus but what has been termed a *prion*. The existence of these diseases has led researchers to consider an underlying infectious process in the etiology of DAT. However, the cumulative evidence to date does not support this hypothesis. Transmission of Alzheimer's disease in experimental animals has been unsuccessful; there have been no reported epidemics; most cases of DAT are sporadic and not familial; and there has been no increased incidence among individuals who care for Alzheimer patients or in individuals who handle pathological specimens (84).

Toxins. High levels of aluminum have been found in the brains of patients with Alzheimer's disease, and it was initially hypothesized that aluminum might be a causative factor (85). However, the results of these early studies have not been consistently replicated (86,87), and it is suggested that the high aluminum levels found in the original studies may have reflected the use of aluminum sulfates in the water treatment plants in the area from which the patient samples were drawn (87,88). It also is now clear that aluminum concentration increases normally with age (87,88). In certain animals, injectable aluminum can stimulate the growth of neurofibrillary tangles, an important histopathological feature of Alzheimer's disease. Despite this suggestive evidence, the etiological role of aluminum in the development of DAT in humans has not been established.

Course of Alzheimer's disease. Alzheimer's disease can be divided into different clinical phases. Reisberg and colleagues (89) have developed a global deterioration scale which encompasses seven levels from stage I in which there is no cognitive decline to stage VII in which impairment is severe. In research studies, these have been correlated with psychometric test performance, CT scan findings and positron emission tomography (PET) scan results. For more clinical purposes, Alzheimer's disease may be separated into three stages: early, middle, and late (90). These stages are summarized in Table 7–4.

Early phase. In the early stages of Alzheimer's disease, family members report that the patient is more irritable and more easily frustrated than usual. Although the individual may not have complained about memory trouble during this period, family or care-

TABLE 7-4 Clinical Features of the Phases of Alzheimer's Disease

Stage	I (early)	II (middle)	III (late)
Duration	2–4 years	3–6 years	Variable
Memory	Predominant symptom Difficulty learning new material Remote mildly impaired	Recent and remote memory more severely impaired	Remote and recent memory profoundly impaired
Visuospatial and temporal orientation	Mild spatial and temporal disorientation May become lost while driving or walking in familiar surroundings 3-D constructions faulty	Worsening disorientation May be disoriented in own home Apraxias Marked deterioration in constructions	Persistently disoriented and confused Unable to recognize familiar faces May be unable to recognize own face
Language	Word-finding problems Circumlocutions Poverty of speech content	Anomia more severe Paraphasias Comprehension impaired May be confabulation Frequent repetition	Dysarthria May be mute

Mood and personality	Denial may begin May be anxiety and depression Loss of pride, self-esteem Suspiciousness Obsessive-compulsive defenses may appear	Paranoid symptoms and hallucinations may occur Prominent denial Irritability Catastrophic reactions	Deterioration of all aspects of previous personality
Behavior	Social behavior usually intact Difficulty adapting to a change in environment or routine	Episodes of socially inappropriate behavior such as denudation, aggression may occur More socially withdrawn, less sensitive to others	Often bed-ridden May have periods of marked agitation
Motor	Loss of spontaneity	Restlessness Agitation Some unsteadiness of gait	Intention tremor Primitive reflexes Extrapyramidal rigidity Myoclonic jerks
Activities of daily living	Usually able to care for self May continue working but with impaired performance	Grooming and hygiene neglected Difficulties dressing self Requires supervision	Requires constant supervision and institutional care Fecal and urinary incontinence

takers notice that the patient has been repeating questions, forgetting names, having problems finding words, relying excessively on lists, and having difficulty remembering the reasons why activities, such as going to the store or bank, were initiated. There may be occasional episodes of becoming lost while driving or walking in familiar surroundings. Social behavior is usually intact in the beginning, although subtle deterioration in dress and grooming may be noted. Multiple somatic complaints are a common initial presentation, and it has been suggested that dementia should be included in the differential diagnosis of any elderly patient presenting in this fashion (14). If the patient is employed, performance at work usually begins to deteriorate. Previously accomplished tasks such as balancing a checkbook or counting change become difficult, and certain activities or social interactions may be avoided in order to conceal the impairments. The world of these patients becomes constricted. Although insight may be lacking in patients with advanced Alzheimer's disease, it is often preserved during the early stages. The awareness of progressive cognitive decline may lead to irritability, depression, and anxiety.

Middle phase. During the middle stage of Alzheimer's disease, as the symptoms progress, memory impairment becomes more prominent. Remote memory now becomes increasingly affected, and the patients may forget aspects of personal history such as their own birthdate and the names of their children. Patients may become disoriented and confused even in familiar surroundings, tolerating any change in routine, physical environment, and caretakers less and less well. There is a growing inability to learn anything new. Language problems including paraphasias and anomias develop and then become more severe such that fluency and spontaneity in speech deteriorate. Comprehension may now become impaired. There is a decline in abstract thinking and problem solving, a growing inability to follow arguments or conversations and a failure of conceptual and metaphorical thinking. Many patients describe feeling most confused in the morning. Dressing and grooming begin to take an inordinately long time as the patient cannot decide what to wear or how to put on certain articles of clothing. Mild disturbances of balance and gait in the form of reduced stride, decreased arm swing, rigidity, and postural instability may be present.

Late Phase. In the late stage of Alzheimer's disease, the patient's memory is so severely impaired that disorientation and confusion are persistent. Familiar faces are not recognized and the patient may not even be able to identify his or her own face. Dysarthria or muteness may be present. If there is some preservation of language, it is often in the form of repetitive words or simple sentences. Eventually the patient may be wheelchair- or bed-ridden with intermittent periods of severe agitation. Parkinsonian symptoms become more prominent, and primitive reflexes as well as focal neurological signs can often be elicited. There is usually significant weight loss. Incontinence of urine and feces is common, and patients require constant supervision and nursing care.

Psychiatric symptomatology during the course of the disease appears to reflect both the patient's response to the illness as well as the disease process itself. In the early stages, anxiety and denial are common and often marked. As the disease progresses, depression, anger, uncontrollable explosive rage, mania, or paranoia are often seen.

Treatment of Alzheimer's disease. No effective treatment exists for Alzheimer's disease. Nevertheless, a wide variety of pharmacological agents have been tried in Alzheimer's patients. The most important of these are listed in Table 7-5.

Vasodilators and anticoagulants. Alzheimer's disease was, at one time, thought to arise from decreased cerebral blood flow presumably due to arteriosclerosis. This notion, since discredited, led to efforts to treat Alzheimer's disease with vasodilators and anticoagulants. Not surprisingly, these therapies were not shown to be beneficial. In fact, harmful effects may have resulted in some patients (91).

Agents promoting neurotransmission. In the past decade, attention has turned to the possibility that Alzheimer's disease may be due to abnormalities of neurotransmission, opening potential new avenues for pharmacotherapy. The discovery of decreased acetylcholine in Alzheimer cortex led to the hope that treatment with agents that enhance or promote cholinergic neurotransmission might be beneficial to Alzheimer's disease patients. To date, many controlled clinical trials have failed to establish the therapeutic efficacy of

TABLE 7-5 Drugs Used in Treatment of Memory Impairment and Dementia

Therapeutic Rationale	Class of Drug	Name of Drug
Increased cerebral blood flow	Vasodilators	Papaverine Isoxuprine Cyclandelate
	Anticoagulants	
Promotion of neurotransmission	Cholinergic agents Precursors	Lecithin (phosphatidylcholine) Choline
	Acetylcholinesterase inhibitors	Physostigmine
	Agonists	Arecholine, Bethanecol
	Noradrenergic agonists	Clonidine
	Serotonergic reuptake inhibitor	Alaproclate
	Neuropeptides	ACTH, ACTH analogs, vasopressin analogs
	Opiate antagonists	Naloxone
CNS activation	Stimulants	Dextroamphetamines, methylphenidate pentylenetetrazol, pipradol, pemoline, centrophenoxine
	Nootropic agents	Piracetam and analogs
CNS metabolic enhancement	Metabolic enhancers	Dihydroergotoxine (Hydergine), Procaine hydrochloride (Gerovital GH$_3$), Pentoxyfylline
Unknown	Calcium-channel blockers	Nimodipine Nifedipine
	Aluminum chelators	Desferrioxamine

cholinergic agents in Alzheimer's disease (92). More recent studies have shown that several other neurotransmitters, such as norepinephrine and serotonin may also be compromised in Alzheimer's disease. These findings have prompted treatment strategies aimed at restoring noradrenergic and serotonergic function. The neuropeptides ACTH and vasopressin which appear to facilitate learning and memory in experimental animals have only modest effects in Alzheimer's patients, principally on mood and attention rather than learning and memory (92). Naloxone, a narcotic antagonist, was shown to improve memory function in patients with mild Alzheimer's disease (93). Follow-up studies, however, have not confirmed these observations (94,95).

Agents associated with CNS functioning and metabolism. Psychomotor stimulants, especially methylphenidate and pentylenetetrazol, which have been approved for treatment of symptoms associated with senile dementia, have not been found to improve memory or cognition, although they may have limited effect upon mood, fatigue, and psychomotor retardation (90,92,96-98). Nootropic agents are analogs of gamma-amino butyric acid (GABA) and are believed to enhance cortical functioning. To date they, too, have not been proven to affect either memory or cognition in Alzheimer's disease (92,99). Dihydroergotoxine, once thought to be a cerebral vasodilator, is now believed to be a general enhancer of metabolism in the CNS. It is a drug widely prescribed for the elderly. More than 33 controlled trials in patients with memory impairment have demonstrated very modest but statistically significant effects on a range of symptoms (92). When cognitive function has been measured directly, effects have not been as apparent suggesting that its effect may be primarily to elevate mood (90,92). Hydergine is usually prescribed in dosages of 3 mg/day although higher doses of up to 6 mg may be more effective. Benefits may not be seen for many months (90,100). Procaine hydrochloride or Gerovital has been used in Europe and Asia for years. In controlled studies, it has been shown to have no effect on memory or cognition but, being a weak monoamine oxidase inhibitor, it may have mood-elevating effects (92).

Pseudodementia

Pseudodementia is a descriptive term used to signify any primary psychiatric illness that clinically resembles dementia but in which the intellectual decline is potentially reversible if the underlying disorder is treated. Historically, the term arose from misdiagnoses of dementia with the psychiatric nature of the illness being recognized only after the patient either unexpectedly recovered or did not show the progressive decline associated with dementia (101,102). It is estimated that psychiatric illness accounts for 10% of cases evaluated for intellectual impairment (27,103,104), making it essential that pseudodementia be considered in the differential diagnosis of memory loss and cognitive impairment.

A wide range of psychiatric illnesses has been implicated in the etiology of pseudodementia. Depression, personality disorder, Ganser's syndrome, hypomania and mania, hysteria, psychosis, schizophrenia, anxiety disorders, and post-traumatic stress disorder have all been associated with cognitive impairment (28,29,101,102,104–107). The most common psychiatric disorders believed to underlie pseudodementia in the elderly are depression and characterological disturbances. There is considerable controversy about the use of the term pseudodementia and to which condition it is most suitably applied. In depressive pseudodementia, for example, the prefix "pseudo" with its implication of false or illusory cognitive change does not do justice to the very real and significant impairment of intellect in these patients. It has been suggested that depressive pseudodementia would be more accurately referred to as the dementia syndrome of depression (108). On the other hand, elderly patients with long-standing character disorders of a passive-dependent or hysterical nature may be more accurately thought of as "burlesques" or "caricatures" of dementia (101). Their poor performance on mental status examination and formal testing is primarily reflective of regression. Overall, the literature on pseudodementia in the elderly is not extensive, and the actual nature of the cognitive impairments in either depressive or characterological pseudodementia has not been carefully studied.

Depressive Pseudodementia

Depression is the psychiatric illness most frequently misdiagnosed as dementia in the elderly (105,108–110) since there is considerable overlap in the clinical presentation of each. This is especially true of patients with severe depression when compared with patients in the early stages of dementia who become dysphoric in response to their intellectual deterioration. The validity of frequently cited clinical features (101) used to distinguish depressive pseudodementia from dementia must be questioned as the data have been derived from patients of all ages with different diagnoses, particularly characterological disturbances.

A careful history from family or friends is invaluable in correctly establishing the diagnosis. The history will usually reveal mood disturbance, social withdrawal, and loss of interest in activities antedating the cognitive impairment. A history of previous episodes of depression, prior spontaneous remissions in the present symptom complex, and recent losses or major changes in the individual's life preceding either mood or cognitive change should prompt consideration of the diagnosis of depressive pseudodementia.

Clinically, a flat or depressed affect may be more typical of a patient with depression than with dementia. Elderly patients with severe depression often do not communicate their depression effectively, and the clinician may not be able to rely upon "empathic detection" of depression as readily in these patients. The chief complaints are often not about sadness, despair, or loss but about physical complaints or cognitive impairment.

The speech of patients with depressive pseudodementia may be slow, hesitant, and hypophonic, but without the language impairments (anomias, paraphasias, and circumlocutions) that one sees in patients with dementia. Patients with depressive pseudodementia are likely to suffer from an appetite disturbance with weight loss as well as disturbed sleep with early morning awakening. Inattention to grooming and hygiene is usually apparent. Psychotic material in the form of nihilistic, guilty, or somatic delusions can often be elicited from patients with depressive pseudodementia and there may be active suicidal ideation.

Insufficient data is available regarding the actual nature of the intellectual deficits in these patients, and it is not clear whether there is a pattern of cognitive impairment specific to depression (111). The memory deficit in depressive pseudodementia can be severe. There is clearly impairment of immediate recall and recent memory related, in part, to inattention, preoccupation, poor concentration, and lack of interest and effort during testing.

The compromise of recent memory function contributes to uncertainties about the date and frank disorientation as well as poor knowledge of current events and difficulty learning new tasks (4, 28, 105). The literature on depressive pseudodementia reports both impaired and unimpaired remote memory. Poverty of content and slow mental processes are reflected in inadequate word lists and picture descriptions, deficient spontaneous elaborations, and omissions of details in copying and drawing. While constructional and visual-spatial impairments are felt to be sensitive indicators of organicity, tests for these impairments may give inaccurate results when a patient is depressed (101,105,111). During testing, depressed patients show a lack of effort and interest, easy fatigability, and a tendency to give up easily. They are often openly self-critical and may view their poor performance as evidence that they are suffering from dementia. The physical examination of patients with depressive pseudodementia should be essentially normal and reveal no apraxia, aphasia, or agnosia.

The dexamethasone suppression test (DST) as well as the TRH stimulation test are not useful in distinguishing depressive pseudodementia from organic dementia since the DST. may be positive in dementia as well as in depression, and in males over 60 the thyroid-stimulating hormone (TSH) response to TRH is normally blunted. The EEG should be normal in patients with depressive pseudodementia. Nuclear magnetic resonance may become a useful procedure in distinguishing dementia from nondementia (32, 33).

In summary, despite the features that may help the clinician to recognize depressive pseudodementia, there is no particular clinical finding, neuropsychological test, or diagnostic procedure that reliably and infallibly separates it from organic dementia. The clinician can only form a global clinical impression and frequently must give an empirical trial of either electroconvulsive therapy (ECT) or an antidepressant to distinguish the two forms of cognitive decline.

Characterological Pseudodementia

Patients with dependent and hysterical character disorders may be vulnerable to the development of pseudodementia as they age (14, 28, 101–106, 108, 112, 113). In fact, they have been described as patients who are "most accurately referred to as [having] pseudodementia" (14) emphasizing the spurious nature of their cognitive impairment. These patients are felt to indulge in the problems of aging to get attention and care. They complain bitterly about dysphoria and memory disturbance. There is both active protest that nothing can be remembered and communication to others of distress and helplessness. In this sense they are more interpersonally engaged and less withdrawn than depressed patients. Communicating helplessness, they implore others to care for them.

The onset of characterological pseudodementia is often gradual, reflecting an exaggeration of lifetime patterns. Vegetative signs and symptoms are usually lacking. The grooming and hygiene of patients with hysterical pseudodementia may be impeccable, and they may have concurrent physical conversion symptoms such as limb anesthesia, dizziness, or difficulty walking.

Mental status and neuropsychological testing are remarkable for verbal expressions of anxiety, lack of effort, and emphasis on deficits. However, while unable to concentrate when being tested, these patients appear alert and attentive to the interviewer. The professed ignorance and poverty of content on formal testing may be contrasted with the rich and meticulous details of discussions in other situations, especially in patients with hysterical pseudodementia. Striking inconsistencies are often noted between the way patients with characterological pseudodementia function during formal testing and the way they are observed to function in other settings. They can accurately balance their checkbooks, find their way around, and remember promises and commitments. During testing they are dysphoric and seem to exaggerate the distress they are in. On formal mental status questions, these patients give many "I don't know" or "I can't remember" answers, but unlike patients with an underlying depression, they resist encouragement and do not respond to greater structure and organization provided by the examiner.

The diagnosis of characterological pseudodementia rests on exclusion of organic dementia and depression. Previous psychiatric history and information from the family concerning the patient's characterological style may be diagnostically helpful. If characterological or behavioral regression is the cause of cognitive impairment, the most effective interventions will be supportive and directed toward helping the patient gradually resume responsibility for daily care and activity. Caretakers will benefit from guidance in learning how to taper interventions that are regressive without provoking feelings of abandonment.

CARING FOR THE DEMENTED PATIENT

The physician who cares for the patient with dementia must remain alert to those aspects of the patient's problems that may require specific treatment. Since demented patients are less likely to complain of the symptoms of an illness, detection is often less prompt. Intercurrent physical illnesses that are common in the elderly (such as dehydration, infection, trauma, heart failure, anemia, thyroid disease, and nutritional deficiencies) are especially likely to occur in demented patients when self-care, institutional care, or family care may be inadequate.

Physical deficits associated with aging may, if treated, maximize or enhance a patient's functional capacity. Reduced visual acuity, auditory impairment, and disruption of eating patterns secondary to poor dentures or loss of teeth are all problems that can be successfully treated. Adequate shoes, canes, or walkers, and other equipment for assisting mobilization may all promote continued physical activity.

Changes and surprises in the patient's world are best kept to a minimum. Attempts should be made to prepare the patient for upcoming changes in the environment through frequent reiteration of what is anticipated and gradual exposure to new situations. Orientation can be enhanced by placing calendars, pictures of family members with names attached, and reminders of future events in the patient's living area. If possible, the family should make changes in the home that will reduce the chance of injuries from falls. Demented patients do not travel well and if the family or caretakers have to be away, it may be preferable to have someone stay with the patient in familiar surroundings rather than to expose the patient to a new, disorienting environment.

Routine daily activities should be maintained whenever possible, although the patient should be asked or encouraged to do only those tasks that can be successfully accomplished without frustration in order to maintain self-esteem. These tasks should be simple, straightforward and time-limited. Family and caretakers must, at the same time, guard against prematurely usurping responsibility for things that the patient can clearly manage. Patients may need to be protected from social events and interactions that will be too demanding intellectually. The disorientation, confusion, and visual-spatial impairments of Alzheimer's disease make it hazardous for the patient with dementia to drive. The physician should take the initiative in discussing this safety issue with the family.

Educating families about dementia and preparing them for progressive deterioration is very important. The diagnosis and various stages of the illness need to be outlined as clearly as possible. It is natural for family members to feel enormous conflict between their wish to provide for the patient and their concern about the effect of the illness on their own lives in terms of time, energy, and financial resources. Caretakers should be advised early on about the eventual need for a nursing home. This is an emotionally evocative issue for most families. Denial, protest, grief, guilt, and anger will surface, and considerable tact, time, and empathy are required to achieve some resolution. Often the physician is unable to provide these services, and, in such instances, caretakers should be referred to appropriate social and counseling services. Legal dimensions, such as guardianship, should be discussed so that decisions about health care can be made when a patient is unable to do so.

Patients with Alzheimer's disease may suffer from a number of secondary psychiatric syndromes that the psychiatrist will be called upon to assess and treat. This is not an easy task for a number of reasons. (a) There is a paucity of good data available on the use of psychotropic medications in the elderly patient with dementia (114). (b) These patients are sensitive to medication side effects, particularly the anticholinergic properties of many psychotropic medications. (c) Information that is available suggests that even when patients appear to be good candidates for treatment, many become worse on medication (115). (d) Finally, the time course of many of the psychiatric syndromes is uncertain. Anecdotal evidence suggests that disturbances of mood, thinking, and behavior are often transient and self-limiting. This makes it difficult to know when to initiate and when to discontinue a medication. Many clinicians err on the side of continuing medications long after they are needed (115). Disturbances of mood (such as depression and anxiety), disturbances in thinking (such as paranoid ideation or misperceptions), and disturbances in behavior (such as agitation, assaultiveness, wandering and insomnia) are all common in dementia. Assessment of these problems begins with a comprehensive medical evaluation. As mentioned earlier, the elderly demented patient is especially vulnerable to the development of delirium. A diagnosis of delirium must be considered whenever an abrupt change in mood, thinking, or behavior occurs and is accompanied by a precipitous deterioration in cognition from the patient's recent baseline. The acute or subacute onset or worsening of disorientation as well as inattention, fluctuations between alertness and drowsiness, delusions, hallucinations, and disorder of the sleep–wake cycle are characteristics of delirium. A careful review of medications should be undertaken since drug effects and toxicity, particularly anticholinergic toxicity, are frequent causes of delirium in the elderly.

If a diagnosis of delirium is made, the underlying causes must be vigorously pursued and treated. In addition to drug toxicities, certain infections, particularly pneumonia and urinary tract infections, electrolyte disturbances, dehydration, uremia, congestive heart failure, and cardiovascular accidents, are commonly associated with delirium in the elderly.

An evaluation of psychosocial stresses should be undertaken whenever there is an acute disturbance of mood, thinking, or behavior. This would include an inquiry into losses, recent trips or exposures to unfamiliar environments, changes in the location of the patient's room or living situation, changes in daily routine, and changes in the patient's caretaking that may be causing excessive or deficient stimulation. Some disturbances of mood, thinking, and behavior are drug related and will improve as drug doses are lowered or medications are discontinued.

Depression

Depression is believed to occur in 10–20% of patients with Alzheimer's disease. It is most apt to occur early in the course of the illness when insight and awareness of failing cognition are intact. Neither diagnosis nor treatment of depression in elderly demented patients is straightforward. Signs and symptoms, such as psychomotor retardation or agitation, inattention to self-care, loss of interest in usual activities, fatigue, feeling worse in the morning, and diminished ability to think and concentrate are common to both dementia and depression. Sudden decrease in appetite, weight loss, and early morning awakening may be more helpful indications of the onset of depression.

Often the only sign of depression is an acute or subacute worsening of the individual's memory and cognitive difficulties that cannot be accounted for by the presence of delirium or other compromise in the patient's medical condition. Similarly, any relatively rapid change in the patient's usual behavior beyond that which has occurred since dementia was diagnosed may suggest depression. For example, a patient who has been verbal and able to express himself/herself reasonably well may become quiet and apprehensive rather suddenly; or a patient who has been socially active may become seclusive and withdrawn over a short period of time. The thought content of demented patients who are depressed may be marked by themes of guilt, self-loathing, pessimism, and suicidal ideation.

Cyclic antidepressants may have some therapeutic usefulness in patients with mild Alzheimer's disease who also have clearly diagnosable major depressive disorders (116). In patients whose depressive symptoms are atypical, or in whom dementia is moderate or severe, tricyclic antidepressants are not therapeutic and may actually worsen agitation, confusion, insomnia, restlessness, and cognitive functions.

If a cyclic antidepressant trial is to be used, a physical examination, EKG and baseline vital signs should be obtained. Elderly patients with dementia are especially prone to the development of anticholinergic toxicity, orthostatic hypotension, and disorientation from sedation. Orthostasis can result in falls, strokes, or heart attacks. The common anticholinergic side effects of antidepressants include dry mouth, constipation, and urinary retention. In an elderly demented patient who cannot communicate these problems and whose self-care may already be compromised, these symptoms can quickly progress to gingivitis, stomatitis, obstipation with gastrointestinal obstruction, and urinary tract infection. The anticholinergic mydriatic action of cyclic antidepressants, causing blurred vision, can lead to falls and can worsen disorientation and confusion in the demented patient.

Since the tertiary amines amitryptyline, imipramine, doxepin, and trimipramine all have strong sedating, orthostatic hypotensive, and anticholinergic side-effects, the secondary amines (nortriptiline or desipramine) are usually the antidepressants of first choice (117). Dosage and serum therapeutic ranges for cyclic antidepressants have not been clearly established for the demented patient. Medications should be started at very low doses, increased slowly, and divided throughout the day as increases are made. A reasonable regimen would be to start with nortriptyline, 10 mg q.i.d. for 1 week with increases of 10 mg every 5-7 days up to a total of approximately 60 mg q.i.d. If desipramine is selected, a starting dose of 10 mg should again be used with a similar schedule for increasing the total amount up to 100-150 mg q.i.d. in divided doses. The patient must be carefully monitored for either side effects or a therapeutic response. If the former occur, the medication should be lowered to the dose at which there were no side effects and, after a longer period, an increase can again be attempted.

The physician will do best if clear target symptoms can be identified and followed clinically. While there is little information available regarding maintenance therapy in patients with dementia, it would seem prudent to continue medication for 4-6 months if it is well tolerated.

If a secondary amine is unsuccessful, the clinician may want to try another medication. However, it must be emphasized that few data are available regarding their use in elderly demented patients.

Maprotiline, a tetracyclic compound, has a therapeutic and side-effect profile similar to nortriptyline, with anticholinergic, hypotensive, and cardiovascular properties. Skin rashes are more common with maprotiline, and grand mal seizures have been reported at dosages greater than 250 mg/day. The recommended therapeutic range for an elderly demented patient would be approximately 50-150 mg q.d. starting with 25 mg.

Amoxapine is an atypical secondary amine that, like maprotiline resembles nortriptyline in therapeutic and side-effects profile. There is no evidence that either maprotiline or amoxapine has an earlier onset of action than other antidepressants. Of concern in using amoxapine in the elderly is that one of its active metabolites, 7-OH-amoxapine, has potent dopamine-blocking effects. Patients taking this drug can develop the full range of neuroleptic side effects including dystonic reactions, akathisia, parkinsonism, and tardive dyskinesia. Amoxapine can be started at 25 mg/day and increased to 150 mg.

Trazodone, a triazolopyridine antidepressant has been suggested for use in the elderly because it is devoid of anticholinergic side effects. However, it has its own profile of side effects that are problematic in these patients including marked sedation, postural hypotension, gastric upset, and, rarely, ventricular arrythmias. A recommended starting dose would be 25 mg q.d. with gradual increases up to 150-200 mg as tolerated.

Bupropion* is a second-generation antidepressant medication that while new, holds promise for the treatment of depression in the elderly. It is reported to be nonsedating, without hypotensive effects, and less anticholinergic. However, it has been associated with headaches, agitation, decreased appetite, and weight loss, and may be more epileptogenic than tricyclic antidepressants (117). The daily dose for the nonelderly, nondemented patient is 150-600 mg. To date, there is little information available about its use in older patients with dementia.

Evidence of increased monoamine oxidase-B activity (118) in the brains of patients with Alzheimer's disease provides a theoretical

---

*Bupropion was removed from the market by the U.S. FDA because of concern about its potential to cause seizures. It is being studied further and may again be released.

basis for the use of monoamine oxidase (MAO) inhibitors to treat depression associated with dementia. However, since the relationship of this increased enzyme activity to clinical depression is unclear, the rationale for using MAO inhibitors in these patients is uncertain. Furthermore, MAO inhibitors cause significant postural hypotension and require that the demented patient be adequately supervised so that the essential dietary restrictions will be followed and drug interactions avoided. Like the cyclic antidepressants, MAO inhibitors commonly cause an increase in agitation, restlessness, insomnia, and confusion in patients with moderate or severe dementia. For these reasons, they should not be used routinely and should be prescribed only by someone experienced with their use and after a trial of a cyclic antidepressant has failed.

If the patient with Alzheimer's disease is suffering from a severe or psychotic depression or is unable to tolerate any medications because of side effects, ECT should be used. To decrease the severity of any confusion or memory loss that may occur during a course of ECT, the frequency of treatments should be decreased, and ECT should be administered to the nondominant cerebral hemisphere.

Methylphenidate and other stimulants are not recommended for patients with Alzheimer's disease, because of the confusion, agitation, and restlessness they can produce.

Anxiety

The patient with early-stage Alzheimer's disease may frequently suffer from anxiety. Sleep, appetite, memory, and cognition can all be adversely effected when anxiety is extreme. Before symptomatic treatment is begun, the clinician should ascertain whether the anxiety is a feature of another psychiatric disorder such as depression or paranoia. Medical causes of anxiety such as hypoglycemia, hypoxia, electrolyte disturbances, pulmonary embolus, and hyperthyroidism as well as cardiac arrythmias should be considered. Nonpharmacological treatments of anxiety may be effective either alone or in conjunction with medications. Supportive meetings with the patient and with family members or caretakers, during which specific fears can be identified and addressed, are helpful. Some patients in the early stages of dementia who spend a great deal of time alone may become much less anxious if they are provided with the companionship of someone who can distract, comfort, orient, and correct misinterpretations of the environment.

If anxiety is severe, a short course of a low-dose benzodiazepine may be indicated. The clinician should watch carefully for evidence of behavioral disinhibition, ataxia, sedation, confusion, and worsening of memory, all of which can occur with benzodiazepine use, particularly in the elderly demented patient. In general, benzodiazepines that are shorter acting and depend for their metabolism on conjugation rather than oxidation, such as oxazepam and lorazepam, are preferable to long-acting benzodiazepines. Accumulation and progressive toxicity are less likely to occur. The initial and maintenance dose should be low, usually one-third to one-half of that used in younger patients (117). Discontinuation of benzodiazepines should be gradual since withdrawal symptoms of tremor, agitation, and seizures have been reported.

Paranoia

Paranoid delusions may be more common than mood changes in the demented patient. Whenever there is impairment in hearing, vision, or cognitive ability as in dementia, paranoid elaboration of perceptual stimuli is likely to occur. Gaps or lapses in memory may be filled in with delusional ideas that often capture the sense of vulnerability these patients feel. Simplifying, clarifying, and routinizing the demented patient's daily schedule may reduce paranoid stimuli, although reassurance is often unhelpful. When paranoia is severe, agitation becomes common, and neuroleptics may be necessary to treat both paranoid thinking as well as to quell the agitation.

Agitation

Agitation is a common problem in the elderly demented individual. Medical illnesses, pain, depression, anxiety, and paranoia as well as medication side effects can all be expressed as agitation. Neuroleptic drugs, even in low doses, can cause agitation secondary to akathesia. If medical or toxic causes can be ruled out, the clinician should conduct a psychosocial assessment of the patient with family or caretakers to determine whether any environmental or personal stresses can be identified that are precipitating or perpetuating episodes of agitation.

The treatment of agitation is sometimes accomplished by simple interventions like distraction, physical soothing, or having the patient return to a familiar setting. When agitation is severe, neuroleptics may be used for behavioral control (116, 117). However, a recent review of the literature reveals that only a minority of patients show dramatic improvement with neuroleptics and many deteriorate (115).

Choice of Neuroleptics

Several types of neuroleptic drugs are available, each with a distinct chemical structure. The largest group consists of the phenothiazines, the prototypic neuroleptic. Other classes are butyrophenones (haloperidol), thioxanthenes (chlorprothixene, thiothixene), indolones (molindone), and dibenzoxazepines (loxapine).

Neuroleptic drugs are therapeutically equivalent and differ only in milligram potency and side-effect profile. Selection of any one neuroleptic in preference to another is based on the pharmacokinetic and side-effect profile of each drug, the patient's history of prior drug response, and the experience of the clinician with each agent. Once treatment has begun, if an older patient does not respond to one neuroleptic, another should be tried, preferably of a different chemical class (117).

Neuroleptic drugs that require relatively few milligrams to produce a clinical effect are termed high potency, in contrast to low-potency agents, which require more milligrams. The use of the term potency in this context, however, refers to relative potency on a milligram-for-milligram basis rather than to differential efficacy. In general, low-potency neuroleptics tend to be strongly sedating, hypotensive, and anticholinergic. Only one neuroleptic, rather than a combination, should be prescribed at a time in order to minimize side effects and to evaluate the individual drug's effectiveness.

Dosage and administration. No particular neuroleptic has been found to be superior to another for the demented patient. Starting dosages should be one-fifth to one-quarter those prescribed for younger nondemented adults, and dosage should be gradually increased or decreased according to clinical response or development of side effects (117). Initially, antipsychotic drugs should be given in divided doses two or three times a day since elderly patients may be less tolerant of a sudden decrease in blood pressure from one large daily dose.

Once dosage is stabilized and clinical response has been achieved with minimal side effects, the total daily dose should be given at one time. For the geriatric patient with nighttime agitation, the daily dose should be given 1–2 hours before the agitation usually occurs to take advantage of the drug's sedating effects. Since agitation and behavioral disturbances may be short-lived, medication should be ordered for brief periods and then reassessed.

Side effects. Common side effects of neuroleptic drugs that are particularly frequent in old people are sedation, orthostatic hypotension, anticholinergic reactions, and extrapyramidal symptoms (Table 7-6). Older, demented patients are more sensitive to the side effects of neuroleptics, which, in turn, are prolonged by age-related pharmacokinetic changes.

Sedation is one of the most common side effects of neuroleptic drugs. Low-potency neuroleptics with sedative side effects are excellent sleep inducers and may be helpful for the elderly patient who has insomnia or who is severely agitated during the day. However, because metabolism and excretion of neuroleptic drugs is delayed in elderly patients, sedation persists for many hours after the drug has been administered. In addition, since regularly prescribed neuroleptic drugs accumulate because of slowed metabolism, sedating effects become progressively extended and ultimately may interfere with the older patient's level of arousal throughout the day. Sedation may impair mental functioning and may increase confusion and disorientation in the older patient with dementia. High-potency neuroleptic drugs with low sedation thus tend to have an advantage for most elderly patients who require sustained neuroleptic treatment. However, even these may cause drowsiness (see Table 7-6).

Orthostatic hypotension during neuroleptic treatment is common and has more serious sequelae in older people. Falls, resulting in bone fractures and head injuries, from which these patients recover poorly, are frequent. Hypotension is secondary to neuroleptic blockade of central vasoregulatory centers and peripheral alpha-adrenergic receptors. Elderly patients with low cardiac output, as well as those receiving additional medications that block alpha-adrenergic receptors, are especially vulnerable.

Neuroleptics, particularly those of low potency such as thioridazine, can produce changes on the EKG. Prolongation of the QT and PR interval as well as T wave and ST segment depression may occur. Usually these changes are of no clinical significance. However, patients with pre-existing cardiac disease should be carefully monitored, and low-potency neuroleptics are best avoided in treating

TABLE 7-6 Relative Incidence of Side Effects of Neuroleptic Drugs

Generic name	Trade name	Approximate dosage range, mg/day	Sedation	Hypotension	Extrapyramidal symptoms	Anticholinergic symptoms
Chlorpromazine	Thorazine Chlor PZ	10–300	Marked	Marked	Moderate	Marked
Chlorprothixene	Taractan	10–300	Marked	Marked	Moderate	Marked
Thioridazine	Mellaril	10–300	Marked	Marked	Mild to moderate	Moderate
Acetophenazine	Tindal	10–60	Moderate	Moderate	Moderate	Moderate
Perphenazine	Trilafon	4–32	Moderate	Moderate	Moderate	Moderate
Loxapine	Loxitane	5–100	Moderate	Moderate	Moderate	Moderate
Molindone	Moban	5–100	Moderate	Moderate	Moderate	Moderate
Trifluoperazine	Stelazine	4–20	Moderate	Moderate	Moderate to marked	Moderate to mild
Thiothixene	Navane	4–20	Moderate	Moderate	Moderate to marked	Moderate to mild
Fluphenazine	Prolixin	0.25–6	Mild	Mild	Marked	Mild
Haloperidol	Haldol	0.25–6	Mild	Mild	Marked	Mild

them. Combinations of neuroleptics and antidepressants can produce additive cardiovascular effects (119).

Elderly patients are especially susceptible to the extrapyramidal symptoms produced by neuroleptic drugs. Low-potency neuroleptics, particularly thioridazine, are likely to produce fewer and less severe extrapyramidal symptoms than the higher-potency drugs.

Akathisia, the most common drug-induced extrapyramidal symptom in elderly patients, with peak incidence in the seventh decade, is characterized by motor restlessness and muscular tension experienced as a compulsion to move. Patients who develop this condition constantly pace and move their legs in a restless manner that is sometimes difficult to differentiate from the more generalized restlessness of agitation or anxiety. Asking the older person manifesting this symptom whether or not his or her leg muscles feel tense, stiff, or jittery—muscular feelings usually reported when akathisia is present—provides the basis for differentiation. When akathisia is confused with agitation and the clinician increases neuroleptic dosages, the condition worsens.

The preferred drug treatment for older persons with akathisia consists of lowering the neuroleptic dosage and using relatively low-potency agents. If these treatment methods prove ineffective, a neuroleptic drug in combination with an antiparkinsonian agent could be used. However, these are often ineffective. Beta blockers such as propranolol in a low dose range of 20–80 mg/day has been recommended for the treatment of akathisia (120) when reduction of the neuroleptic is impossible. However, the use of multiple drugs in patients with brain disease who are extremely sensitive to medication side effects is best avoided. Akinesia, sometimes considered part of the Parkinson-like side-effect syndrome, is not uncommon in older patients. It is characterized by a lack of energy, decreased spontaneous movements, and a blank or sometimes sad expression on the patient's face. Because this side effect resembles psychomotor retarded depression, it may be incorrectly diagnosed as part of a depressive disorder.

The anticholinergic side effects of neuroleptic drugs in the presence of age-related decreased cholinergic functioning in the body can lead to serious problems in the elderly patient. The likelihood of anticholinergic toxicity increases when anticholinergic drugs are used to treat extrapyramidal symptoms produced by neuroleptics. In addition, because older patients are also more likely to be taking antiparkinsonian drugs and other medications that produce anticholinergic side effects concomitantly with neuroleptics, the risk of severe toxicity is further increased.

Treatment with propranolol. Propranolol, a non-neuroleptic drug that blocks postsynaptic beta-adrenergic receptor sites, has been reported to successfully treat agitation, assaultiveness, and explosive outbursts of rage in patients with organic brain disease of various etiologies (121–123).

The mechanism of this therapeutic effect is unknown. Propranolol may be preferable to neuroleptics for some older patients because it does not cause extrapyramidal or anticholinergic symptoms or lead to longer-term risk of tardive dyskinesia. However, there no data from well-controlled prospective studies concerning its use in agitated demented patients.

Dosages of propranolol vary considerably in older patients, depending on the pharmacokinetic parameters of the drug in older people and the clinical condition of the patient. Starting dosages should be 10 mg, two or three times a day, with increases of 10 mg each day thereafter. When no toxic effects occur or in cases of severe agitation, more rapid dosage increments may be necessary. The therapeutic range of propranolol in most cases seems to be between 80 and 200 mg/day. The appearance of clinical effects usually correlates with a slowing of the pulse rate, indicating effective beta-receptor blockade.

The major side effects of propranolol are hypotension, bradycardia, and decreased cardiac output. Asthma and chronic obstructive lung disease can also be exacerbated. Because depression has been associated with its use, it is essential to evaluate mood as well as the cardiovascular and respiratory status of the patient prior to instituting propranolol therapy. Once such therapy is instituted, vital signs must be taken regularly, and cardiovascular functioning must be monitored.

REFERENCES

1. Jarvik, L. (1982). Aging and psychiatry. *Psychiatric Clinics of North America* 5:5–9.
2. Wells, C. (1981). A deluge of dementia. *Psychosomatics* 22:837–838.

3. Gurland, B. J., and Cross, P. S. (1982). Epidemiology of psychopathology in old age. *Psychiatric Clinics of North America* 5:11–26.
4. Cummings, J. L., and Benson, F. D. (1983). *Dementia: A Clinical Approach.* Boston: Butterworth.
5. Strub, R. L., and Black, F. W. (1977). *The Mental Status Examination in Neurology.* Philadelphia: F. A. Davis.
6. Geschwind, N. (1975). The apraxias: neural mechanisms of disorders of learned movement. *American Scientist* 63:188–195.
7. Hachinski, V. C., Iliff, L. D., and Zalkha, E. (1975). Cerebral blood flow in dementia. *Archives of Neurology* 32:632–637.
8. Rosen, N. G., Terry R. D., Fuld, P. A., et al. (1980). Pathological verification of ischemia score in differentiation of dementia. *Annals of Neurology* 7:486–488.
9. Blessed, G., Tomlinson, B. E., and Roth, M. (1968). The association between quantitative measures of dementia and of senile change in the cerebral grey matter of elderly subjects. *British Journal of Psychiatry* 114:797–811.
10. Folstein, M. F., Folstein, S. E., and McHugh, P. R. (1975). Mini-mental state: a practical method for grading the cognitive state of patients for the clinician. *Journal of Psychiatric Research,* 12:189–198.
11. Kral, V. A. (1967). Senescent forgetfulness: benign and malignant. *Canadian Medical Association Journal* 86:257–260.
12. Reisberg, B. (1985). Alzheimer's disease update. *Psychiatric Annals* 15:319–322.
13. Albert, M. (1984). Cognitive function assessment in the elderly. *Psychosomatics* 25:310–317.
14. Wells, C. (1985). Organic mental disorders. In *Comprehensive Textbook of Psychiatry,* ed. V. I. Kaplan and B. J. Sadock. Baltimore, MD: Williams & Wilkins.
15. Lipowski, Z. J. (1983). Transient cognitive disorders (delirium, acute confusional states) in the elderly. *American Journal of Psychiatry* 140:1426–1436.
16. *Diagnostic and Statistical Manual of Mental Disorders,* 3rd ed. (1980). Washington, DC: American Psychiatric Association.
17. Liston, E. H. (1982). Delirium in the aged. *Psychiatric Clinics of North America* 5:49–65.
18. Adams, M. V., and Victor, M. (1981). *Principles of Neurology,* 2nd ed. New York: McGraw-Hill.
19. Lipowski, Z. V. (1980). *Delirium: Acute Brain Failure in Man.* Springfield, IL: Charles C Thomas.
20. Chien, C. P., Townsend, E. J., and Ross-Townsend, A. (1979). Substance use and abuse among the community elderly: the medical aspect. In *Drug Use Among the Aged,* ed. D. M. Peterson, pp. 357–372. New York: Spectrum.
21. Salzman, C., ed. (1984). *Clinical Geriatric Psychopharmacology.* New York: McGraw-Hill.
22. Salzman, C. (1985). Geriatric psychopharmacology. *Annual Review of Medicine* 36:217–228.
23. Katzman, R. (1976). The prevalence and malignancy of Alzheimer's disease. *Archives of Neurology* 33:217–218.

References

24. Terry, R. D., and Katzman, R. (1983). Senile dementia of the Alzheimer type. *Annals of Neurology* 14:497-506.
25. McKann, G. (1984). Clinical diagnosis of Alzheimer's disease: report of the NINCDS-ADRDA workgroup under the auspices of health and human services task force on Alzheimer's disease. *Neurology* 34:939-944.
26. National Institute on Aging Task Force Report (1980). Senility reconsidered: treatment possibilities for mental impairment in the elderly. *Journal of the American Medical Association* 244:259-263.
27. Marsden, C. D., and Harrison, M. J. G. (1972). Outcome of investigation of patients with presenile dementia. *British Medical Journal* 2:249-252.
28. Nott, P. N., Fleminger, J. J. (1975). Presenile dementia: the difficulties of early diagnosis. *Acta Psychiatrica, Scandinavica* 51:210-217.
29. Ron, M. A., Toone, B. K., Garralda, M. E., and Lishman, W. A. (1979). Diagnostic accuracy in presenile dementia. *British Journal of Psychiatry* 134:161-168.
30. Hachinski, V. C. (1974). Multi-infarct dementia: a cause of mental deterioration in the elderly. *Lancet* 2:207-210.
31. Fisher, C. M. (1982). Lacunar strokes and infarcts: a review. *Neurology* 32:871-876.
32. Besson, J. A. O., Corrigan, F. M., Foreman, E. I., et al. Differentiating senile dementia of Alzheimer type and multi-infarct dementia by proton NMR imaging. *Lancet* 2:789.
33. Besson, J. A. O., Corrigan, F. M., Foreman, E. I., et al. (1985). Nuclear magnetic resonance (NMR): II imaging in dementia. *British Journal of Psychiatry* 146:31-35.
34. Wells, C. E. (1977). *Dementia.* New York: Davis.
35. Seltzer, B., and Sherwin, I. (1978). Organic brain syndromes: an empirical study and critical review. *American Journal of Psychiatry* 135:13-21.
36. Cutting, J. (1978). The relationship between Korsakov's syndrome and alcoholic dementia. *British Journal of Psychiatry* 132:240-251.
37. Lishman, W. A. (1981). Cerebral disorders in alcoholism. *Brain* 104:1-20.
38. Carlen, P. E., et al. (1978). Reversible cerebral atrophy in recently abstinent chronic alcoholics measured by computed tomography scan. *Science* 200:1076-1078.
39. Fisher, C. M. (1982). Hydrocephalus as a cause of disturbances of gait in the elderly. *Neurology* 32:1358-1363.
40. Butters, N., Sax, D., Montgomery, K., and Tarlow, S. (1978). Comparison of the neuropsychological deficits associated with early and advanced Huntington's disease. *Archives of Neurology* 35:585-589.
41. Martin, J. B. (1984). Huntington's disease: new approaches to an old problem. *Neurology* 34:1059-1072.
42. Boller, F. (1983). Alzheimer's disease and Parkinson's disease: clinical and pathological associations. In *Alzheimer's Disease: The Standard Reference*, ed. B. Reisberg. New York: The Free Press.
43. Hakim, A. M., and Mathieson, G. (1978). Basis of dementia in Parkinson's disease. *Lancet* 2:729.
44. Lieberman, A., Dziatolowski, M., and Kupersmith, M. (1979). Dementia in Parkinson's disease. *Annals of Neurology* 6:355-359.

45. Cummings, J. L., and Duchen, L. W. (1981). Kluver-Bucy syndrome in Pick disease: clinical and pathological correlations. *Neurology* 31:1415–1422.
46. Berg, L. (1985). Does Alzheimer's disease represent an exaggeration of normal aging? *Archives of Neurology* 42:737–739.
47. Khatchaturian, Z. S. (1985) Diagnosis of Alzheimer's disease. *Archives of Neurology* 42:1097–1105.
48. Heston, L. L., and White, J. (1978). Pedigrees of 30 families with Alzheimer's disease: associations with defective organization of microfilaments and microtubules. *Behavior Genetics* 4:315–331.
49. Heston, L. L. (1977). Alzheimer's disease, trisomy 21 and myeloproliferative disorders association suggesting a genetic diathesis. *Science* 196:322–323.
50. Seltzer, B., and Sherwin, I. A. (1983). A comparison of clinical features in early and late-onset primary degenerative dementia: one entity or two? *Archives of Neurology* 40:143–146.
51. Breitner, J. C. S., and Folstein, M. F. (1984). Familial Alzheimer dementia: a prevalent disorder with specific clinical features. *Psychological Medicine* 14:63–80.
52. Mohs, R. C., Silverman, M. A., Greenwald, B. S., and Davis, K. L. (1984). A study of familial Alzheimer's disease (abstract). Los Angeles: American Psychiatric Association.
53. Chiu, H. C., Teng, E. L., Henderson, V. W., and Moy, A. C. (1985). Clinical subtypes of dementia of the Alzheimer's type. *Neurology* 35:1544–1550.
54. Bondareff, W., Mountjoy, C. Q., and Roth, M. (1981). Selective loss of neurones of origin of adrenergic projection to cerebral cortex (nucleus locus coeruleus) in senile dementia. *Lancet* 1:783–784.
55. Pierce, J. (1974). The extrapyramidal disorder of Alzheimer's disease. *European Neurology* 12:94–103.
56. Molsa, P. K., Marttila, R. J., and Rinne, U. K. (1984). Extrapyramidal signs in Alzheimer's disease. *Neurology* 34:1114–1116.
57. Mayeaux, R., Yaakov, S., and Sano, M. (1985). Psychosis in patients with dementia of the Alzheimer type (abstract). Annual meeting of the American Neurological Association, Chicago.
58. Whitehouse, P. J., Price, D. L., Struble, R. G., et al. (1982). Alzheimer's disease and senile dementia: loss of neurons in the basal forebrain. *Science* 215:1237–1239.
59. Bondareff, W., Mountjoy, C. Q., and Roth, M. (1981). Selective loss of neurones of origin of adrenergic projection to cerebral cortex (nucleus locus coeruleus) in senile dementia. *Lancet* 1:783–784.
60. Tomlinson, B. E., Irving, D., and Blessed, C. (1981). Cell loss in the locus coeruleus in senile dementia of the Alzheimer type. *Journal of the Neurological Sciences* 49:419–428.
61. Curcio, C. A., and Kemper, T. (1984). Nucleus raphe dorsalis in dementia of the Alzheimer type: neurofibrillary changes and neuronal packing density. *Journal of Neuropathology and Experimental Neurology* 43:359–368.
62. Yamamoto, T., and Hirano, A. (1985). Nucleus raphe dorsalis in Alzheimer's disease: neurofibrillary tangles and loss of large neurons. *Annals of Neurology* 17:573–577.

63. Tomlinson, B. E. (1982). Plaques, tangles and Alzheimer's disease. *Psychological Medicine* 12:449–459.
64. Hirano, A., and Zimmerman, H. M. (1962). Alzheimer's neurofibrillary changes. *Archives of Neurology* 7:227–242.
65. Tomlinson, B. E., and Kitchner, D. (1972). Granulacuolar degeneration of hippocampal pyramidal cells. *Journal of Pathology* 106:165–185.
66. Bowen, D. M., Smith, C. B., White, P., and Davison, A. N. (1976). Neurotransmitter-related enzymes and indices of hypoxia in senile and other abiotrophies. *Brain* 99:459–498.
67. Davies, P., and Maloney, A. J. (1976). Selective loss of central cholinergic neurones in Alzheimer's disease. *Lancet* 2:1403.
68. Francis, P. T., Palmer, A. M., Neil, R. S., et al. (1985). Neurochemical studies of early-onset Alzheimer's disease: possible influence on treatment. *New England Journal of Medicine* 313:7–11.
69. Adolfsson, R., Gottfries, G. C., Roos, B. E., and Winblad, B. (1979). Changes in brain catecholamines in patients with dementia of Alzheimer type. *British Journal of Psychiatry* 135:216–223.
70. Beal, M. F., Mazurek, M. F., Tran, V. T., et al. (1985). Somatostatin receptors are reduced in cerbral cortex in Alzheimer's disease. *Science* 229:289–291.
71. Davies, P., Katzman, R., and Terry, R. D. (1980). Reduced somatostatin-like immunoreactivity in cerebral cortex from cases of Alzheimer's disease and Alzheimer senile dementia. *Nature* 288:270–280.
72. Roberts, G. W., Crow, T. J., and Polak, J. M. (1985). Location of neuronal tangles in somatostatin neurones in Alzheimer's disease. *Nature* 314:92–94.
73. Morrison, J. H., Rogers, J., Scherr, S., et al. Somatostatin immunoreactivity in neuritic plaques of Alzheimer's patients. *Nature* 314:90–92.
74. Ferrier, I. N., Crow, T. J., and Adrian, T. E. (1983). Neuropeptides in Alzheimer type dementia. *Journal of the Neurological Sciences* 62:159–170.
75. Kazniak, A. W., Garron, D. C., Foz, J. H., et al. (1979). Cerebral atrophy, EEG slowing, age, education and cognitive functioning in suspected dementia. *Neurology* 78:182–186.
76. Donaldson, A. A. (1979). CT scan in Alzheimer pre-senile dementia. In *Alzheimer's Disease: Early Recognition of Potentially Reversible Deficits*, ed. A. I. Glen and L. J. Whalley, pp. 97–101. New York: Churchill Livingston.
77. Yamaguchi, F., Myer, J. S., Yamamoto, M., et al. (1980). Noninvasive regional cerebral blood flow measurements in dementia. *Archives of Neurology* 37:410–418.
78. Benson, D. F., Kuhl, D. E., Hawkins, R. A., et al. (1981). Positron computed tomography in the diagnosis of dementia. *Annals of Neurology* 10:76.
79. Wurtman, J. H. (1985). Alzheimer's disease. *Scientific American*, 62–74.
80. Cook, R. H., Ward, B. E., and Austin, J. H. (1979). Studies in aging of the brain: IV familial Alzheimer's disease—relation to transmissible dementia aneuploidy and microtubular defects. *Neurology* 229:1402–1412.
81. Heston, L. L., Mastri, A. R., Anderson, V. E., and White, J. (1981). Dementia of the Alzheimer type. *Archives of General Psychiatry* 38:1985–1990.
82. Heyman, A., Wilkinson, W. E., Hurwitz, B. J., et al. (1983). Alzheimer's dis-

ease: genetic aspects and associated clinical disorders. *Annals of Neurology* 14:507–515.
83. Rossor, M. N. (1982). Neurotransmitters and CNS disease. *Lancet* 2:1200–1204.
84. Pruisner, S. B. (1984). Some speculations about prions, amyloid and Alzheimer's disease. *New England Journal of Medicine* 310:661–663.
85. Crapper, D. R., Krishman, S. S., and Dalton, A. J. (1973). Brain aluminum distribution in Alzheimer's disease and experimontal neurofibrillary degeneration. *Science* 180:511–513.
86. McDermott, J. R., Smith, Iqbal, K., and Wisniewski, H. M. (1979). Brain aluminum in aging and Alzheimer's disease. *Neurology* 29:809–814.
87. Markesbury, W. R., Ehmann, W. D., Hossain, T. I. M., et al. (1981). Instrumontal neuron activation analysis of brain aluminum in Alzheimer's disease and aging. *Annals of Neurology* 10:511–516.
88. Katzman, R. (1986). Alzheimer's disease. *New England Journal of Medicine* 314:964–973.
89. Reisberg, B., et al. (1982). The global deterioration scale for assessment of primary degenerative dementia. *American Journal of Psychiatry* 139:1136–1139.
90. Goodnick, P., Gershon, S., and Salzman, C. (1984). Dementia and memory loss in the elderly. In *Clinical Geriatric Psychopharmacology*, ed. C. Salzman. New York: McGraw-Hill.
91. Cook, P., and James, I. (1981). Cerebral vasodilators. *New England Journal of Medicine* 305:1508–1513.
92. Crook, T. (1985). Clinical drug trials in Alzheimer's disease. *Annals of the New York Academy of Sciences*, 428–436.
93. Reisberg, B., Ferris, S., DeLeon, M. J., and Crook, T. (1982). The global deterioration scale for assessment of primary degenerative dementia. *American Journal of Psychiatry* 139:1136–1139.
94. Panella, J. S., and Black, J. P. (1984). Lack of clinical benefit from naloxone in a dementia day hospital. *Annals of Neurology* 15:308.
95. Blass, J. S., Drachman, D., Katzman, R., and Spar, J. E. (1983). Naloxone in dementia (letter). *New England Journal of Medicine* 309:556.
96. Crook, T. (1979). Central nervous system stimulants appraisal of use in geropsychiatric patients. *Journal of the American Geriatrics Society* 27:476–477.
97. Salzman, C. (1981). Stimulants in the elderly. In *Age and the Pharmacology of Psychoactive Drugs*, ed. A. Raskin, D. S. Robinson, and J. Levine, pp. 171–180. New York: Elsevier.
98. Branconnier, R. S., and Cole, J. O. (1980). The therapeutic role of methylphenidate in senile organic brain syndrome. In *Psychopathology in the Aged*, ed. J. O. Cole, pp. 183–194. New York: Raven Press.
99. Growdon, J. H., Corkin, S., and Huff, F. J. (1985). Clinical evaluation of compounds for the treatment of memory dysfunction. *Annals of the New York Academy of Sciences*, 428–436.
100. Yesavage, J. A., Hollister, L. E., and Burian, E. (1979). Dihydroergotoxine: 6-mg versus 3-mg dosage in the treatment of senile dementia (preliminary report). *Journal of the American Geriatrics Society* 27:80–82.

References

101. Wells, C. E. (1979). Pseudodementia. *American Journal of Psychiatrics* 136:845-900.
102. Kiloh, L. G. (1961). Pseudo-dementia. *Acta Psychiatrica Scandinavica* 37:336-351.
103. Freeman, F. R. (1976). Evaluation of patients with progressive intellectual deterioration. *Archives of Neurology* 33:658-659.
104. Smith, J. S., and Kiloh, L. G. (1981). The investigation of dementia: results in 200 consecutive admissions. *Lancet* 1:824-827.
105. Caine, E. D. (1981). Pseudodementia. *Archives of General Psychiatry* 38:1359-1364.
106. Good, M. I. (1981). Pseudodementia and physical findings masking significant psychopathology. *American Journal of Psychiatry* 138:811-814.
107. Seltzer, B., and Sherwin, T. (1978). Organic brain syndromes: an empirical study and critical review. *American Journal of Psychiatry* 135:13-21.
108. Folstein, M. F., and McHugh, P. R. (1978). Dementia syndrome of depression. In *Alzheimer's Disease: Senile Dementia and Related Disorders*, ed. R. Katzman and K. L. Bick, pp. 87-93. New York: Raven Press.
109. McAllister, T. W. (1983). Overview: pseudodementia. *American Journal of Psychiatry* 140:528-533.
110. Post, E. (1965). *The Clinical Psychiatry of Late Life*. Oxford: Pergamon Press.
111. McAllister, T. W. (1981). Cognitive function in the affective disorders. *Comprehensive Psychiatry* 22:572-586.
112. McEvoy, J. P., and Wells, C. E. (1979). Case studies in neuropsychiatry: II conversion pseudodementia. *Journal of Clinical Psychiatry* 40:447-449.
113. Mersky, H. (1979). *The Analysis of Hysteria*. London: Bailliere Tindall.
114. Winograd, C. H., and Jarvik, L. F. (1986). Physician management of the demented patient. *Journal of the American Geriatrics Society* 34:295-308.
115. Risse, S., and Barnes, R. (1986). Pharmacologic treatment of agitation associated with dementia. *Journal of the American Geriatrics Society* 34:368-376.
116. Spira, N., Dysken, M. W., Lazarus, L. W., et al. (1984). Treatment of agitation and psychosis. In *Clinical Geriatric Psychopharmacology*, ed. C. Salzman, pp. 49-76. New York: McGraw-Hill.
117. Gelenberg, A. J. (1985). Bupropion: the second generation continues. *Biological Therapies in Psychiatry* 8:17.
118. Oreland, L. (1985). Monoamine oxidase in normal aging and in ad-sdat. In *Normal Aging, Alzheimer's Disease and Senile Dementia: Aspects on Etiology, Pathology, Diagnosis and Treatment*, ed. C. G. Gottfries, pp. 129-134. Bruxelles: Editions de l'Université de Bruxelles.
119. Gelenberg, A. J. (1983). Psychosis. In *The Practitioner's Guide to Psychoactive Drugs*, ed. E. L. Bassuk, S. C. Schoonover, and A. J. Gelenberg, pp. 115-165. New York: Plenum.
120. Lipinski, J. F., Zubenko, C. S., Cohen, B. M., and Barreira, P. J. (1984). Propranolol and the treatment of neuroleptic-induced akathisia. *American Journal of Psychiatry* 141:412-415.
121. Greendyke, R. M., Schuster, B., Worten, S. A. (1984). Propranolol in the

treatment of assaultive patients with organic brain damage. *Journal of Clinical Psychopharmacology* 4:282.
122. Petrie, W. M., and Ban, T. A. (1981). Propranolol in organic agitation (letter). *Lancet* 1:324.
123. Yudofsky, S., Williams, D., and Gorman, J. (1981) Propranolol in the treatment of rage and violent behavior in patients with chronic brain syndrome. *American Journal of Psychiatry* 138:218.

8

Child Psychiatry Problems

Barbara J. Coffey, M.D.

GENERAL APPROACHES TO DRUG THERAPY

Advances in the use of medication in the child and adolescent population have been among the most exciting developments in the field of child psychiatry in the 1970s and 1980s. Although psychopharmacological agents have been used to treat children's disorders for many years, only recently has the era of modern scientific pediatric psychopharmacology begun.

Today's child psychiatrist can choose from all of the categories of psychotropic agents available to the adult psychiatrist. Knowledge of formal and informal indications for drug use, drug categories, and side-effect profiles in childhood and adolescence is mandatory for all up-to-date clinicians.

Despite widespread use of these agents, however, there exists very little good research. Diagnostic imprecision in child psychiatry has also contributed to the lack of scientific data on uses of these agents.

Indications

Despite recent advances in research strategies and methodology in pediatric psychopharmacology, there are still few formal indications for psychoactive drug use in childhood and adolescence. Drugs, like all forms of therapy in child psychiatry, are to be used to promote optimal development and maturation, or to assist in the removal of obstacles for development to proceed onward in an adaptive fashion. In most cases, drug therapy represents one component of a total treatment plan for the child, including other forms of therapy. Quite frequently, medication can be used to help make the disturbed child more responsive to other forms of therapy, such as psychodynamic and/or psychoeducational approaches. Medication cannot, however, create new skills or improve intellectual potential alone but must be used in conjunction with other treatments.

Established indications are discussed in the section on specific agents. General indications for drug therapy include the following categories of disturbance:

1. childhood and adolescent psychosis,
2. severe behavioral disturbance accompanying mental retardation or child psychiatric emergencies,
3. Gilles de la Tourette's disorder,
4. enuresis,
5. attention-deficit disorder with hyperactivity,
6. some forms of sleep disturbance.

Other conditions in which indications are informally established at present but are potentially drug responsive include:

1. childhood depression,
2. separation anxiety disorder,
3. anxiety states,
4. borderline states,
5. sleep arousal disorders.

Although there are few formal indications for which drug therapy has been established in pediatric psychopharmacology, the U.S. Food and Drug Administration (FDA) does allow and expect that practitioners will use approved drugs for indications that are not technically approved for advertising. An example is the use of tricyclic antidepressants for the treatment of childhood major depression, which is a frequent practice in child psychiatry at this time, despite lack of FDA approval for marketing of these agents.

GENERAL GUIDELINES TO DRUG THERAPY IN CHILDHOOD AND ADOLESCENCE

Children and adolescents are not frequently self-referred for psychiatric intervention; often they are not even willing patients. In most cases, the child's behavior or emotional state is disturbing to someone else in the environment, usually an adult such as a parent or teacher. The parent's attitude toward the use of medication and ability to work with the doctor and child is extremely important. A parent is a necessary source of information about the child's functioning and response to medication. The parent (and often the teacher) needs to be informed about the reasons for the drug therapy, the likely therapeutic effects, side effects, and toxicities. A child with an unreliable parent who cannot observe, administer, and monitor the medication may not be treatable with pharmacotherapy.

As there are few formal diagnostic indications for pharmacotherapy in childhood and diagnostic criteria themselves such as DSM-III have some limitations in applicability in child psychiatry, it is useful to approach drug therapy on a problem-oriented or target-symptom basis. Although establishing a diagnosis is important for each child, it is frequently the target symptom that will guide the clinician as to choice of agent. The clinician should, in a cohesive and relevant way, draw up a list of problems or target symptoms with which the child presents. Common target symptoms that are potentially drug responsive include attentional difficulties, hyperactivity, enuresis, tics, and sleep disturbance such as insomnia or night terrors.

Children differ significantly from adults in their pharmacokinetic capacities. Children have relatively large liver size in proportion to body weight when compared with adults, and after about one year of age reach adult glomerular filtration rates; therefore, they seem to function metabolically more efficiently with regard to drug handling. Children often tend to need higher doses relative to body weight when compared with adults (1).

In addition, evidence suggests that children tend to have less adipose tissue and less protein binding when compared to adults and may have more drug available for bioactivity and, potentially, side effects (2).

Growth and development itself are associated with changes in organ size and proportion and in tissue mass, particularly water and adipose tissue. These changes may have significant effects on drug handling. Adolescents approach adults in their metabolic and pharmacokinetic parameters.

Appropriate drug selection requires comprehensive information about the child, his or her history and current functioning, family history, and medical history. Criteria for drug selection are based on a combination of diagnosis and target symptomatology and are not always clearly defined in this young population.

Dosage regulation requires time and experience. Few guidelines are available in the literature (3). In general, calculating initial dose and ceiling dose on a milligram per kilogram basis is useful, particularly with the antidepressants and psychostimulants. Plasma levels of some drugs can be readily obtained, and therapeutic ranges similar to those of adults have been identified such as with the tricyclic antidepressants and lithium. In general, except in emergencies, it is best to start with a low dosage and raise by standardized increments every 2–3 days until therapeutic effect or range is reached or until the onset of side effects. Often it is necessary to push the dosage up to the point of development of side effects in order to explore the optimal range. Frequently the dosage can then be gradually lowered to find a balance between the minimum necessary for therapeutic effect and minimal possibility of side effects.

In the case of the acutely psychotic child with target symptoms of motor overactivity, delusional thinking or hallucinations, and agitation, or the acutely assaultive child in an emergency state, medication can be given more frequently until the child is sedated or calmed. In this situation, oral concentrates can be given every 1–2 hours until a therapeutic effect is achieved.

Side effects are not infrequent in childhood and adolescence, although they may be transient or of little clinical significance. Many of the side effects of neuroleptics, antidepressants, and lithium seen in adult patients can be seen in children and adolescents. Of particular concern are the anticholinergic and cardiovascular side effects of the tricyclic antidepressants and the extrapyramidal side effects of the neuroleptics, including dyskinesias (4, 5).

Duration of treatment will depend upon the target symptom, the age of the child, the kind of psychotropic agent, and the unique features of the clinical situation. There are few fixed guidelines as to length of time on medications, drug holiday programs, and indications for stopping. In general, if a child has not responded to an agent within 4 weeks while in the therapeutic range, it is unlikely he or she will respond at a later date. A rational approach to this situation would be to switch to another drug in the same category or to another category altogether if indicated and possible.

Most children with a therapeutic response to medication will need a trial of 3–6 months depending on the clinical situation. Some will require a longer period of time. In general, no child or adolescent should remain on any agent for more than a year without at least a 1- to 2-month drug holiday.

Periodic drug holidays are indicated for all psychotropic agents for two reasons: (a) to reassess the child's need for the agent at regular intervals and (b) to monitor for the development of side effects such as growth changes or dyskinesias.

The frequency and timing of drug holidays should be geared to the individual child. Most children should have attempted holidays at approximately 6-month intervals. There is controversy in the adult literature regarding the frequency of holidays and the incidence of tardive dyskinesia, but there is little information on this subject with children and adolescents.

CLINICAL GUIDELINES

Preliminary Drug Evaluation

All child and adolescent patients who are candidates for psychopharmacological agents should undergo a thorough medical and psychiatric evaluation. Data of particular importance in the evaluation of children include a medication history for family members with psychiatric illness, with responses to medication, and information from teachers regarding classroom performance and behavior.

Data with regard to cognitive-intellectual function can be documented with psychometric testing. The role of projective testing is controversial with regard to its usefulness in differential diagnosis; however, these can be helpful in decision making as to class of medication if the child has a constellation of target symptoms that can potentially be treated with more than one type of agent. For example, a child with attentional difficulties and hyperactivity with much depressive affect on projective testing should probably be tried on imipramine first, rather than a stimulant.

Complete physical examination prior to starting medication is of paramount importance. First, for differential diagnostic purposes, physical assessment is necessary to rule out organic sources of the child's disturbance, such as temporal lobe seizures or hyperthyroidism. There are a number of pediatric disorders that can present with psychiatric symptoms. For example, chronic lead intoxication can result in motor overactivity and learning and academic difficulty. Signs and symptoms of anorexia nervosa can be due to underlying endocrinopathy or malabsorption syndrome. Second, all of the agents can have physical effects on the child, such as alterations in blood pressure, pulse, or weight. Height, weight, blood pressure, temperature, pulse, and respiration should be noted. It is important that growth and development be monitored with height and weight parameters and yearly physical exams throughout the course of treatment.

A screening neurological examination should be performed on all patients who are candidates for psychotropic agents. Before medication is started, note should be made as to the presence or absence of unusual movements, tics, or stereotypic behaviors. These are commonly seen in psychotic youngsters and need to be noted before pharmacotherapy to enable identification of medication-related dyskinesias (6).

Children with special problems, such as heart conditions or seizure disorders, may need consultation with a specialist prior to drug therapy.

A minimal laboratory work-up for all children who are candidates for medication includes:

- complete blood count (CBC) and differential;
- urinalysis;
- blood urea nitrogen (BUN), creatinine, electrolytes;
- height, weight, and growth chart;
- pregnancy test where appropriate, in sexually active female adolescents;

- toxic screen where appropriate, in substance users;
- lead level in the child who presents with hyperactivity.

Additional Considerations

For children who are candidates for tricyclic antidepressants the following are useful baseline parameters:

- thyroid function tests: T_3, T_4, T_4I, thyroid-stimulating hormone (TSH);
- SMA12 including liver function tests (LFTs): protein, albumin, bilirubin (direct and indirect); alkaline phosphatase, SGOT, SGPT, lactic dehydrogenase (LDH), creatine phosphokinase (CPK);
- electrocardiogram (EKG);
- electroencephalogram (EEG) may be useful and necessary in the child with pre-existing seizure disorder, family history of seizures, or previous abnormal EEG;
- blood pressure (BP) and pulse, sitting and standing.

For children who are candidates for neuroleptics (antipsychotics):

- Add SMA12 including LFTs as above;
- Abnormal Involuntary Movement Screen (AIMS);
- BP and pulse.

For children who are candidates for psychostimulants:

- add Conners checklist for attention-deficit disorder with hyperactivity before, and it can be repeated after medication. Both parents and teacher can fill out the checklist for 5-7 days prior to drug therapy for baseline, then after the child has reached therapeutic range. These can provide useful quantitative data in determining drug response.
- add BP, pulse, height, weight, and growth chart.

For children who are candidates for lithium carbonate add:

- SMA12 including LFTs and calcium;
- thyroid function tests as for tricyclics;
- creatinine clearance can be helpful, but not mandatory, if urinalysis, BUN, and creatinine have been obtained on at least two or three occasions and averaged.

The role of specialized tests studied in adult psychiatry, such as the dexamethasone suppression test, urinary catecholamines, sleep architecture studies, and hypothalamic-pituitary stimulation tests have not been clarified for routine clinical use in this age group despite some evidence that they may have some value as research tools.

Written and informed consent of the parent(s) or legal guardian and assent of the child may be useful in some cases in which the indications for drug therapy are not formally established, such as use of tricyclic antidepressants for children under 12 years of age with major depression or separation anxiety disorder. But, in general, informed consent is a process that takes place in an ongoing dialogue between doctor, parent(s), and child. The parent and child have a right to know expected therapeutic and adverse effects and relative risks versus benefits. Discussion of these issues in a straightforward, simple fashion can facilitate ongoing communication in most cases. Clear documentation of the rationale for drug selection, response, adverse effects, and changes in dosages or drugs is required.

Drug Maintenance and Monitoring

Children and adolescents usually need to be seen at regular and frequent intervals during the initiation of drug therapy, at least once a week. Close communication is necessary with the parent(s) during this time as well. Parents should be encouraged to call the doctor if any questions arise about medication.

Once the child has been stabilized, usually after several weeks, on his/her maintenance dosage, a drug maintenance program can begin. Children can generally be seen less frequently, such as monthly, to review therapeutic response and development of side effects. Information from teachers and other clinicians involved in the child's care must be regularly communicated to the prescribing physician.

All children on all pharmacotherapy should have at least one yearly drug holiday to reassess need for the drug and to monitor for the development of side effects. The duration and timing of the drug-free period will vary with the individual child, type of drug, and clinical situation.

Periodic laboratory screening should be done on a regular basis during the entire duration of drug therapy. It is judicious practice to repeat CBC and differential, urinalysis, and basic chemistry screening at 3 months and every 6 months for each of the medications. Certain specific procedures, such as EKG monitoring, are discussed in the section on specific agents.

In general, it is very useful to record weight and height on a monthly or quarterly basis, as many of these agents can cause weight gain, or in some cases, weight loss. Keeping a growth chart, such as that provided by the National Center for Health Statistics, can provide the clinician easy access to growth parameters over an extended period of time.

SIDE EFFECTS AND DRUG INTERACTIONS

Despite their drug-handling efficiency, children and adolescents are no less at risk for the development of adverse effects of these agents (Table 8-1). This has both physiological and practical significance; clinicians must be acquainted with the side-effect profiles of the drug(s) they prescribe and must know how to manage adverse effects should they arise. In addition, children and adolescents are particularly prone to sensitivities about their bodies and how they work and often get quite frightened or suspicious if a sudden change or dysfunction occurs in the context of drug therapy. Such feelings can interfere with compliance.

In general, the best therapy for adverse effects is preventive; that is, if at all possible, it is best to avoid high doses, polypharmacy, sudden withdrawal of drugs, or challenging a child with a drug to which he or she has previously demonstrated hypersensitivity.

TABLE 8-1 Side Effects and Their Management

Drug Category	Common Adverse Effects	Clinical Management
Neuroleptics (antipsychotics)	*Short Term:*	
	Autonomic Nervous System	
	dry mouth	in general, lower dosage if possible or switch drug if persistent; child may "equilibrate" after several weeks
	urinary retention	Bethanechol chloride only if severe and persistent
	constipation	Docusate sodium (Colace) tablets or bisacodyl (Dulcolax) suppositories
	orthostatic hypotension	avoid sudden postural changes; reduce dosage if severe
	Extrapyramidal	
	acute dystonic reaction	IM diphenhydramine or benztropine, then switch to oral form
	parkinsonism	anticholinergic/antiparkinsonian medication on an as-needed basis
	Other:	
	akathisia	lower dosage; sometimes anticholinergic can help
	hypersensitivity/rash	discontinue drug
	drowsiness	child usually becomes tolerant; if persistent switch to less sedating class of drugs
	photosensitivity	avoid sun exposure
	increased levels in LFTs	may not have clinical significance
	Long Term:	
	weight gain	lower dosage; consider switch to another class of drugs
	dyskinesias (tardive and withdrawal)	prevention is best; use lowest possible dose for maintenance

Psychostimulants	*Short Term:* anorexia, nausea, abdominal pain	reduce dose; give most of dosage in A.M.; consider switch
	insomnia	move P.M. dose to earlier in the day; reduce dosage; then reintroduce
	dysphoria	consider another stimulant, if persistent, or imipramine
	Long Term: weight loss	institute drug holidays or change of drug
	tics/Tourette's syndrome	discontinue immediately and avoid rechallenge
TCAs	*Autonomic Nervous System*	see neuroleptics
	Cardiovascular (increases in BP, pulse, and PR; T wave changes, arrhythmias)	monitor EKGs serially with dosages 3.5 mg/kg; most changes have little clinical significance in healthy child
	CNS (seizures)	discontinue medication gradually; EEG; may need anticonvulsant
Anxiolytics- Sedative hypnotics antihistamines	oversedation	decrease total dosage, administer most at bedtime
	rash	discontinue medication
benzodiazepines	disinhibition	discontinue medication
	GI: nausea, vomiting, abdominal pain, diarrhea, metallic taste	consider dose reduction if persistent
Lithium	CNS: tremor, memory lapses, fatigue	consider dose reduction if persistent
	Endocrine: goiter, increased Ca++	discontinue medication and follow with lab studies
	Renal: polyuria/polydipsia	monitor BUN, creatinine, electrolytes and urinalysis on a regular basis (every 2–3 months)
	Hematologic: leukocytosis	monitor; may not be of clinical significance

Guidelines to avoid possible adverse effects include:

1. Use the lowest possible maintenance dose in the therapeutic range once it has been established.
2. Try to avoid prescribing more than one drug at a time in a given child. For example, it is best to try lowering the dosage of a neuroleptic slightly for parkinsonism or akathisia if at all possible, rather than adding an antiparkinsonian agent.
3. In most cases, drugs should be tapered gradually, both for physiological and psychological purposes. This provides more opportunity for the reestablishment of equilibrium.
4. Never give an agent to a child who had demonstrated previous sensitivity to it, such as tics on stimulants or dyskinesias on phenothiazines.

Common Drug Interactions in Children and Adolescents

Drug interaction occurs when one agent alters the therapeutic or adverse effects of another agent (Table 8-2). Interactions can occur at any phase in a drug treatment plan. Common instances when such alterations occur include:

1. in absorption, such as in the gastrointestinal tract;
2. in distribution, such as competition for binding sites;
3. in metabolism, such as effects upon liver enzyme functions;
4. in excretion;
5. in receptor site function (7).

Children and adolescents are no less prone to drug interaction effects than are adults. The best rule of thumb is to try to avoid interactive effects by avoiding polypharmacy where at all possible. However, if at times it becomes necessary to prescribe two or more agents simultaneously, the clinician should be alert to possible interactions.

SPECIFIC AGENTS

Neuroleptic (Antipsychotic) Drugs

Formal indications for use of neuroleptics include symptoms of (a) childhood and adolescent psychoses and pervasive developmental disorders such as agitation, stereotypies, and social withdrawal; (b) severe behavior disturbance as accompaniment to mental retardation, such as self-destructive or assaultive behavior; (c) psychiatric emergencies, including acute homicidal behavior; and (d) Gilles de la Tourette's disorder (Table 8-3). Informal indications include attention-deficit disorder with hyperactivity and mania.

These medications are effective in children with such target symptoms as auditory hallucinations or delusions. In addition, they can decrease severe agitation and motor overactivity, stereotypic movements and postures, and render an apathetic, socially nonrelated psychotic child more amenable to his/her environment (8).

In general, neuroleptics tend to be chosen for their side-effect profile rather than their clinical effects which are approximately equal with comparable doses.

Neuroleptics can be administered in one to two daily doses, as in adults, due to their relatively long half-lives, although there is little information in the literature regarding pharmacokinetics in children.

Infantile autism is a pandevelopmental disorder affecting cognition, behavior, and social relatedness that occurs in the first 3 years of life. Etiology is not well understood, but it is likely that there is an underlying neurobiological basis. Neuroleptic drugs have been used in this population, particularly haloperidol, for such target symptoms as agitation, stereotypies, and social withdrawal. In addition, there have been recent investigations into the use of fenfluramine in the population including a U.S. multicenter study. There appears to be a subgroup of autistic children whose behavior, relatedness, and cognitive function improves on this agent. An agitated child with stereotypic behaviors generally responds more successfully to a sedating neuroleptic, whereas an anergic, withdrawn child should probably be treated with a less sedating drug. Sedation effects must be monitored though, as an oversedated child cannot learn. There is some evidence that low-dose neuroleptic drugs such as haloperidol can, in fact, facilitate learning in simple discrimination tasks in some very young autistic children.

TABLE 8-2 Common Drug Interactions in Child and Adolescent Psychiatry

	Neuroleptics	Stimulants	Antidepressants	Sedative/Hypnotics Anxiolytics	Lithium
Neuroleptics	—				neuroleptics can suppress nausea secondary to lithium toxicity
Stimulants	Thioridazine increases methylphenidate effects in hyperactives	—			
Antidepressants	TCAs potentiate anticholinergic effects; both lower seizure threshold	Methylphenidate increases effects of TCAs and blood levels; MAOI and stimulants to be avoided	TCA-MAOI combination problematic	potentiates anticholinergic effects of MAOI	
Sedative-Hypnotics/ Anxiolytics	neuroleptics potentiate CNS depressants	stimulants may oppose hypnotic effects	—	—	—
Lithium	some reports of neuroleptic–haloperidol neurotoxicity	—	—	—	

224

Others:

Anticonvulsants	can increase sedation but not anticonvulsant effect	—	—	barbiturates decrease TCA blood levels	—
Anticoagulants	phenothiazines decrease effect	Methylphenidate potentiates effect of coumarin preparations	Chloral hydrate decreases effects of coumarin preparations	—	—
Anti-inflamatory Agents	—	Methylphenidate inhibits action of phenylbutazone	—	—	—
Vasopressors	neuroleptics block effect of epinephrine and decrease BP	—	—	—	—
Antihelmintics	piperazine and phenothiazines cause seizures	—	—	—	—
Diuretics	can cause decreased BP	—	—	—	decreases lithium clearance and increases lithium toxicity

TABLE 8-3 Neuroleptics (Antipsychotics) for Children Older than 6 Years

Generic Name	Trade Name	Indications	Range of Oral Dosages, mg	Common Side Effects Short Term	Common Side Effects Long Term
Phenothiazines:				*Autonomic nervous system* (esp. with low-potency drugs): sedation, dry mouth, orthostatic hypotension, urinary retention, blurring of vision	
Chlorpromazine[a]	Thorazine	PDD and psychoses, acute or chronic; severe behavioral problems assoc. with mental retardation; psychiatric emergencies; acute agitation	10–300		
Thioridazine[a]	Mellaril		10–300		
Trifluoperazine	Stelazine		1–20		
Fluphenazine[b]	Prolixin		1–10		
Perphenazine[b]	Trilafon		2–24		
Butyrophenones:					
Haloperidol[a]	Haldol	Tourette's Disorder (Haldol is useful)	1–16	EPS (esp. with high-potency drugs): acute dystonic reaction, akathisia, parkinsonism	withdrawal and tardive dyskinesias
Thioxanthenes:					
Thiothixene[b]	Navane	→	2–20	Endocrine: increased prolactin, menstrual irregularities	weight gain
Dibenzoxazepine:					
Loxapine[c]	Loxitane		5–60	Hypersensitivity: rash, blood dyscrasias, elevated liver functions	
Dihydroindolones:					
Molindone[b]	Moban		10–50	CNS: seizures, behavioral reactions	

Guidelines for Treatment of Psychosis/Pervasive Developmental Disorders:
For children older than 6 years (for children younger than 6 years halve the doses)

Chlorpromazine: p.o. tablets or concentrate
start with 0.5–1.0 mg/kg.
acutely: give 0.5–2.0 mg/kg every 2–4 hours until therapeutic response or side effects; usually 3 or 4 doses will have therapeutic effect
daily maintenance dose range: 3–10 mg/kg.

Haloperidol: p.o. tablets or concentrate
start with 0.5 mg.
acutely: give 0.01–0.10 mg/kg every 2–4 hours until therapeutic response or side effects; usually 3 or 4 doses will have therapeutic effect
daily maintenance dose range: 0.1 mg–0.5 mg/kg.

For treatment of agitation/anxiety—psychiatric emergencies (aggressive behavior):
Follow the acute recommendations as above; discontinue medication when feasible. In some cases hydroxyzine can be used (see Table 8–6).

For treatment of Tourette's disorder:
Haloperidol:
start with 0.25 mg. for 3–4 days, then increase by 0.25 mg. every 5–7 days;
daily maintenance dose is usually 1.5 to 10 mg. daily

---

[a]FDA approved for advertising < 6
[b]FDA approved for advertising > 12
[c]FDA approved for advertising > 16

Children and adolescents who present with acutely disorganizing aggressive behavior or acute psychosis can be treated with a nonsedating neuroleptic such as haloperidol, 0.5 mg by mouth, every 1–2 hours or until therapeutic response is reached, usually within several hours.

Patients with Tourette's syndrome (motor–verbal–tic disorder) can be successfully treated with haloperidol starting at 0.5 mg daily with gradual increments to about 6–8 mg. Doses above this are often limited by the presence of significant side effects such as lethargy, weight gain, or depression. A new neuroleptic, pimozide (Orap) has recently been approved for use in Tourette's syndrome, but should be used at this time only after more traditional approaches have been tried such as haloperidol and clonidine.

Children and adolescents are like their adult counterparts in that they are at risk for development of autonomic nervous system and extrapyramidal side effects.

There is growing evidence that adolescents and even young children can develop neuroleptic-related dyskinesias. Some studies (9) have indicated that children are more likely to develop withdrawal emergent dyskinesias that are more reversible upon discontinuation of the medication than tardive or late-appearing dyskinesias; nevertheless, tardive dyskinesia has been reported in young children as well as in adolescents (10). Abnormal movements often present in these disturbed children prior to drug treatment must be differentiated from any that develop after drug treatment.

In general, it is good practice to prescribe the lowest possible effective dose for maintenance and to attempt to take the child off the neuroleptic at least every 6 months to once yearly in the case of a chronic psychosis or severe behavioral disturbance associated with mental retardation. In the case of a psychiatric emergency, such as acute agitation or assaultive behavior, the child should be taken off medication as quickly as possible following return of psychic, family, and environmental equilibrium.

Antiparkinsonian Agents

The psychopharmacological treatment of extrapyramidal symptoms as side effects of neuroleptic therapy in childhood follows guidelines used for adults. In general, except for the acute dystonic reactions, it is best to try to decrease neuroleptic dosage before

Specific Agents

adding an antiparkinsonian agent. If decreasing neuroleptic dosage is not possible, then antiparkinsonian treatment is indicated.

In general, our practice is to avoid prophylactic antiparkinsonian medication despite the controversy in the literature. In our experience, choosing a neuroleptic less likely to cause extrapyramidal side effects (EPS) (see previous section) and using lowest possible maintenance dosages lessens the possibility of EPS development. Should the symptoms develop, however, an antiparkinsonian agent can be readily added.

In the case of acute dystonic reaction, treatment with intramuscular diphenhydramine or benzotropine mesylate is indicated. The child can then be maintained on oral forms for 2–4 weeks and then have it discontinued; any recurrence of EPS symptomatology is indication for further treatment.

Psychostimulants

The psychostimulants are some of the most widely prescribed and best studied psychotropic agents in child psychiatry and pediatrics. Methylphenidate (Ritalin), dextroamphetamine (Dexedrine), and magnesium pemoline (Cylert) are the agents available for use in this country (Table 8–4). These drugs are indicated in the treatment of attention-deficit disorder with hyperactivity (minimal brain dysfunction, hyperkinesis in past) and they help these children to focus their attention more clearly, to slow down their motor activity, and to become less distractible. They have also been used with some conduct disorders and attention-deficit disorder without hyperactivity, although their use in these conditions is less well studied. Their effect actually does not appear to be paradoxical (11) in that adult males and normal boys also appear to increase concentration and focusing when given a single dose of dextroamphetamine. Stimulants appear to achieve their effects by short-term improvement of attentional difficulties and concentration; they have not been shown to have any long-term effects by themselves on achievement or cognition.

Dextroamphetamine and methylphenidate have a relatively short duration of action with peak effects between 1 and 3 hours and so must be administered in divided doses twice a day or so (12). They are typically given at breakfast and at noontime (or early afternoon). As this may necessitate the child receiving the medication in school, it

TABLE 8-4 Psychostimulants for Children Older than 6 Years

Generic Name	Trade Name	Indications	Dosages, range (mg)	Common Side Effects	
				Short Term	Long Term
Dextroamphetamine[a]	Dexedrine	Attention-deficit disorder with hyperactivity	10–40	insomnia	multiple tics (Tourette's)
	Dexedrine Spansule (long acting)			dysphoria	
Methylphenidate	Ritalin		20–80	anorexia, nausea, abdominal pain, headaches	weight loss and/or diminished growth
	Ritalin S-R (slow release)				
Pemoline Magnesium	Cylert		37.5–112.5		↑ SGPT, SGOT

Suggested treatment regimen for attention-deficit disorder with hyperactivity:

Dextroamphetamine: for child older than 6 years start with 5 mg in A.M. for 2–3 days, 5 mg in A.M. and noon every 2–3 days; add 5-mg increments until response; range 0.15–0.50 mg/kg.

Methylphenidate: start with 10 mg in A.M. for 2–3 days, increase by 10 mg every 2–3 days; range 0.3–1.0 mg/kg.

Pemoline Magnesium: start with 37.5 mg in A.M. for 2–3 days, increase by 18.75 mg every 2–3 days; range 0.5–2.0 mg/kg.

[a]FDA approved for advertising for children younger than 6 years.

Specific Agents

may sometimes be easier to give it to the child immediately after school as long as it does not interfere with sleep. This may save the child some embarrassment in school from having to go to the school nurse's office everyday for his or her "pill". Pemoline, with a longer duration of action and said to have less side effects, can be given once a day before school. There are also slow-release forms available for dextroamphetamine and methylphenidate.

The Conners Scale is an instrument that has been used in many pharmacotherapy studies and is particularly useful for working with the child with attention-deficit disorder with hyperactivity in the clinical setting. There is a long form and a shorter, ten-item version that is administered to the child's parents and teacher(s) simultaneously. Ratings of such items as fidgetiness, impulsivity, and mood lability are quantified. Clinicians can administer the form before and after a drug trial so as to better quantitate the child's response to medication.

One study indicates a differential effect of dosage of methylphenidate on cognitive performance and behavioral symptomatology, with cognitive performance optimal at lower dosages (0.3 mg/kg) than behavior (1.0 mg/kg) (13).

Common side effects include nausea, abdominal discomfort, anorexia, and insomnia. There have been some reports of adverse effects on growth parameters that are reversible with discontinuation of the medication (14, 15), but other evidence has been contradictory. A potentially serious side effect is the development of Tourette's disorder in the vulnerable child, so that a pre-existing tic and/or family history of tics is in most cases a contraindication for use. Stimulants may precipitate psychotic symptomatology, including hallucinosis, in children at risk. Methylphenidate seems to be less likely than dextroamphetamine to produce side effects.

All drugs in this group should generally be given on a drug holiday basis to mitigate the potential for side effects. Weekends, school vacation, summer vacations, and the first months of school in the fall should be drug-free periods.

Antidepressants

The use of tricyclic antidepressants (TCAs) in child psychiatry has grown in the past few years; they now appear to have widespread use in several conditions, though still largely deserving further study (Table 8–5).

TABLE 8-5 Antidepressants for Children Older than 12 Years

Generic Name	Trade Name	Indications	Dosage, range (mg)	Common Side Effects
Imipramine[a]	Tofranil	Enuresis; ↑ hyperactivity/ ↑ attention–deficit disorder;	25–125 mg (imipramine)	*Autonomic nervous system:* dry mouth, orthostatic hypotension, urinary retention, blurred vision
Amitriptyline	Elavil	↑	25–100 (imipramine)	
Desipramine	Norpramin	depression; ↑	100–300 (imipramine)	*CNS:* seizures, precipitate mania/psychosis
Nortriptyline	Aventyl	separation anxiety (school refusal) ↑	100–200 (imipramine)	*Cardiovascular:* alterations in conduction, pulse, BP; prolonged PR, QRS; arrhythmias

Others:
Doxepin (Sinequan), Maprotiline (Ludiomil)[b], Amoxapine (Asendin)[c], Trazodone (Desyrel)[b]

Suggested treatment regimen for enuresis:
start with 0.5 mg/kg of imipramine for 2–3 nights
increase by 25 mg or 0.5 mg/kg every 2–3 nights until therapeutic response
daily maintenance dose range: 0.5–2.5 mg/kg.

Suggested treatment regimen for hyperactivity–attention-deficit disorder:
start with 0.5 mg/kg imipramine
increase by 25 mg or 0.5 mg/kg every 5–7 days until therapeutic response or side effects
daily maintenance dose range: 0.5–4.0 mg/kg.

Suggested treatment regimen for childhood depression:
start with 0.5 mg/kg imipramine for 2–3 days
increase by 0.5 mg/kg every 3–4 days
daily maintenance dose range: 3–5 mg/kg.

[a]FDA approved for advertising for children older than 6 years for enuresis, older than 12 years for depression
[b]FDA approved for advertising for patients older than 18 years only
[c]FDA approved for advertising for children older than 16 years only

The TCAs are established for use in children with enuresis and hyperactivity/attention-deficit disorders; in addition TCAs have been studied for use in conduct disorders, childhood depression, and school refusal based on separation anxiety (16). The TCAs have also been used in sleep arousal disorders such as somnambulism and *pavor nocturnus* (night terrors), eating disorders, obsessive-compulsive disorders, and many other clinical situations. Tricyclics such as desipramine (Norpramin), amitriptyline (Elavil), and nortriptyline (Aventyl) have been used in this age group but not as widely as imipramine.

Enuretic and hyperactive children tend to respond to imipramine within days of beginning drug therapy, whereas school refusers and depressed children tend to require several weeks to respond.

Studies seem to indicate that imipramine's effectiveness in enuresis is not related to its anticholinergic properties or its effects on sleep architecture but perhaps through some direct effects on bladder muscles (17).

The mechanism of action in school refusers has not been clearly elucidated at this time. In one placebo-controlled study (18), 35 school-age children who had failed to return to school through behavior modifications returned with imipramine treatment on an average dosage of 150 mg/day. This study has not been replicated, however.

There has been increasing interest in recent years in childhood depression, and evidence has accumulated that both adolescents and prepubertal children can meet adult research criteria or DSM-III criteria for major depression.

Some investigators are currently studying biological parameters of depression in prepubertal adolescents, such as cortisol hypersecretion, growth hormone response to insulin-induced hypoglycemia, and sleep architecture. Evidence has accumulated suggesting neuroendocrine dysfunction in some major depressive disorders, particularly in endogenous subtypes, similar to that found in adults (19).

Studies have shown (20) that some of these depressed children are responsive to TCA treatment in fairly high dose ranges, 3–5 mg/kg (see Table 8-5).

Newer antidepressants, such as trazodone (Desyrel) and maprotiline (Ludiomil), have had some informal use in this country, but no controlled studies in this age group have been performed to date.

Experience in this country with monoamine oxidase (MAO) inhibitors in this age group is extremely limited, particularly in the prepubertal child. Due to their potential for toxicity, these are difficult to prescribe for most youngsters. Some adolescents with atypical depressive features and/or phobias may be candidates.

Tricyclic antidepressants in general must be administered to prepubertal children 2–3 times a day and to adolescents once or twice daily; this schedule takes into account prepubertal children's shorter half-lives, more efficient clearance of the drug, and mitigates the potential of toxicity. Children with enuresis typically respond to 25–100 mg daily, those with attention-deficit disorder with hyperactivity to 2–5 mg/kg daily, and childhood depression 3–5 mg/kg daily.

Side effects of TCAs are primarily anticholinergic, cardiovascular, and effects on the central nervous system (CNS). Lowering of seizure threshold is of significant concern. Cardiovascular effects include increased pulse, PR interval prolongation, arrhythmias and decreased BP. Serial EKG monitoring should take place with doses above 3.5 mg/kg/day, with each incremental change. Monitoring can take place in this age group with the use of plasma levels (21).

Anxiolytics and Sedative-Hypnotics

Despite widespread use in pediatric practice, anxiolytics and sedative-hypnotics have not been well studied in this population. Due to their safety and nonspecificity of action, these medications have been used for a number of childhood and adolescent conditions, such as night terrors, insomnia, anxiety, and hyperactivity (Table 8-6).

There are two classes of medication in this category that are useful in a number of clinical situations: (a) antihistamines, such as hydroxyzine (Vistaril, Atarax) or diphenhydramine (Benadryl), and (b) benzodiazepines, such as diazepam (Valium) and chlordiazepoxide (Librium). Experience with other sedative hypnotics, such as barbiturates and propanediols for anxiolysis, is limited in this age group.

The antihistamines are useful for anxiolysis in the nonpsychotic, mild-to-moderately disturbed population of children and for sedation/hypnotic effects in the preschool through adolescent age groups. Sleep disturbances such as inability to fall asleep due to restlessness, fearfulness, or hyperactivity in the young child are likely to respond to an antihistamine.

Night terrors is a particular form of sleep disturbance seen in young children during N-REM sleep, frequently upon arousal from stage III or IV to lighter sleep stages. Characteristically, the child awakens in a terror, screaming, with signs of physiological arousal,

TABLE 8-6 Anxiolytics and Sedative Hypnotics for Children Older than 6 Years

Generic Name	Trade Name	Indications	Dosages, mg (range)	Common Side Effects
Antihistamines:				
Diphenydramine[a]	Benadryl	Bedtime sedation	25–500	Oversedation hypersensitivity: skin rash, dryness of mucous membranes
Hydroxyzine[a]	Vistaril Atarax	Anxiety states, agitation, bedtime sedation	25–500	
Benzodiazepines:				
Diazepam[a]	Valium	Night terrors: exogenous anxiety	1–20 2–10	drowsiness paradoxical agitation or excitement Withdrawal reactions
Chlordiazepoxide	Librium	Night terrors: exogenous anxiety	10–100	
Alprazolam[b]	Xanax	Separation anxiety	0.25–5	
Flurazepam[c]	Dalmane	Bedtime sedation	15–30	Daytime sedation
Miscellaneous:				
Chloral hydrate	Noctec	Bedtime sedation	500–1000	

Suggested treatment regimen for *Sleep Induction*: children older than 6 years

Diphenydramine or Hydroxyzine:

Start with 25–50 mg at bedtime; **increase** every 2 days by 25 mg until therapeutic effect daily **maintenance** range 25–500 mg at bedtime or 2.0–5 mg/kg.

Chloral Hydrate:

500–1000 mg at bedtime

Suggested treatment regimen for *Pavor Nocturnus* (night terrors) with *Diazepam*:

Start at 1 mg at bedtime, then **increase** by 0.5 mg every 2–4 days until therapeutic response

Daily **maintenance** dose range 1–20 mg at bedtime

Suggested treatment regimens for *Anxiety*/Agitation

Diphenydramine or Hydroxyzine:

Acute: **Start** with 25–50 mg, then repeat dose every 2–4 hours until therapeutic effect

Non-acute: **Start** with 25–50 mg, then **increase** by 25 mg every 2–3 days

Daily **maintenance** dose range: 75–500 mg or up to 5 mg/kg/day.

Chlordiazepoxide:

Start with 5–10 mg, then **increase** by 5–10 mg every 3–4 days until response

Daily **maintenance** dose range: 45–90 mg.

---

[a]FDA approved for advertising for children younger than 6 years.
[b]FDA approved for advertising for patients older than 18 years.
[c]FDA approved for advertising for adolescents older than 15 years.

and is inconsolable during the episode for which he or she is amnestic. Diazepam in small doses administered at bedtime for several weeks can be useful for this particular problem.

Benzodiazepines have been found to be generally safe and effective anxiolytics for adult patients. There are few studies of such use in the pediatric population in this country. There have been some reports of paradoxical reactions or disinhibition to these drugs in young patients such as pathological aggression or excitement; perhaps this has limited their practical use and investigation. Another dilemma for the pediatric practitioner has been the confusion and lack of validated criteria for defining anxiety and its manifestations in this age group.

DSM-III-defined anxiety disorders in childhood include separation anxiety disorder, overanxious disorder, and post-traumatic stress disorder. Children are also found to suffer from phobias and other symptoms of anxiety that can range across diagnostic categories. There is extremely little in the scientific literature regarding the pharmacotherapy of such conditions in childhood and adolescence. Antihistamines have been more commonly used in the very young population than benzodiazepines, perhaps because of their traditional use as nonspecific sedatives and low side-effect profile. Hydroxyzine is thought to be less sedative than diphenhydramine and more anxiolytic.

In the nonpsychotic, nonsubstance-using adolescent population, benzodiazepines can be useful in limited quantities for anxiety that threatens to interfere with daily functioning. Chlordiazepoxide, lorazepam, and diazepam have found some usefulness in this situation. In some adolescents with early and middle insomnia, flurazepam (Dalmane) or triazolam (Halcion) can be used for limited periods of time. Chloral hydrate is also a safe and effective nighttime sedative for this population.

Interest has increased recently in the use of a newer anxiolytic, alprazolam (Xanax), in the child or adolescent with separation anxiety–panic disorder symptomatology, paralleling its uses in adults with panic disorders (see Table 8-6).

Side effects with both of these classes of medication are relatively infrequent, particularly for the antihistamines.

Lithium

Interest in and experience with lithium in the child and adolescent population has increased significantly in the past several years (Table 8-7).

TABLE 8-7 Lithium for Children Older Than 6 Years

Generic Name	Trade Name	Indications	Dosages (range)	Common Side Effects
Lithium carbonate[a]	Eskalith Lithobid	Bipolar and some recurrent unipolar affective disorders; some behavior disorders	150 mg and higher	*GI:* Nausea, vomiting, diarrhea, abdominal distress *CNS:* tremor, memory lapses, fatigue *Renal:* polyuria, polydipsia, tubular changes *Hematological:* leukocytosis *Endocrine:* Increase in calcium levels, goiter

Suggested Treatment Regimen for Childhood/Adolescence
Bipolar/Periodic Disorders and Aggressive Behavior: children older than 6 years **start** with 150 mg every 3–4 days until blood levels are in range of 0.8–1.5 mEq/L. Some adolescents may require higher doses approaching 2.0 mEq/L. Daily **maintenance** dose range: 300–2,400 mg daily.

[a]FDA approved for advertising only for children older than 12 years.

While lithium has been clearly found effective for treatment of acute mania and prophylaxis for bipolar disorders in the adult population, these disorders are rarely found in the pediatric population in the adult form. Nevertheless, studies suggest that some adolescents with bipolar disorders and children with certain kinds of behavior disorders or variants of bipolar disorder can be treated effectively with lithium despite lack of any formal indications for use in this age group.

It appears that children with periodic or cyclic disturbances of behavior and mood, children with such disturbances with relatives who have been lithium responsive, and children with severely aggressive behavior disorders are potentially responsive to lithium (22–24). Investigators in the past decade or two have used lithium for children and adolescents for a wide range of indications, although there have been very few double-blind, placebo-controlled studies.

Perhaps because of lithium's antiaggressive action in animals and in some adult populations, several investigators have used it in chronically impulse-ridden, aggressive children and adults as well as in the aggressive, behaviorally disturbed mentally retarded population. One group has studied lithium, regardless of target symptomatology, in children of lithium-responsive parents. Results have been mixed.

Thus, the child or adolescent with bipolar disorder is certainly a candidate for lithium; other potential candidates, particularly where other treatments have failed, include the child with recurrent, cyclic disturbances of mood or activity without overt mania, and the child with severe and chronic aggression. Studies are ongoing in this area and promise a potentially exciting and useful approach to some of the most difficult patients in the child psychiatric population.

Children and adolescents run the same risks for side effects and toxicities as do their adult counterparts, so they must be carefully worked up and monitored. Common short-term effects include gastrointestinal distress, tremor, fatigue, polyuria and polydipsia. Long-term effects can include hypothyroidism, alteration of bone density, weight gain, and possibly renal deficiency.

Medication can be administered in two or three daily doses and should be adjusted according to blood levels. In general, prepubertal children can be started with 300 mg in divided doses and postpubertal children with 300–600 mg.

Specific Agents

Plasma levels should be obtained to monitor clinical effects on a regular basis. Saliva levels are an alternative to venipuncture for the younger child. During initiation of treatment, twice weekly levels are called for, which can be followed by weekly and then approximately monthly levels once equilibrium and steady state has been reached. Levels of 0.6–1.6 mEq/L are within the therapeutic range, but some patients may require up to 1.8–2.0 mEq/L to attain therapeutic efficacy. Kidney, endocrine, and cardiac function must be monitored on a regular basis (see Table 8–7).

Other Drugs

In recent years, other drugs available to the adult practitioner have gained informal or experimental use in the pediatric and adolescent population. The beta-adrenergic blocker propranolol (Inderal) is used in some young patients with uncontrollable aggressive behavior (25), those with lithium-induced tremors, and those with certain anxiety states manifest by physiological symptomatology. They are contraindicated in diabetics, asthmatics, and patients with cardiac disease. Their use is still experimental in this age group at this time.

Clonidine has enjoyed increasing clinical use and has been found in some studies to be a useful alternative to treatment of Tourette's disorder with haloperidol. It can be used in combination with haloperidol in low doses or as a primary drug therapy. Some evidence indicates that it has been useful for both the motor and verbal tics that characterize the disorder, but it is also useful in modifying the behavioral concomitants that often accompany the tics, such as attention problems, hyperactivity, and lability of mood (26).

Blood pressure and pulse must be closely monitored during treatment since the blood pressure may be reduced and the pulse slowed.

Anticonvulsants have had a long-standing role in pediatrics for the treatment of seizure disorders, including grand mal and complex partial seizures. Carbamazepine (Tegretol) is gaining favor in psychiatric populations as an alternative treatment for affective disorders such as bipolar illness and behavioral disorders (Table 8–8) (27).

TABLE 8-8 Anticonvulsant Medications

Medication	Dosage mg/kg/day	Therapeutic Serum Concentration, g/ml	Type of Seizures	Common Side Effects
Carbamazepine (Tegretol)	10–30	4–12	All except petit mal and infantile spasms, especially valuable in complex partial seizures	Dose Related: drowsiness, ataxia, dysarthria Other: gastrointestinal upset, leukopenia, thrombocytopenia, elevation of liver enzymes
Clonazepam (Klonopin)	0.01–0.15	0.015–0.06	Petit mal, minor motor; adjunctive therapy in major motor	Dose Related: sedation, dizziness Other: behavioral effects including: impulsivity, irritability, sleep disturbance, inattentiveness
Chlorazepate (Tranxene)	0.3–1.0	0.05–0.075	Adjunctive therapy for generalized and partial seizures, especially complex partial	Dose Related: sedation, dizziness Other: elevation of liver enzymes, gastrointestinal distress
Ethosuximide (Zarontin)	20–40	40–120	Petit mal; adjunctive for refractory seizures	Dose Related: sedation Other: nausea, vomiting, irritability, sleep disturbance, leukopenia, pancytopenia
Phenobarbital	2–6	20–40	All except petit mal and infantile spasms	Dose Related: sedation, ataxia, irritability Other: hyperactivity, irritability, depressed affect, attention deficit disorder, hypocalcemia
Phenytoin (Dilantin)	5–10	10–20	All except petit mal and infantile spasms	Dose Related: nystagmus, ataxia, irritability Other: depressed affect, gum hypertrophy, hirsutism, tremor, fever, lymphadenopathy, choreoathetosis; thickened facial features

REFERENCES

1. Briant, R. H. (1978). An introduction to clinical pharmacology. In: *Pediatric Psychopharmacology: The Use of Behavior Modifying Drugs in Childhood*, ed. J. Werry. New York: Brunner/Mazel, pp. 3–28.
2. Rapaport, J., and Mikkelson, E. (1978). Antidepressants. In: *Pediatric Psychopharmacology: The Use of Behavior Modifying Drugs in Childhood*, ed. J. Werry. New York: Brunner/Mazel, pp. 208–233.
3. Popper, C., and Famularo, R. (1983). Child and adolescent psychopharmacology. In: *Developmental Pediatrics*, ed. M. D. Levine, M. A. Crocker, R. Gross, W. B. Carey. Philadelphia: W. B. Saunders, pp. 1138–1159.
4. Klein, D., Gittelman, R., Quitkin, F., and Rifkin, A. (1980). Diagnosis and drug treatment of psychiatric disorders: adults and children. Second edition. Baltimore: Williams and Wilkins.
5. Gualtieri, C., Barnhill, J., McGimsey, J., and Schell, D. (1980). Tardive dyskinesia and other movement disorders in children treated with psychotropic drugs. *Journal of the American Academy of Child Psychiatry* 19:491–510.
6. Campbell, M., Gregs, D., Green, W., and Bennett, W. (1983). Neuroleptic-induced dyskinesias in children. *Clinical Neuropharmacology* 6(3):207–222.
7. Campbell, M., Shapiro, T. (1975). *Manual of Psychiatric Therapeutics*, ed. R. Shader. Boston: Little, Brown, pp. 137–162.
8. Polizos, P., Englehardt, D., Hoffman, S., and Waizer, J. (1973). Neurological consequences of psychotropic drug withdrawal in schizophrenic children. *Journal of Autism and Childhood Schizophrenia* 3:247–253.
9. Gualtieri, C. T., Quade, D., Hicks, R., Mayo, J., and Schroeder, S. (1984). Tardive dyskinesia and other clinical consequences of neuroleptic treatment in children and adolescents. *American Journal of Psychiatry* 141:20–23.
10. Cantwell, D., and Carlson, G. (1978). Simulants. In: *Pediatric Psychopharmacology: The Use of Behavior Modifying Drugs in Childhood*, ed. J. Werry. New York: Brunner/Mazel, pp. 171–207.
11. Rapoport, J., Buschbaum, M., Weingartner, H., Zahn, T., Ludlow, C., and Mikkelson, E. (1980). Dextroamphetamine: Its cognitive and behavioral effects in normal and hyperactive boys and normal men. *Archives of General Psychiatry* 37:933–943.
12. Shaywitz, S., Hunt, R., Jatlow, P., Cohen, D., Young, J., Pierce, R., Anderson, G., and Shaywitz, B. (1982) Psychopharmacology of attention deficit disorder. *Pediatrics* 69(6):688–694.
13. Sprague, R., and Sleator, E. (1977). Methylphenidate in hyperkinetic children: Differences in dose effects in learning and social behavior. *Science* 198:1274–1276.
14. Safer, D., Allen, R., and Barr, E. (1972) Depression of growth in hyperactive children on stimulant drugs. *New England Journal of Medicine* 287:217–220.
15. Mattes, J., and Gittelman, R. (1983). Growth of hyperactive children on maintenance regimen of methylphenidate. *Archives of General Psychiatry* 40:317–321.

16. Rapoport, J., and Mikkelsen, E. (1978). Antidepressants. In: *Pediatric Psychopharmacology: The Use of Behavior Modifying Drugs in Childhood*. ed. J. Werry. New York: Brunner/Mazel, pp. 208–233.
17. Rapoport, J., Mikkelsen, E., Nee, L., Gruenau, C., et al. (1980). Childhood enuresis I and II. *Archives of General Psychiatry* 37:1139–1152.
18. Gittleman-Klein, R. (1975). Pharmacotherapy and management of pathological separation anxiety. *International Journal of Mental Health* 4:255–271.
19. Puig-Antich, J. (1984). Growth hormone secretion in prepubertal children with major depression. *Archives of General Psychiatry* 41:455–460, 463–466, 471–475, 479–483.
20. Puig-Antich, J. (1980). Affective disorders in childhood: A review and perspective. *Psychiatric Clinics of North America* 3(3):403–424.
21. Weller, E. (1983). Childhood depression: Imipramine levels and response. *Psychopharmacology Bulletin* 19(1):59–62.
22. DeLong, R. (1977). Lithium carbonate treatment of select behavior disorders in children suggesting manic-depressive illness. *Journal of Pediatrics* 93:689–699.
23. Youngerman, J., and Cannino, I. (1978). Lithium carbonate use in children and adolescents. *Archives of General Psychiatry* 35:216–224.
24. Campbell, M., Cohen, I., and Small, A. (1982). Drugs in aggressive behavior. *Journal of the American Academy of Child Psychiatry* 21(2):107–117.
25. Williams, D., Mehl, R., Yudofsky, S., and Adams, D. (1982). The effects of propranolol on uncontrolled rage outbursts in children and adolescents with organic brain dysfunction. *Journal of the American Academy of Child Psychiatry* 21(2):129–135.
26. Cohen, D., Detlor, J., Young, J., and Shaywitz, B. (1980). Clonidine ameliorates Gilles de la Tourette syndrome. *Archives of General Psychiatry* 37:1350–1357.
27. Stores, G. (1978). Antiepileptics. In *Pediatric Psychopharmacology: The Use of Behavior Modifying Drugs in Childhood*, ed. J. Werry. New York: Brunner/Mazel, pp. 274–315.

9

Eating Disorders

Harrison G. Pope, Jr., M.D.
James I. Hudson, M.D.

For many years, the two primary eating disorders—anorexia nervosa and bulimia—have been treated primarily with various forms of psychological therapy, including individual psychotherapy, family psychotherapy, group psychotherapy, and behavioral therapy. Unfortunately, these techniques have not as yet produced clearly documented benefit in patients with eating disorders; there is, to our knowledge, no available methodologically sound study, using a parallel control group, showing any form of psychological therapy to be effective in anorexia nervosa or bulimia (1,2). Admittedly, some uncontrolled reports of these techniques show promise, but adequately controlled data are yet to be obtained (3–7). As a result, there has been increasing interest in the possibility that some form of biological treatment might be helpful in these disorders. The present status of this rapidly evolving field follows.

ANOREXIA NERVOSA

A number of different families of agents have been tried in the treatment of anorexia nervosa. These include antipsychotic medications, 9-tetrahydrocannabinol, naloxone, L-dopa, zinc, cyroheptadine, lithium carbonate, and various antidepressant medications.

Uncontrolled reports have suggested that phenothiazines, such as chlorpromazine, may be useful in the treatment of anorexia nervosa (8-14). However, to our knowledge only one placebo-controlled double-blind study has examined an antipsychotic drug in this disorder: Vandereycken and Pierloot (15), using pimozide, found a trend in favor of a drug effect, but this did not reach statistical significance. When it is considered that most antipsychotic drugs have a large array of side effects—some of which may be particularly severe in cachectic patients with anorexia—it appears that these drugs do not presently offer much promise.

A second, rather unusual agent to be tried in the treatment of anorexia nervosa is 9-tetrahydrocannabinol, the active principal in marijuana and hashish. Gross and colleagues (16) tested tetrahydrocannabinol in a placebo-controlled double-blind study, in the hopes that the appetite-stimulant properties of the drug might be beneficial for anorexic patients. Unfortunately, in this study no significant benefit was found; several patients found the effects quite unpleasant because of the "paranoid" feelings induced by the drug. One possible explanation for the failure of tetrahydrocannabinol is that it is merely an appetite stimulant; yet, most anorexic patients do not describe an actual loss of appetite, but rather a fear of gaining weight and getting fat. Therefore, giving an appetite stimulant to such patients may not be effective for the core symptomatology of anorexia nervosa.

Naloxone, an opiate antagonist, was found of some benefit for anorexic patients in a nonblind and largely uncontrolled preliminary study (17). However, interpretation of the findings of the study is compromised by the fact that all of the patients in the study were simultaneously treated with low doses of antidepressants. Thus, we must await a controlled study using naloxone alone before drawing further conclusions.

L-dopa has been tried in an uncontrolled study of nine anorexic patients in a hospital clinical research center (18,19). Five of the nine patients gained more than 3 kg within 19-27 days. Controlled trials with this agent have not appeared.

Some recent reports have suggested that zinc deficiency may be involved in the pathogenesis of anorexia nervosa (20, 21). One recent case report found dramatic improvement in an anorexic patient following initiation of zinc therapy (22). However, to our knowledge, larger studies with zinc have not been published.

A somewhat more promising agent in the treatment of anorexia nervosa has been cyproheptadine. This drug has now been the subject of four placebo-controlled double-blind studies. The first study, examining ten anorexic patients receiving cyproheptadine as compared to ten receiving placebo, found that patients assigned to active drug gained significantly more weight during the course of the study period (23). However, in two subsequent studies, both using larger samples, this finding could not be replicated (24, 25). On the other hand, a more recent study, using somewhat larger doses of cyproheptadine, has found a modest, but significant difference in favor of cyproheptadine, suggesting that the drug may have at least some value in certain anorexic patients (26–28). The investigators in this most recent study have suggested that cyproheptadine may have antidepressant properties. Although patients responding to cyproheptadine in the study demonstrated improvement in their mood, it is difficult to ascertain whether cyproheptadine acted primarily as an antidepressant, primarily as an appetite stimulant, or by some other mechanism. To our knowledge, there are no studies of cyproheptadine in nonanorexic patients with major depression. Thus, assessing its antidepressant properties, if any, is difficult.

The last two categories of agents to be tested in anorexia nervosa—lithium carbonate and antidepressants—would seem promising on the basis of evidence linking anorexia nervosa to major affective disorders. For example, studies of the phenomenology of anorexic patients have shown that many display either major depression or bipolar disorder, or at least symptoms suggestive of major affective disorder, at some time in their lives (1, 29–36). Family history studies, similarly, have shown a much higher than expected prevalence of major affective disorder among the first-degree relatives of anorexic patients (30, 36–38). In fact, in one study (36), the prevalence of affective disorder in the relatives of the anorexic patients actually exceeded the prevalence of affective disorder in the relatives of depressed controls and closely approached the prevalence found in the relatives of controls with bipolar disorder. If, as these findings suggest, anorexia nervosa is in some way related to major affective disorder, then it would seem reasonable that medications used in the treatment of major affective disorder might benefit anorexic patients.

Several preliminary findings with such medications have now appeared. In one uncontrolled report, two anorexic patients treated with lithium carbonate were reported to have gained 20 and 26 pounds respectively within a period of 6 weeks (29). Even more importantly, they were found to have maintained their weight after 1 year of follow-up. Two subsequent case reports have also described encouraging results with lithium in individual patients (39, 40). These findings prompted a subsequent placebo-controlled double-blind study of lithium in anorexia nervosa (41). In this study, Gross and colleagues assigned eight anorexic patients to treatment with lithium and eight to placebo. Significant differences between lithium and placebo emerged by the third week of the 4-week study, with the lithium group gaining an average of about 15 pounds while the placebo group gained an average of about 11.4 pounds. This difference, although modest, was statistically significant.

Although the study was well designed, it should be noted that the eight patients treated with lithium weighed slightly more at the outset of the study and were initially eating more calories per day than the group assigned to placebo. Although the study offers some evidence that lithium was effective even if we correct for this difference, the question remains as to whether a lithium effect would hold up in a study using larger and more closely matched groups. To our knowledge, however, no subsequent studies of lithium carbonate in anorexia nervosa have as yet appeared.

Antidepressant medications have been reported effective in several uncontrolled reports describing small numbers of patients (42–46). However, in the three available controlled studies to date, the results have been less encouraging. In the first study, Lacey and Crisp (47) used clomipramine, 50 mg/day, versus placebo in a small sample of anorexic patients. No difference was found between active drug and placebo. However, given that the dose of clomipramine used was very low, and likely to produce plasma levels below the therapeutic range even in low-weight patients, it is difficult to be certain that this study represented an adequate trial of the antidepressant.

In the second study, using amitriptyline, a very slight difference was found in favor of drug, but it did not reach statistical significance (26–28). However, since plasma levels of amitriptyline were not monitored, some question can be raised as to whether adequate doses of the drug were used in the study. In the third controlled study of tricyclic antidepressants in anorexia nervosa (48), amitriptyline was again found to show no significant superiority to placebo. This lack of significant differences persisted even when the authors examined the relationship between antidepressant plasma levels and outcome.

In summary, therefore, tricyclic antidepressants appear unpromising in anorexic patients. However, it seems possible that better results might be obtained if anorexic patients were treated with adequate doses of these agents, documented with plasma levels, for an adequate period of time. This is more easily said than done, however, given that emaciated patients may be particularly susceptible to hypotension, anticholinergic effects, and sedation with large doses of tricyclic antidepressants. Thus, even if tricyclics theoretically would have some advantage in anorexia nervosa, they may be rather impractical drugs for most patients.

One recent uncontrolled study has addressed the possibility that other families of antidepressant agents—particularly monoamine oxidase (MAO) inhibitors and trazodone—might be more acceptable in the treatment of anorexia nervosa, since they have less prominent anticholinergic side effects (49). Among ten patients treated with various antidepressants in this study, several experienced improvement with tranylcypromine or trazodone. Nevertheless, a majority of the patients in this study failed to show a marked and persistent response.

In summary, pharmacological treatments for anorexia nervosa have yielded, to date, rather unimpressive findings. It appears that cyproheptadine may benefit some patients, and that antidepressant agents and lithium may also be of value in certain cases. However, none of these agents has been shown to have a clear and substantial effect in the overall population of patients with anorexia nervosa. Thus, these agents are at best ancillary treatments to be used in conjunction with an overall program for the treatment of anorexia nervosa.

There presently is no way to predict which patients with anorexia nervosa are most likely to respond to cyproheptadine, lithium, or antidepressants. However, these drugs should probably not be reserved only for anorexic patients who are clearly manic or depressed, since, in the related disorder (bulimia), antidepressants appear at least as effective for bulimic patients who are not depressed as for those who are. More detailed studies will be required to assess whether there are specific subpopulations of anorexic patients who are particularly likely to benefit from available pharmacological treatments.

BULIMIA

Studies of pharmacotherapy in bulimia have produced more consistent results. Over the past decade or so, more than thirty reports, nine of which are placebo-controlled double-blind studies, have described the use of various types of medications in bulimic patients. Most of these medications have been thymoleptics (agents known to affect manic or depressive symptoms) or at least agents that are believed to possess thymoleptic properties.

Interestingly, the first studies of pharmacological treatment in bulimia employed phenytoin, a drug normally considered an anticonvulsant rather than a thymoleptic agent. An initial report found that nine of ten patients with "compulsive eating disorders" improved with phenytoin (50). Most of these patients were also found to have various electroencephalographic (EEG) abnormalities. Subsequent uncontrolled reports continued to report success in some bulimic patients treated with phenytoin but found smaller numbers of drug responders and fewer patients who had clear EEG abnormalities (51–55). Finally in 1977, a placebo-controlled double-blind study of phenytoin appeared (56). In this study, ten subjects were treated with phenytoin for 6 weeks, followed by 6 weeks of placebo, while the other ten received placebo followed by phenytoin. Although there was a statistically significant difference in favor of phenytoin in terms of frequency of binge eating, the difference was relatively modest. Only one of the twenty subjects experienced a remission of her bulimia on phenytoin and only five others (26%) experienced a decrease of greater than 75% in their frequency of binge eating. Furthermore, of the four "marked" responders followed long-term on phenytoin, two relapsed within the first 2 months despite their continuing to take the medication. Thus, the results seem unpromising.

It is also of interest in this study that the authors did not find a correlation between either phenytoin blood levels or EEG abnormalities and response to the drug. These findings may argue against the possibility that phenytoin affects bulimia as a result of its anticonvulsant action. In fact, the authors suggest that phenytoin "is reported to have a wide variety of properties other than anticonvulsant action that might play an important role . . ." (p. 1252). It is worth noting, in this connection, that phenytoin's other properties may include a weak thymoleptic effect (57–59).

In short, although phenytoin may benefit certain individuals with bulimia, it does not appear to be very effective for a majority of patients. If it is effective in certain patients, it is also unclear whether it is effective as a result of its anticonvulsant action or as a result of some other property. In any event, it does not appear that phenytoin has survived well in the "marketplace" of clinical practice; to our knowledge, only one additional case report of phenytoin treatment of bulimia has appeared in the last 5 years (60).

More promising findings have now emerged from studies using antidepressant medications. Between 1977 and 1982 several individual case reports described patients with bulimic symptoms that improved during treatment with tricyclic antidepressants or MAO inhibitors (43, 61, 62). In two cases, interestingly, the symptoms of binge eating and self-induced vomiting recurred promptly when the antidepressant agents were stopped and then remitted again when antidepressants were resumed. In 1982, two small series of bulimic patients treated with antidepressants were described. In one series of eight patients, treated primarily with imipramine or desipramine, six experienced at least a 50% decrease in their frequency of binge eating (63). In a second series of six patients treated with MAO inhibitors, four experienced a complete remission of binge eating and the remaining two reduced their frequency of binge eating to only once or twice per month (64). Within the following year, several other anecdotal reports described similarly encouraging results in bulimic patients treated with various types of antidepressants (65–67).

These encouraging but uncontrolled findings prompted a series of placebo-controlled double-blind studies using various antidepressant agents in bulimia. Five such studies, to our knowledge, have now appeared.

Sabine and colleagues (68) used the antidepressant mianserin (a drug not approved for commercial use in the United States) in a double-blind study of fifty patients with "bulimia nervosa." Curiously, in this study, both the patients assigned to mianserin and those assigned to placebo improved significantly on most measures, including ratings of depression and anxiety and a bulimia-rating scale of the authors' own design. However, the frequency of binge eating and vomiting did not change in either the drug group or the placebo group during the 8-week study period.

It is not clear how best to interpret these findings. It does appear from the study that bulimic patients may improve with brief office visits and placebo alone. In this connection, the authors of the study stressed that their contact with the subjects during the study "in no way would have met the criteria of insight-directed psychotherapy" (p. 200S). They add, "many of the subjects entering the trial had been struggling secretly for long periods with their bingeing and vomiting and associated feelings of guilt and loss of control. Entry into the trial represented for many of them the first attempts to seek help for their distressing condition" (p. 200S).

We would emphasize, in passing, that these observations underline the need for skepticism when evaluating any uncontrolled reports of treatment of bulimic patients. Given that many patients, particularly those who are seeking treatment for the first time, may be particularly "primed" or motivated to improve, a control group is necessary to allow for the placebo effect.

However, we still must note that neither the mianserin group nor the placebo group in this study experienced an improvement in their frequency of binge eating. Although it may be that mianserin is simply ineffective for bulimia, such an interpretation may not be correct. First, the dose of mianserin used was only 60 mg/day. This may be too low, given that one American study required doses of up to 150 mg/day for an adequate effect (69). In addition, since the study subjects were generally engaging in self-induced vomiting or laxative abuse, it is possible that these behaviors may have interfered with adequate absorption of the drug, further reducing its effect. Thus, it would have been of interest to document actual plasma levels of mianserin in each subject in order to ascertain whether these levels were adequate. Pending a study that documents adequate plasma levels, it may be premature to pass judgment on the efficacy of mianserin in bulimia.

In a second placebo-controlled double-blind study, Pope and colleagues (70) compared imipramine with placebo in twenty-two subjects with chronic bulimia. These subjects were required to have been ill for at least one year and to be displaying at least two episodes of binge eating per week. All were between 80 and 120% of ideal body weight at the time of their entry into the study. At the end of the 6-week study period, the frequency of binge-eating episodes in the imipramine group had declined by about 70%, but was virtually unchanged in the placebo group, a significant difference. Significant improvement also occurred on Hamilton Rating Scale scores for depression and on various subjective measures of eating behavior, such as preoccupation with food, self-control with relation to food, intensity of binge eating, and subjective global improvement. The study also found a significant correlation between the improvement in depression and the decrease in the frequency of binge eating at the end of 6 weeks.

Placebo subjects were offered antidepressant treatment at the end of the blind phase of this study. On follow-up of 1-8 months, 90% of the twenty subjects showed at least some improvement and seven (35%) had achieved a remission.

More recently, Pope and colleagues (71) presented additional follow-up data on the same twenty subjects. Of the twenty subjects, eleven were followed for a period of 2 years or more; eight of these (73%) were in remission from bulimia at the end of the 2-year period; two (18%) were moderately or markedly improved; and one (9%) was unimproved. Of the remitted patients, three had been able to discontinue their antidepressant agent at some point during the follow-up, but five still required antidepressants to maintain remission. Of the nine patients followed less than 2 years, two (22%) were in remission at time of last follow-up, and the remaining seven (78%) were either moderately or markedly improved. These results suggest that the beneficial effects of antidepressants in bulimia persist over the long term. The authors noted, however, that antidepressant treatment was often complicated in their subjects, requiring considerable experimentation with different drugs and dosages from time to time.

In a third placebo-controlled double-blind study, Walsh and colleagues (72) treated twenty-five bulimic patients with the MAO inhibitor phenelzine versus placebo. Phenelzine proved significantly superior to placebo both in decreasing the frequency of binge eating and in decreased scores on the Eating Attitudes Test (EAT) (73). Of the nine study "completers" assigned to phenelzine, five attained a remission of their bulimia within a matter of a few weeks; the remaining four experienced at least 50% improvement of their bulimic symptoms. Long-term follow-up of these patients was not presented.

In the fourth study, Hughes and colleagues (74) assigned twenty-two bulimic patients, comparable to those of the previous studies in terms of severity and chronicity of illness, to desipramine versus placebo. In this study, bulimic patients who had a current diagnosis of major depression were excluded. Although this criterion was not applied in the three previous placebo-controlled double-blind studies described above, it does not appear to represent a major departure from them; only one of the twenty phenelzine subjects of Walsh and colleagues and only seven of the nineteen imipramine subjects of Pope and colleagues displayed current major depression. In the Hughes study, on all four measures used (including frequency of binge-eating episodes per week), the Zung Self-Rated Depression Scale (75), and two scales of the authors' own design, desipramine was significantly superior to placebo. At the end of the 6-week study period, subjects were offered an open trial of desipramine. After ten weeks, fifteen (68%) of the total group of twenty-two subjects had attained a remission of binge eating. In this study, as in the previous double-blind studies, no ancillary therapy other than the drugs was provided.

Unlike the investigators in the previous studies, Hughes and colleagues obtained antidepressant plasma levels. Of twenty subjects tested, fourteen were found to be outside of the postulated therapeutic range of desipramine (125–275 mg/ml at the Mayo Clinic laboratories). Ten of the fourteen subjects were below the lower limit of the therapeutic range; four were already in remission from bulimia and, therefore, their dosages were not increased. In the remaining six, however, the dosages of desipramine were increased in order to attain therapeutic plasma levels. Four of these six subjects then achieved remission; one subject ultimately required 350 mg of desipramine per day. In the four subjects whose desipramine plasma levels were initially found to be too high the dosage was reduced, with considerable improvement in side effects and no deterioration of clinical response.

These findings would suggest that adequate plasma levels of medications are critical in the treatment of bulimia. It seems possible that since bulimic patients are often young, they probably metabolize antidepressant medication more rapidly than do older patients. Furthermore, their purging behavior may additionally compromise the degree of drug absorption. Thus it is not surprising that unusually high doses of antidepressants may be required in some bulimic patients in order to produce adequate plasma levels.

Finally, in a fifth placebo-controlled double-blind study, Mitchell and Groat (76) treated 32 bulimic patients with either amitriptyline (150 mg/day) or placebo. At the end of the study, amitriptyline was significantly superior to placebo on one of the depression rating scales (the Hamilton) but not on the other (the Zung). Interestingly, both the amitriptyline group and the placebo group improved on all of the four measures of bulimic symptoms. On each of these measures, amitriptyline was superior to placebo, but the differences did not reach statistical significance. Two of the differences, however, approached significance ($p < 0.10$).

The modest findings of this study may again be related to inadequate drug plasma levels. When the investigators measured the levels of amitriptyline plus nortriptyline in eight of the subjects on active drug, they found that one subject had a plasma level of zero and three others had amitriptyline plus nortriptyline levels that were less than 75 mg/ml. Thus, four of the eight subjects tested had levels below the therapeutic range that has been suggested by most studies with amitriptyline (77–79). Since the authors measured plasma levels near the end of the study, they were unable to correct the dosage in the manner of the Hughes study just cited. Thus, as the authors themselves point out, "as many as one-half of the subjects may have received inadequate doses of the drug" (p. 192).

In summary, of the five placebo-controlled double-blind studies testing antidepressant medications in bulimia to date, three have produced clearly positive findings, one a weakly positive finding, and one a negative finding. However, there is considerable reason to believe that the subjects in the latter two studies may in many cases have received inadequate doses of medication.

Three other double-blind studies, involving other medications, have also appeared. In one, Ong and colleagues (80) administered 15 mg of methamphetamine intravenously on one day and a placebo on another day, separated by a 1-week interval, to eight inpatients with bulimia. Episodes of binge eating were significantly reduced after methamphetamine, as was caloric consumption.

In a similar study (81) 60 mg of fenfluramine was administered orally as a single dose versus placebo, again separated by a 1-week interval, to fifteen individuals with bulimia. Fenfluramine also was associated with reduced caloric consumption and fewer episodes of binge eating during the test period after drug administration.

It is unclear in these two studies, whether the antibulimic effects of methamphetamine and fenfluramine are attributable to their anorexigenic properties or whether they may be attributable to the thymoleptic properties of the agents. Both methamphetamine and fenfluramine, in recent studies, have been shown to possess antidepressant properties in addition to their anorexigenic properties (82, 83). It is also unclear, on the basis of these single-dose studies, whether either of these agents would offer any long-term benefit in the treatment of bulimia. Obviously, methamphetamine is an impractical drug to use in the treatment of bulimia, due to its potential for abuse. Fenfluramine may have more promise, but has not been formally tested in a long-term study. In seven bulimic patients whom we treated (Pope et al., unpublished observations), a 2- to 4-week trial of 60 mg/day of fenfluramine produced only transient improvement.

In the last placebo-controlled study, Kaplan and colleagues (84) used carbamazepine, an agent effective in some patients with bipolar disorder (85), to treat six individuals with bulimia. All of the bulimic patients had normal EEGs. Although five patients showed little improvement with carbamazepine, one displayed a virtual remission of her bulimic symptoms with carbamazepine and relapsed when switched to placebo. She also displayed prominent affective symptoms, described by the authors as "cyclothymic if not bipolar mood disorder." These symptoms also declined markedly with carbamazepine.

In addition to the above double-blind studies, there have been various uncontrolled reports of other medications in bulimia.

Trazodone

Although one study has reported improvement in eight bulimic patients treated with trazodone (86), the same authors reported three cases of delirium in bulimic patients receiving this agent (87). Another report described worsening of depression and bulimic symptoms in three patients who were switched to trazodone after having been treated with tricyclic antidepressants or lithium carbonate (88). In all cases, these patients improved when they were resumed on their previous medications. Thus, there is little clear evidence to suggest that trazodone would be the agent of choice for bulimic patients.

Monoamine Oxidase (MAO) Inhibitors

In addition to the data with phenelzine, cited earlier, there is an additional report from the Columbia University group, describing an expanded open trial of MAO inhibitors in twelve bulimic patients (89). The results of this report were substantially the same as those of the uncontrolled report of six patients cited earlier.

Kennedy and colleagues (90) have performed an open trial of another MAO inhibitor, isocarboxazid, in fourteen subjects with eating disorders. Eight of these displayed current bulimic symptoms. During the course of the study, three of the eight remitted, three were at least 50% improved, and two were unimproved. Although the predrug versus postdrug difference did not reach significance in this study (possibly because of the small sample size), the measure of "urges to binge" did reach significance.

Lithium Carbonate

Hsu (91) treated fourteen bulimic women with lithium carbonate at standard serum levels. Twelve of the fourteen patients experienced either a remission or at least a 75% improvement in their frequency of binge-eating episodes. Most subjects maintained their improvement throughout follow-up periods which ranged from 6 to 16 months; seven of the fourteen patients were able to discontinue lithium at some time during the follow-up interval without a relapse.

Chevlen (92) added lithium carbonate to other antidepressants in seven bulimic individuals who had shown an inadequate response to the antidepressants alone. One achieved a remission of her symptoms and two others about a 50% improvement after the addition of lithium; the remaining four patients apparently did not respond.

Bupropion

Horne (93) used bupropion (removed from the market by the USFDA but continues to have research programs associated with it) to treat seventeen patients with bulimia and major depression. Doses were 450–600 mg/day. It is notable that all of these patients had failed to respond to previous antidepressants. After 1 month, 41% of the patients were in remission, 47% showed at least a 50% decrease in binge-eating episodes, and 12% were unimproved. After 6 months, four patients had dropped out of the study, but all others maintained their degree of improvement.

Nomifensine

Pope and colleagues (94) treated twelve consecutive bulimic patients with nomifensine in doses of 150–300 mg/day. Two patients developed fevers, a previously described allergic reaction (95), and were withdrawn. Of the remaining ten patients, three experienced a remission of bulimic symptoms, six moderate or marked improvement, and one, no improvement.*

Sodium Valproate

Sodium valproate, like carbamazepine, may be effective both acutely and prophylactically in the treatment of bipolar disorder (96, 97). Herridge and Pope (98) described one woman with a history of both rapid cycling bipolar disorder and bulimic symptoms who displayed a striking response to sodium valproate. During the course of her treatment, she experienced two recurrences of her bulimic and affective symptoms; both of these recurrences coincided with a drop in her plasma valproate level to less than 50 mg/ml. When her valproate dosage was increased, her symptoms remitted again, suggesting that her improvement was indeed attributable to valproate.

Studies Using Various Antidepressants

Two other uncontrolled studies have described experience with pooled samples of bulimic patients treated with several different categories of antidepressants. Pope and colleagues (99) described sixty-five consecutive patients treated at their center. Most were treated with tricyclics initially and then switched to an MAO inhibitor if the tricyclics had failed. A few other patients were treated with trazodone, lithium carbonate, carbamazepine, or magnesium pemoline. When the authors scored the eventual response of patients to whatever antidepressant had proved most effective in a sequence of drug trials, it was found that twenty-two (33.8%) of the 65 had achieved remission, twenty-five (38.5%), marked improvement, twelve (18.5%), moderate improvement, and six (9.2%), no improvement. Although these results appeared encouraging, the authors cautioned that considerable experi-

---

*Nomifensine was withdrawn from the market after a few cases of fatal hemolytic anemia were reported.

mentation was often necessary in some subjects to achieve optimum response. They also found that unusually high doses of tricyclic antidepressants or MAO inhibitors were often necessary in order to achieve adequate plasma levels [an impression consistent with the findings of two of the double-blind studies cited earlier (74,76)]. Some putative "nonresponders" to antidepressants, when assessed for plasma drug levels or platelet MAO levels in this study, proved simply to be undertreated.

In a second study, Brotman and colleagues (100) described twenty-two patients treated with antidepressants at their center. Only five (23%) of the patients were considered "true responders" who remained essentially in remission from their bulimia throughout a 6-month follow-up. However, these modest results may be due to several methodological problems in the study, since the authors (a) used low and probably inadequate doses of antidepressants in most of their subjects; (b) failed to obtain plasma levels of tricyclic antidepressants or platelet MAO levels in any subject treated; and (c) generally failed to try a second or third antidepressant when a first one was unsuccessful. To give one example of these problems, Brotman and colleagues defined 125 mg/day of a tricyclic antidepressant to be an adequate dose. Yet in the study of Hughes and colleagues, cited above (74), it was found that even 200 mg of desipramine per day produced *inadequate* plasma levels in 50% of subjects and that one subject required 350 mg. Thus, some of the subjects in the study of Brotman and colleagues may have been undertreated by as much as a factor of three. This accumulation of methodological problems severely limits interpretations of the findings of the study. Similar criticisms of the study have been published by Walsh and colleagues (101).

In summary, although these latter studies are uncontrolled, they seem consistent with the results of the double-blind studies cited earlier in finding that a wide range of thymoleptic medications—including not only antidepressants, but lithium carbonate, carbamazepine, sodium valproate, and other agents—appear effective in the treatment of bulimia. Most of the studies have found that a majority of bulimic patients experience either a remission from their bulimic symptoms or at least a marked improvement in their urge to binge-eat with such agents. These data stand in contrast to the data for anorexic patients, presented earlier, where antidepressants have shown a much more equivocal effect.

The available studies of thymoleptic treatment of bulimia suggest several other tentative impressions. First, there do not appear to be any specific subgroups of bulimic patients who are, or are not, candidates for thymoleptic agents. There appears to be no evidence, nor even a visible trend in the evidence, to suggest that bulimic patients with major depression, those with other concomitant psychiatric diagnoses, those with positive family histories for affective disorder or other disorders, or those with positive dexamethasone suppression tests are more likely to respond to thymoleptic agents than are bulimic patients who lack these attributes. It should be particularly noted that antidepressants appear at least as effective in bulimic patients who are not depressed as in those who are. In fact, in the one study which excluded bulimic patients with major depression, that of Hughes and colleagues (74), the response to antidepressants was, if anything, slightly better than in other double-blind studies. Therefore, there appears to be no basis for withholding antidepressants from bulimic patients who do not display major depression.

Second, many studies have indicated that adequate plasma levels of antidepressant agents are critical in order to achieve optimum results in bulimia. In studies that have used apparently inadequate plasma levels of drugs in some of their subjects (68,76,100), the results have been less satisfactory than found in studies that specifically assessed plasma levels (74,99). It seems important, therefore, particularly when treating bulimic patients with self-induced vomiting or laxative abuse, to take unusual care to achieve adequate antidepressant levels.

Third, the evidence tentatively suggests that antidepressants may benefit bulimic symptoms via the same mechanism as they do depression. Some writers have questioned this hypothesis, pointing out that there are certain bulimic patients in whom depressive symptoms improve but bulimia does not, or in whom bulimia improves but depression does not (100). However, such an observation does not necessarily imply two separate mechanisms of action for antidepressants. In congestive heart failure, for example, digitalis may be effective for edema but relatively ineffective for dyspnea in certain patients, while having a reverse effect in other patients. Yet the anti-edema and anti-dyspnea effects of digitalis do not represent different mechanisms of action of the drug.

In favor of the possibility that antidepressants benefit bulimia and depression by a similar mechanism, several observations have accumulated: (a) comparable plasma levels of the various drugs are required in the treatment of both syndromes (74,76,84,91,98,99), (b) the time course for the antidepressant and antibulimic effects is roughly similar (70,72,74,76), and (c) in the one study where it was assessed, a highly significant correlation was found between decrease in depression scores and decrease in frequency of binge eating (70). We must add a fourth observation that not one but virtually all of the major thymoleptic agents currently in use have been shown to be of at least some benefit in bulimia. The converse also seems to apply: there is little evidence that nonthymoleptic drugs benefit bulimia. Phenytoin and fenfluramine may represent possible exceptions to this rule. However, in the only double-blind study of phenytoin available (56), the drug had at best a weak effect, and what effect it did have may have been unrelated to its anticonvulsant properties. Furthermore, phenytoin may have weak thymoleptic effects of its own (57,59). Similarly, fenfluramine has been shown to have antidepressant effects in at least one placebo-controlled double-blind study (83). Thus, neither drug seems to represent a convincing counterexample to the hypothesis that antidepressants benefit depression and bulimia via similar mechanisms.

Further, we must consider the nonpharmacological body of evidence suggesting that bulimia may be closely related to major affective disorder. Like anorexia nervosa, discussed earlier, bulimia appears related to major affective disorder on the basis of phenomenological observations (34,101–105) and family history studies (37,105,106).

The foregoing evidence appears consistent with the hypothesis that bulimia and major affective disorder may be caused, at least in part, by the same underlying abnormality, and that antidepressants and other thymoleptic agents may benefit both disorders via their effect on this common abnormality. Although each piece of evidence might be individually explained with alternate hypotheses, it would seem difficult to construct an alternate hypothesis that would explain the entire body of evidence with an equal degree of parsimony (107).

The question remains open, however, as to why anorexia nervosa, a disorder that also appears related to major affective disorder, does not respond equally well to the same agents. Whether this is attributable to psychological factors, sociocultural factors, or to some biological difference between anorexic and bulimic patients remains to be elucidated.

REFERENCES

1. Pope, H. G., Jr., and Hudson, J. I. (1984). *New Hope for Binge Eaters.* New York: Harper and Row.
2. Agras, W., and Kraemer, H. (1983). Anorexia nervosa: Treatment and outcome. In *Eating and Its Disorders*, ed. A. J. Stunkard. New York: Raven Press.
3. Boskind-Lodahl, M., and White, W. C. (1978). The definition and treatment of bulimarexia in college women—a pilot study. *Journal of the American College Health Association* 27:84–86.
4. Fairburn, C. G. (1981). A cognitive behavioral approach to the management of bulimia. *Psychological Medicine* 11:707–711.
5. Lacey, J. H. (1983). Bulimia nervosa, binge eating, and psychogenic vomiting: A controlled treatment study and long-term outcome. *British Medical Journal* 286:1609–1613.
6. Liebman, R., Minuchin, S., and Baker, L. (1974). An integrated treatment program for anorexia nervosa. *Psychiatry* 131:532–536.
7. White, W. C., and Boskind-White, M. (1981). An experiential-behavioral approach to the treatment of bulimarexia. *Psychotherapy: Theory, Research, and Practice* 4:501–507.
8. Dally, P. J., Oppenheim, G. B., and Sargant, W. (1958). Anorexia nervosa. *British Medical Journal* 2:633.
9. Dally, P. J., and Sargant, W. (1960). A new treatment of anorexia nervosa. *British Medical Journal* 1:1770–1771.
10. Crisp, A. H., and Roberts, F. J. (1962). A case of anorexia nervosa in a male. *Postgraduate Medical Journal* 38:350–353.
11. Crisp, A. H. (1965). Some aspects of the evolution, presentation, and follow-up of anorexia nervosa. *Proceedings of the Royal Society of Medicine* 58:814–820.
12. Crisp, A. H. (1965). A treatment regime for anorexia nervosa. *British Journal of Psychiatry* 112:505–512.
13. Plantley, F. (1977). Pimozide in the treatment of anorexia nervosa (letter). *Lancet* 1:1105.
14. Hoes, M. J. (1980). Copper sulfate and pimozide for anorexia nervosa. *Journal of Orthomolecular Psychiatry* 9:48–51.
15. Vandereycken, W., and Pierloot, R. (1982). Pimozide combined with behavior therapy in the short-term treatment of anorexia nervosa: A double-blind placebo-controlled crossover study. *Acta Psychiatrica Scandinavica* 60:446–451.
16. Gross, H., Ebert, M. H., Faden, V. B., and Goldberg, S. C. (1983). A double-blind trial of 9-tetrahydrocannabinol in primary anorexia nervosa. *Journal of Clinical Psychopharmacology* 3:165–171.
17. Moore, R., Mills, I. H., and Forster, A. (1981). Naloxone in the treatment of anorexia nervosa: Effect on weight gain and lipolysis. *Journal of the Royal Society of Medicine* 74:129–131.
18. Johanson, A. J., and Knorr, N. J. (1974). Treatment of anorexia nervosa by levodopa. *Lancet* 1:591.

References

19. Johanson, A. J., and Knorr, N. J. (1977). L-Dopa as treatment for anorexia nervosa. In *Anorexia Nervosa*, ed. R. A. Vigersky, pp. 363-372. New York: Raven Press.
20. Bakan, R. (1979). The role of zinc in anorexia nervosa: Etiology and treatment. *Medical Hypotheses* 5:731-736.
21. Esca, S. A., Brenner, W., Mach, K., and Gschnait, F. (1979). Kwashiorkor-like zinc deficiency syndrome in anorexia nervosa. *Acta Dermato-Venereologica (Stockholm)* 59:361-364.
22. Safai-Kutti, S., and Kutti, J. (1984). Zinc and anorexia nervosa (letter). *Annals of Internal Medicine* 100:317-318.
23. Zubiate, T. N. (1970). Tratamiento de la anorexia nervosa con una associacion cyproheptadina-vitaminas. *Revista Medica de la Caja Nacional de Segura Social* 19:147-153.
24. Vigersky, R. A., and Loriaux, D. L. (1977). The effect of cyproheptadine in anorexia nervosa: A double-blind trial. In *Anorexia Nervosa*, ed. R. A. Vigersky, pp. 349-356. New York: Raven Press.
25. Goldberg, S. C., Halmi, K. A., Eckert, E. D., Casper, R. C., and Davis, J. M. (1979). Cyproheptadine in anorexia nervosa. *British Journal of Psychiatry* 134:67-70.
26. Halmi, K. A. (1982). Cyproheptadine for anorexia nervosa. *Lancet* 1:1357-1358.
27. Halmi, K. A., Eckert, E. D., and Falk, J. R. (1983). Cyproheptadine, an antidepressant and weight-inducing drug for anorexia nervosa. *Psychopharmacology Bulletin* 19:103-105.
28. Halmi, K. A., Eckert, E., LaDu, T. J., and Cohen, J. (1986). Anorexia nervosa: treatment efficacy of cyproheptadine and amitriptyline. *Archives of General Psychiatry* 43:177-181.
29. Barcai, A. (1977). Lithium in adult anorexia nervosa. *Acta Psychiatrica Scandinavica* 55:97-101.
30. Cantwell, D. P., Sturzenberger, S., Burroughs, J., Salkin, B., and Green, J. (1977). Anorexia nervosa: An affective disorder? *Archives of General Pscyhiatry* 34:1087-1093.
31. Eckert, E. D., Goldberg, S. C., and Halmi, K. A. (1982). Depression in anorexia nervosa. *Psychological Medicine* 12:115-122.
32. Garfinkel, P. E., Moldofsky, M., and Garner, D. M. (1980). The heterogeneity of anorexia nervosa: Bulimia as a distinct subgroup. *Archives of General Psychiatry* 37:1036-1040.
33. Hendren, R. L. (1983). Depression in anorexia nervosa. *Journal of the American Academy of Child Psychiatry* 22:59-62.
34. Hudson, J. I., Pope, H. G., Jr., Yurgelun-Todd, D., and Jonas, J. M. (1983). Phenomenologic relationship of eating disorders to major affective disorder. *Psychiatry Research* 9:345-354.
35. Kron, L., Katz, J. L., Gorsynski, G., and Weiner, H. (1978). Hyperactivity in anorexia nervosa: A fundamental clinical feature. *Comprehensive Psychiatry* 19:433-440.
36. Gershon, E. S., Hamovit, J. R., Schreiber, J. L., Dibble, E. D., Kaye, W., Nurnberger, J. I., Andersen, A. E. (1984). Clinical findings in anorectics and affective illness in their relatives. *American Journal of Psychiatry* 141:1419-1422.

37. Hudson, J. I., Pope, H. G., Jr., Jonas, J. M., and Yurgelun-Todd, D. (1983). Family history study of anorexia nervosa and bulimia. *British Journal of Psychiatry* 142:133–138.
38. Winokur, A., March, V., and Mendels, J. (1980). Primary affective disorder in relatives of patients with anorexia nervosa. *American Journal of Psychiatry* 137:695–698.
39. Reilly, P. P. (1977). Anorexia nervosa. *Rhode Island Medical Journal* 60:419–422.
40. Stein, G. S., Hartshorne, S., Jones, J., et al. (1982). Lithium in a case of severe anorexia nervosa. *British Journal of Psychiatry* 140:526–528.
41. Gross, H. A., Ebert, M. H., and Faden, V. B. (1981). A double-blind controlled trial of lithium carbonate in anorexia nervosa. *Journal of Clinical Psychopharmacology* 1:376–381.
42. Mills, I. H. (1976). Amitriptyline therapy in anorexia nervosa (letter). *Lancet* 2:687.
43. Moore, D. C. (1977). Amitriptyline therapy in anorexia nervosa. *American Journal of Psychiatry* 134:1303–1304.
44. Needleman, H. L., and Waber, D. (1976). Amitriptyline therapy in patients with anorexia nervosa (letter). *Lancet* 2:580.
45. Needleman, H. L., and Waber, D. (1977). Amitriptyline in anorexia nervosa. In *Anorexia Nervosa*, ed. R. A. Vigersky, pp. 357–362. New York: Raven Press.
46. White, J. H., and Schnaultz, N. L. (1977). Successful treatment of anorexia nervosa with imipramine. *Diseases of the Nervous System* 38:567–568.
47. Lacey, J. H., and Crisp, A. H. (1980). Hunger, food intake, and weight: The impact of clomipramine on a refeeding anorexia nervosa population. *Postgraduate Medical Journal* 56:79–85.
48. Biederman, J., Herzog, D. B., Rivinus, T. M., Harper, G. P., Ferber, R. A., Rosenbaum, J. F., and Harmatz, J. S. (1985). Amitriptyline in the treatment of anorexia nervosa: A double-blind placebo-controlled study. *Journal of Clinical Psychopharmacology* 5:10–16.
49. Hudson, J. I., Pope, H. G., Jr., Jonas, J. M., and Yurgelun-Todd, D. (1985). Treatment of anorexia nervosa with antidepressants. *Journal of Clinical Psychopharmocology* 5:17–23.
50. Green, R. S., and Rau, J. H. (1974). Treatment of compulsive eating disturbances with anticonvulsant medication. *American Journal of Psychiatry* 131:428–432.
51. Weiss, T., and Levitz, L. (1976). Diphenylhydantoin treatment of bulimia (letter). *American Journal of Psychiatry* 133:1093.
52. Greenway, F. L., Dahms, W. T., and Brag, D. A. (1977). Phenytoin as a treatment of obesity associated with compulsive eating. *Current Therapeutic Research* 21:338–342.
53. Green, R. S., and Rau, J. H. (1977). The use of diphenylhydantoin in compulsive eating disorders: Further studies. In *Anorexia Nervosa*, ed. R. A. Vigersky, pp. 377–382. New York: Raven Press.
54. Rau, J. H., and Green, R. S. (1978). Soft neurological correlates of compulsive eating. *Journal of Nervous and Mental Disease* 166:435–437.

References

55. Rau, J. H., Struve, F. A., and Green, R. S. (1979). Electroencephalographic correlates of compulsive eating. *Clinical Electroencephalography* 10:180–188.
56. Wermuth, B. M., Davis, K. L., Hollister, L. E., and Stunkard, A. J. (1977). Phenytoin treatment of the binge-eating syndrome. *American Journal of Psychiatry* 134:1249–1253.
57. Bogoch, S., and Dreyfus, J. (1970). *The Broad Range of Use of Diphenylhydantoin: Bibliography and Review*, Vol 1. New York: Dreyfus Medical Foundation.
58. Bogoch S., and Dreyfus, J. (1975). *DPH 1975* (a supplement to *The Broad Range of Use of Diphenylhydantoin: Bibliography and Review*), Vol. 2. New York: Dreyfus Medical Foundation.
59. Stephen, J. H., and Shaffer, J. W. (1973). A controlled replication of the effectiveness of diphenylhydantoin in reducing irritability and anxiety in selected neurotic outpatients. *Journal of Clinical Pharmacology* 13:351–356.
60. Moore, S. L., and Rakes, S. M. (1982). Binge eating—therapeutic response to diphenylhydantoin: Case report. *Journal of Clinical Psychiatry* 43:385–386.
61. Rich, C. L. (1978). Self-induced vomiting: Psychiatric considerations. *Journal of the American Medical Association* 239:2688–2689.
62. Shader, R. I, and Greenblatt, D. J. (1982). The psychiatrist as mind sweeper. *Journal of Clinical Psychopharmacology* 2:233–234.
63. Pope, H. G., Jr., and Hudson, J. I. (1982). Treatment of bulimia with antidepressants. *Psychopharmacology* 78:167–179.
64. Walsh, B. T., Stewart, J. W., Wright, L., Harrison, W., Roose, S. P., and Glassman, A. H. (1982). Treatment of bulimia with monoamine oxidase inhibitors. *American Journal of Psychiatry* 139:1629–1630.
65. Mendels, J. (1983). Eating disorders and antidepressants (letter). *Journal of Clinical Psychopharmacology* 3:59.
66. Roy-Byrne, P., Gwirtsman, H., Edelstein, C. K., Yager, J., Gerner, R. H. (1983). Eating disorders and antidepressants (letter). *Journal of Clinical Psychopharmacology* 3:60–61.
67. Jonas, J. M., Pope, H. G., Jr., and Hudson, J. I. (1983). Treatment of bulimia with monoamine oxidase inhibitors (letter). *Journal of Clinical Psychopharmacology* 3:59–60.
68. Sabine, E. J., Yonace, A., Farrington, A. J., Barratt, K. H., and Wakeling, A. (1983). Bulimia nervosa: A placebo-controlled double-blind therapeutic trial of mianserin. *British Journal of Clinical Pharmacology* 15:195S–202S.
69. McGrath, P. J., Quitkin, F. M., Stewart, J. W., Liebowitz, M., Fyer, A., and Davies, S. (1981). An open clinical trial of mianserin. *American Journal of Psychiatry* 138:530–532.
70. Pope, H. G., Jr., Hudson, J. I., Jonas, J. M., and Yurgelun-Todd, D. (1983). Bulimia treated with imipramine: A placebo-controlled double-blind study. *American Journal of Psychiatry* 140:554–558.
71. Pope, H. G., Jr., Hudson, J. I., Jonas, J. M., and Yurgelun-Todd, D. (1985). Antidepressant treatment of bulimia: A two-year follow-up study. *Journal of Clinical Psychopharmacology* 5:320–327.
72. Walsh, B. T., Stewart, J. W., Roose, S. P., Gladis, M., and Glassman, A. H. (1984). Treatment of bulimia with phenelzine: A double-blind, placebo-controlled study. *Archives of General Psychiatry* 41:1105–1109.

73. Garner, D. M., and Garfinkel, P. E. (1979). The eating attitudes test: An index of the symptoms of anorexia nervosa. *Psychological Medicine* 9:273-279.
74. Hughes, P. L., Wells, L. A., Cunningham, C. J., and Ilstrup, D. M. (1986). Treating bulimia with desipramine: A placebo-controlled double-blind study. *Archives of General Psychiatry* 43:182-186.
75. Zung, W. W. K. (1965). A self-rating depression scale. *Archives of General Psychiatry* 12:63-70.
76. Mitchell, J. E., and Groat, R. (1984). A placebo-controlled, double-blind trial of amitriptyline in bulimia. *Journal of Clinical Psychopharmacology* 4:186-193.
77. Braithwaite, R. A., Goulding, R., Theano, G., Bailey, J., and Coppen, A. (1972). Plasma concentration of amitriptyline and clinical response. *Lancet* 1:1297-1300.
78. Zeigler, V. E., Clayton, P. J., and Biggs, J. T. (1977). A comparison study of amitriptyline and nortriptyline with plasma levels. *Archives of General Psychiatry* 34:607-612.
79. Kupfer, D. J., Hanin, I., Spiker, D. G., Grau, T., and Coble, P. (1977). Amitriptyline plasma levels and clinical response in primary depression. *Clinical Pharmacology and Therapeutics* 22:904-911.
80. Ong, Y. L., Checkley, S. A., and Russell, G. F. M. (1983) Suppression of bulimic symptoms with methylamphetamine. *British Journal of Psychiatry* 143:288-293.
81. Robinson, P. H., Checkley, S. A., and Russell, G. F. M. (1985). Suppression of eating by fenfluramine in patients with bulimia nervosa. *British Journal of Psychiatry* 146:169-176.
82. Costa, E., and Garattini, S., eds. (1970). *International Symposium on Amphetamines and Related Compounds.* New York: Raven Press.
83. Lechin, F., Van der Dijs, B., Gomez, F., Arocha, L., Acosta, E., and Lechin, E. (1983). Distal colon motility as a predictor of antidepressant response to fenfluramine, imipramine, and clomipramine. *Journal of Affective Disorders* 5:27-35.
84. Kaplan, A. S., Garfinkel, P. E., Darby, P. L., and Garner, D. M. (1983). Carbamazepine in the treatment of bulimia. *American Journal of Psychiatry* 140:1225-1226.
85. Ballenger, J. C., and Post, R. M. (1980). Carbamazepine in manic-depressive illness: A new treatment. *American Journal of Psychiatry* 137:782-790.
86. Damlouji, N. F., and Ferguson, J. M. (1984). Trazodone in the treatment of bulimic patients. Presented at the First International Conference on Eating Disorders, New York, April.
87. Damlouji, N. F., and Ferguson, J. M. (1984). Trazodone-induced delirium in bulimic patients. *American Journal of Psychiatry* 141:434-435.
88. Wold, P. (1983). Trazodone in the treatment of bulimia (letter). *Journal of Clinical Psychiatry* 44:275-276.
89. Stewart, J. W., Walsh, B. T., Wright, L., Harrison, W., Roose, S. P., and Glassman, A H. (1984). An open trial of MAO inhibitors in bulimia. *Journal of Clinical Psychiatry* 45:217-219.
90. Kennedy, S. H., Piran, N., and Garfinkel, P. E. (1985). Monoamine oxidase inhibitor therapy for anorexia nervosa and bulimia—a preliminary trial of isocarboxazid. *Journal of Clinical Psychopharmocology* 5:279-285.

References

91. Hsu, L. K. G. (1984). Treatment of bulimia with lithium. *American Journal of Psychiatry* 141:1260-1262.
92. Chevlen, E. M. (1984). The adjunctive use of lithium carbonate in the management of bulimia resistant to antidepressant therapy. Presented at the First International Conference on Eating Disorders, New York, April.
93. Horne, R. L. (1984). Bupropion in the treatment of bulimia. Presented at the First International Conference on Eating Disorders, New York, April.
94. Pope, H. G., Jr., Herridge, P. L., and Hudson, J. I. (1985). Treatment of bulimia with nomifensine. Presented at the Annual Meeting, American Psychiatric Association, May.
95. Pitts, F., ed. (1984). Nomifensine. *Journal of Clinical Psychiatry* 45(4) (section 2):4-105.
96. Emrich, H. M., Von Zerssen, D., and Kissling, W. (1980). The effect of sodium valproate on mania: The GABA hypothesis of affective disorder. *Archiv für Psychiatrie und Nervenkrankheiten* 229:1-16.
97. Puzynski, S., and Klosiewicz, L. (1983). Valproic acid amide (VAA) in the therapy of affective disorder. Presented at the Seventh World Congress of Psychiatry, Vienna, July.
98. Herridge, P. L., and Pope, H. G., Jr. (1985). Treatment of bulimia and rapid-cycling bipolar disorder with sodium valproate: A case report. *Journal of Clinical Psychopharmacology* 5:229-230.
99. Pope, H. G., Jr., Hudson, J. I., and Jonas, J. M. (1983). Antidepressant treatment of bulimia: Preliminary experience and practical recommendations. *Journal of Clinical Psychopharmacology* 3:274-281.
100. Brotman, A. W., Herzog, D. B., and Woods, S. W. (1984). Antidepressant treatment of bulimia: The relationship between binging and depressive symptomatology. *Journal of Clinical Psychiatry* 45:7-9.
101. Walsh, B. T., Roose, S. P., Glassman, A. H., et al. (1985). Bulimia and depression. *Psychosomatic Medicine* 47:123-131.
102. Herzog, D. B. (1984). Are anorexic and bulimic patients depressed? *American Journal of Psychiatry* 141:1594-1597.
103. Hatsukami, D., Eckert, E. D., Mitchell, J. E., and Pyle, R. (1984). Affective disorder and substance abuse in women with bulimia. *Psychological Medicine* 14:701-714.
104. Hudson, J. I., Pope, H. G., Jr., Yurgelun-Todd, D., Jonas, J. M., and Frankenburg, F. R. (1987). A controlled study of lifetime prevalence of affective and other psychiatric disorders in bulimic outpatients. *American Journal of Psychiatry* 144:1283-1287.
105. Hudson, J. I., and Pope, H. G., Jr. (1987). Depression and eating disorders. In: *Presentations of Depression: Depressive Symptoms in Medical and Other Psychiatric Disorders*, ed. O. G. Cameron, pp. 33-66. New York: John Wiley & Sons.
106. Hudson, J. I., Pope, H. G., Jr., Jonas, J. M., Yurgelun-Todd, D., Frankenburg, F. R. (1987). A controlled family history study of bulimia. *Psychological Medicine* 17:883-890.
107. Pope, H. G., Jr., Hudson, J. I. (1988). Is bulimia a heterogeneous disorder? Reflections from the history of medicine. *International Journal of Eating Disorders* 7:155-166.

10

Treatment-Resistant Problems

David N. Osser, M.D.

Most patients at some point are difficult or treatment resistant to some extent. The clinician may be stuck, confused, or frustrated, and wonder what is wrong. Is it a true treatment-resistant case, or has the diagnosis somehow been missed, or is it a typical unconscious resistance common to psychotherapy, which must be explored and worked through? This thinking is part of the daily experience of most of us practicing the inexact science and art of psychiatry.

Psychopharmacology consultation is sought as a consequence of at least four circumstances:

1. through the initiative of the primary psychiatrist,
2. through the initiative of a collaborating clinician or therapist,
3. when requested by patient or family members,
4. when an outside clinician or agency makes contact with the patient and perceives the need.

These four situations result from progressive increases in anxiety for both physician and patient because the psychiatrist may feel in each case more vulnerable to an attack on his or her sense of competency and narcissism (1). There may have been little positive feedback around the work with the patient so far, and to have to be exposed to possible criticism from a reputable colleague might seem like more than can be endured! Experience suggests that more than half of consults are not initiated by the primary psychiatrist and are thus likely to involve these higher levels of anxiety. A primary factor in persistence of treatment resistance, therefore, may be delayed use of consultation due to the short supply of psychopharmacology consultants with whom physicians can have a consultee–consultant relationship in which there is mutual respect and trust.

In this chapter, the essence of strategies most frequently recommended in psychopharmacology consultations are conveyed. This chapter reviews three common, treatment-resistant problems: (a) depression and dysphoria, (b) manic, schizo-affective, and atypical psychoses, and (c) schizophrenia. The aim is to help the reader evaluate difficult patients through the application of step-by-step formats similar to those used by experienced consultants. Reference to the literature and especially review articles cited here will provide additional aid in deciding how to proceed, particularly when considering using unusual combinations of agents or application of drugs for indications not yet approved by the U.S. Federal Drug Administration (FDA). These materials will also be helpful in discussing the options with the patient and family and obtaining appropriate informed consent for treatment.

Nevertheless, having the patient seen directly by another psychiatrist with a fresh perspective is still one of the most valuable ways to resolve treatment-resistant problems. The critical issues often turn out to be diagnostic in origin and not in the treatment approach. This tends to make the brief "hallside" consultation less valuable than generally thought. One look by the consultant can be worth more than a thousand words of (biased) description.

TREATMENT-RESISTANT DEPRESSION AND DYSPHORIA

In order to deal with this large and extremely heterogeneous group of patients, it is first useful to classify the individual into one of five diagnostic categories on the basis of course and symptoms of the disorder. Then, after some subclassification, the various treatment options may be pinpointed.

It is assumed that the clinician has ruled out or dealt with the medical illnesses that could be causing or exacerbating the condition. The large number of physical ailments and drug toxicities to be considered have been outlined in numerous publications and will not be reviewed here (2). However, it is notable that in doing consultations on treatment-resistant patients, it is very common to find overlooked abnormal laboratory tests or omission of consideration of the medical differential diagnosis, including potential drug toxicities. For example, some depressions will not respond until certain drugs, like propranolol and alcohol, have been removed. Special mention should be made of new evidence that a large number of depressed patients may have a subtle form of thyroid disorder, responsive to thyroid hormone treatment, in which the only laboratory or clinical abnormality is an abnormal response to a thyrotropin-releasing hormone (TRH) stimulation test (3).

Obtaining the critical historical data (such as exact premorbid personality characteristics, family history of mental illness [always of interest], response to treatment in the past, adequacy of previous medication trials, and interepisode functioning) is easier said than done, and consequently it is often not done. Time and economic factors seem paramount; there is no system of payment for the time spent obtaining these facts. Yet, most of the time, a clear, accurate history leads straightforwardly to what would be the reasonable next treatment alternative. Thus, it is strongly recommended that the clinician telephone key previous clinicians and family members and obtain the information that is not available from the patient and medical records before proceeding.

The five major categories of depression or dysphoria, along with their typical courses and symptoms, are shown in Table 10-1. These were developed originally by Schildkraut and Klein (4) and have been modified over the years by subsequent research. Each type will be reviewed and a treatment strategy proposed.

UNIPOLAR DEPRESSION

While perhaps comprising a minority of all patients with complaints of depression, this group is important to identify in that a high response rate to somatic treatment (90% or better) may be expected. As noted in the table, the average age of onset of this disorder is

TABLE 10–1 Five Categories of Depression-Dysphoria

	Unipolar	Bipolar	Characterological	Schizophrenia Related	Schizo-affective
Usual age of onset	30s and older	20s	Childhood, with adult exacerbations	Teens and 20s	Teens and 20s
Course and history	Episodic, median 8 months. Normal self between episodes. If lasts 1 year, prognosis is worse	History of hypomania, mania, drug-induced mania, cyclothymia or family history of bipolar disorder	Usually chronic or present to some degree	Schizotypal premorbid or postmorbid personality; May be episodic or chronic	No schizotypal personality; may be episodic or chronic. Psychotic symptoms precede the depressive or dominate the clinical picture
Symptoms	Lack of reactivity, partial or complete; anergy; excessive guilt; anhedonia; motor and psychic retardation (young patients), motor and psychic agitation (older patients)	Same as unipolar except psychomotor retardation and hypersomnia more common	Reactive or hyperreactive. Intense dysphoria, crying. Anger and dissatisfaction with others prominent. Dramatic attention-seeking behavior. Somatization. Mentally sharp; highly attuned interpersonally	Variable; includes spectrum from anhedonia and anergy to intense dysphoria and demoralization	Same as schizophrenia related

272

Associated features	Vegetative symptoms; work and social function impaired	Same as unipolar	Work function often not impaired. Substance abuse. Syndrome may persist as residual symptoms following successful treatment of unipolar disorder (double depression).	Functioning extremely impaired. Substance abuse.	May function well even when psychotic symptoms present.
Subtypes to be differentiated before choice of treatment	Delusional Nondelusional	Same as unipolar	Panic Disorder Borderline Personality Disorder Atypical Depression Eating Disorder Post-traumatic Stress Disorder		

relatively late, that is, the 30s and older. The typical patient is in his/her 40s or 50s with two previous episodes. Younger patients will usually, though not always, fit diagnostically into one of the other categories (5,6).

The episodic course, with normal intermorbid functioning, is fundamental to this diagnosis and often can only be established by consulting with others who have known the patient during those times. The single most characteristic symptom is lack of reactivity. Often one finds partial degrees of this, where the patient is less reactive than usual to the things that normally stimulate him. The latter is highly characteristic of this diagnosis and predictive of good drug–treatment response. Other key symptoms include anergia, anhedonia, excessive guilt, and motor abnormalities (agitation or retardation). Vegetative symptoms are often present, though they are somewhat less predictive of drug response than the preceding and are much less syndromally specific than previously thought (7,8). Work and social function are usually impaired.

Next, the treatment strategy is chosen based on the critical determination of whether there are delusions present.

Nondelusional Unipolar Depression

The standard treatment here is a cyclic antidepressant (CA). Thus, it should first be determined whether an adequate trial of one or more of these drugs has been offered. Several of the drugs have fairly well-established blood levels associated with optimum therapeutic response (imipramine, nortriptyline, and desipramine); consequently, when possible, these drugs should be used if there is still a question about whether the patient has had an adequate trial in the past. Studies have shown that more than half of nonresponders in this diagnostic group will get significantly better if their blood levels are adjusted to the therapeutic range. Nortriptyline is particularly useful in elderly patients and others who get severe postural hypotension, since it has the least of this particular side effect (9). When hypotension remains a problem and the therapeutic range cannot be reached, it may be worthwhile to try enhancing the tricyclic with 10–25 mg/day of methylphenidate, if there are no contraindications (10). The increased adrenergic tone from the stimulant may counteract the blood pressure difficulties as well as boost the blood level of the CA. Among the CAs, desipramine has the least anticholinergic properties, although for sensitive patients there may still be problems in this respect (11).

The milligrams of oral medication taken are not well correlated with blood levels for any of the antidepressants. Side effects are also not a useful guide as to when therapeutic levels have been reached. For example, anticholinergic effects appear and sometimes reach their peak well below the dose required for antidepressant efficacy (12). In treatment-refractory cases, it is common to find that extremely low or extremely high doses are needed to get effective blood levels. Also, the clinician must be prepared to wait 4–6 weeks for the full effect (13), although some improvement in symptoms usually occurs in the first week or two (for *all* antidepressants) when the patient is on the way to a response. There is evidence that rapid initial dosaging (if the patient can tolerate it) leads to faster improvement (14).

If an adequate CA trial (15) as described briefly above has failed, there are several options available depending on factors such as the urgency and severity of the situation, the patient's likelihood of experiencing particular side effects, and patient compliance and consent. They are listed in Table 10-2 (16-37). As can be seen, the choices will probably be dictated by the circumstances. Even patients with chronic presentations (2–20 years) have been shown to be capable of full recovery with vigorous pharmacotherapy, although probably less frequently than those with episodic courses (38). Therefore, one is usually justified in strongly recommending pursuing these potentially toxic and inconvenient drug combinations for the refractory unipolar patient.

Maintenance treatment, if indicated, should initially be with the medications associated with the clinical response. Then it is often possible in future months (or years) to gradually reduce or eliminate elements of the treatment program if full remission is achieved.

Delusional Unipolar Depression

The weight of evidence suggests that delusional unipolar depression is a separate entity from the nondelusional variety (39). The delusions are affect-consonant (40) and include somatic, nihilistic, and paranoid delusions, and they typically occur late in the progression of an episode of the depressive illness rather than as the initial symptoms. The latter course puts the patient in the schizo-affective category, in this classification.

TABLE 10-2 Treatment Alternatives for Refractory Nondelusional Unipolar Depression

Treatment	Comment	References
Adding lithium to CA (0.5–1.0 mEq/L)	Often rapid response in 2–14 days. May also augment a monoamine oxidase inhibitor (MAOI) or nontypical antidepressant	12–15
Adding triiodothyronine T3 (25–50 micrograms in A.M.)	Said to be particularly useful if pretreatment elevated thyroid-stimulating hormone (TSH) and/or low normal T4 in female patients, but this is unclear	16, 17
Trial of different antidepressant	If initial trial with heterocyclic with good levels, try nontypical such as trazodone or fluoxetine	18, 19
Substituting an MAOI	Often effective. Diet a problem for many patients. Many problem drug interactions: patients should wear medical alert identification. Do not switch to another MAOI without waiting 2 weeks. Tranylcypromine may be preferred, especially in the elderly.	20–23
Electroconvulsive Therapy (ECT)	Most effective, but must still find drug treatment maintenance in many cases. Lithium and MAOIs recommended in refractory cases.	24, 25
Combining MAOI and CA	Should not use imipramine or desipramine. Probably can be done safely, though back-up consultation needed to justify. Superiority to others in table questionable.	26
Adding L-tryptophan to CA	4–6 g/day in divided doses between meals or with carbohydrate meal; or with 0.5–1.0 g nicotinic acid.	27, 28
Adding methylphenidate, 10–25 mg/day to CA or MAOI	Tolerance may develop after a few weeks; attempt to withdraw at that point if positive response. May be useful if childhood history of attention deficit disorder (speculation).	29, 30

TABLE 10-2 (*continued*)

Treatment	Comment	References
Alprazolam	High urinary 3-methoxy 4-hydroxy-phenylglycol (MHPG) may predict response.	31, 36
Carbamazepine	Better in bipolars; occasionally works dramatically in unipolars. Might work as an enhancer with tricyclics.	37

Delusional depression tends to recur. Thus, subsequent episodes of depression in a patient with a *clear* history of *delusional* depression, nondelusional should probably be treated as delusional.

Cyclic antidepressants are generally ineffective in delusional depression, although amitriptyline alone may be effective in some patients (41). Table 10-3 shows the treatment choices available (16, 19, 33, 35-50). In the acute phase, delusional depression is more severe. Though electroconvulsive therapy (ECT) is the most rapid and effective treatment, other alternatives are available. Determination of the most effective maintenance program is very necessary and advised since delusional depression carries a higher risk for relapse or ongoing impaired functioning (45), so the least morbidity is associated with finding and then staying with an effective maintenance drug regimen. There is evidence that at least one drug, generally ineffective in acute treatment of unipolar depression (lithium), can nevertheless be of value for maintenance following ECT (46). This effect was mostly seen in the second 6 months of the 1-year follow-up, and the patients were not ECT-refractory cases. Intuition suggests that for any individual patient, it would be better to select a maintenance regimen from among potentially beneficial but untried acute treatments, rather than choosing a drug that was tried in the past and found clearly ineffective during a symptomatic phase.

TABLE 10-3 Treatment Alternatives for Unipolar Delusional Depression

Treatment	Comment	References
ECT	80%–90% effective; must estimate maintenance treatment, but lithium is suggested	42, 43
Antipsychotic and CA	Effective in up to 80%. Takes 4–5 weeks. Perphenazine and amitriptyline most widely used. Full doses of both drugs optimum	41
CA and lithium	Suggestive evidence only	16
Antidepressant and methylphenidate	One study plus anecdotal experience	33, 44
MAOI and lithium	Recent report	18, 19
Antipsychotic, CA, and lithium	May only work in bipolar depressives	48, 49
Carbamazepine	Recent case report	50

In using combination antipsychotic and antidepressant therapy, better results were reported when perphenazine was used in doses averaging 50 mg/day. When other antipsychotics are used, an equivalent amount should probably be employed, if one can generalize from a recent study. Amitriptyline doses needed to be in the 200-mg range with blood levels over 180 ng/ml, for best results. Other CAs should be used in comparable doses. One must be prepared to wait longer than with nondelusional patients for the clinical results, usually 4 or 5 weeks.

Maintenance treatment involving an antipsychotic is a concern because of tardive dyskinesia. It would seem plausible that the combination treatment, if needed to treat the patient acutely, will probably also be needed for maintenance. Yet, because of the risks of tardive dyskinesia, some have recommended that these patients be offered a CA alone to see if that will be effective (47). An alternative might be lithium plus an antidepressant, although there is only suggestive evidence of such a combination being effective acutely. The patient may well consent to continued use of the combination of antipsychotic and antidepressant in order to have the best chance of minimizing recurrence of this severe illness. For delusional patients who fail to respond to combination therapy, addition of lithium as a third drug has been

BIPOLAR DEPRESSION

Treatment strategies for refractory bipolar depression differ somewhat from unipolar, so it is important to correctly diagnose this condition (50) (see Table 10-1). It is characterized by a younger average age of onset, although many cases begin in adolescence and there is often a family history of bipolar disorder. The diagnosis is made by the history of spontaneous or drug-induced periods of hypomania or mania. Psychomotor retardation and hypersomnia have been reported to be characteristic symptoms in bipolar depressives. Low urinary 24-hour MHPG levels are very highly associated with this diagnosis and probably as well with schizo-affective depression as defined in this classification (51).

The biggest problem with these patients is finding ways to treat their depression without inducing more rapid cycling. Studies have shown as many as 69% of female bipolar depressives may become manic if treated with a cyclic antidepressant (52). Yet maintenance treatment with lithium alone is often less successful for the depressed phase than for the manic phase (53). Neuroleptic use during the manic phase also seems to induce more depression (54).

Therefore, in attempting to treat refractory bipolar depression, it is suggested that antidepressant therapy be maintained at a lower dose or removed following acute use. However, the same alternatives suggested in Table 10-2 for unipolars may still be used. For nonpsychotic bipolars, antipsychotics should be removed if possible. By contrast, they will usually be needed for psychotically depressed bipolars, just as with delusional unipolar patients. Lithium or some other antimanic treatment (such as carbamazepine, clonidine, valproic acid, or verapamil) will need to be included in the regimen.

It is interesting that the antidepressant bupropion may become an option for treating depression in sensitive bipolar patients, since it is reported to also have prophylactic effects upon mania and not induce manic breakthrough (55).* However, similar early claims for

---

*Bupropion has been removed from the market by USFDA but continues to have reasearch programs associated with it.

trazodone seem not to have been realized with subsequent experience, so enthusiasm must be guarded.

Maintenance ECT at approximately monthly intervals has anecdotal support for effectiveness in sustaining the euthymic state (56). Lithium must be stopped at least 48 hours before each ECT, and anticonvulsants regimens probably should be held overnight to avoid interference with the ECT convulsion (57).

The options for treating rapid cyclers and refractory manic-depressive patients is reviewed in more detail in the section on treatment-resistant psychoses.

CHARACTEROLOGICAL DEPRESSION

This very large group of patients comprises some of the toughest problems for clinicians and their consultants because of their generally less satisfactory response to drug treatment and, indeed, to treatment in general. Some dramatic results do occur with certain subgroups, but with most, the effect of drugs, if any, is to reduce the intensity of their dysphoria or overreactivity rather than eliminate it. Consequently, excessive expectations for medication, or hostile antitherapeutic transference attitudes on the part of the patient, can mask or undermine drug effects that actually are in a positive direction. The clinician must carefully negotiate the drug treatment and do psychotherapeutic work around the patient's attitude toward his or her illness and medications in order to achieve maximum benefits. When the therapist is not the prescribing physician, the potential for these problems increases because of the frequently distorted attitudes that a nonmedical therapist may have about medication, which may make it difficult for him or her to explore the patient's covert attitudes objectively. Thus, diagnosis of the characterological subtype must be made early in the consultation in order to be able to approach these treatment-difficult depressions in the appropriate comprehensive manner.

As shown in Table 10-1, the history, course, and symptoms contrast significantly with the unipolar and bipolar groups. These patients are chronically depressed by their own report, but only intermittently depressed by objective observation. Their extreme reactivity to environmental events on a moment-to-moment basis is the key symptom characteristic. Following a disappointment, criticism, or rejection, they may experience intense, painful dysphoria and despair, only to have this clear in moments on receiving a kindly word or glance from someone important to them. Even while suffering, they are able to state what would make them feel better, unlike truly anhedonic patients. Often they feel considerable anger at those whom they see as withholding what would make them happy. This can certainly include the psychopharmacologist; thus prescribing zeal has to be tempered by concern about the potential for the patient to overdose in a fit of rage or disappointment. Their mental alertness and intensity, picking up on every clue from their environment that could signal loss or potential gratification of their needs, also contrasts with the psychic dullness or confusion of unipolar patients when depressed.

Other characteristics, including relatively good work functioning, tendency to employ substances abusively to deal with dysphoria, and the common co-occurrence of this syndrome with more drug-responsive symptoms of unipolar depression ("double depression") (58) are also noted in Table 10-1.

Identification of certain subtypes of characterological depression may point to specific drug treatments that can be extremely effective, so a first step should be to review the differential diagnostic list, which includes panic disorder, borderline personality disorder, atypical depression, eating disorders, and post-traumatic stress disorder.

Panic Disorder

The disabling effects of this condition leads to depressive preoccupations, demoralization, and secondary characterological-pattern depressive symptoms that can mask the primary problem of an anxiety disorder. A careful history focusing on the initial onset of symptoms, as well as the *most* distressing present symptomatology will often lead to this diagnosis and more specific pharmacotherapy such as an MAOI, imipramine, clonazepam, or alprazolam (59,60). The benzodiazepines are probably less useful when the panic is accompanied by the depressive symptoms of unipolar disorder. Other CAs and trazodone may also be useful, although this is much less well documented.

Borderline Personality Disorder

Even with DSM-III criteria, this is a heterogenous group of patients (61). Some clearly are subsyndromal affective disorder or cyclothymic patients who should be tried on lithium (62). Others, who have a soft-core thought disorder with features like blocking, slightly loose associations, and paranoid ideation, may benefit from low doses of an antipsychotic (63). Those with transient psychotic (primarily paranoid) experiences, not secondary to substance abuse, probably meeting criteria of Gunderson (64) although not of DSM-III, could be tried on either lithium or an antipsychotic. Low-dose lithium (serum level 0.2–0.5 mEq/L) has anecdotally been found more useful than "standard" doses in this patient group. Monoamine oxidase inhibitors are also sometimes helpful, although CAs are frequently disappointing. Another portion of these patients may have an organic impairment with subictal limbic seizure activity, which produces sharply delineated episodes (lasting up to hours) of fear, anger, depression, panic-anxiety, and occasionally eroticism (65). Neurological consultation and electroencephalograms (EEGs) (especially sleep-deprived or with nasopharyngeal leads) sometimes help confirm the diagnosis, but often it must be made on clinical grounds. Useful drugs include clorazepate (most benign) (66), clonazepam, carbamazepine (most effective), and valproic acid (65).

All drug treatments are to be used with great caution in borderline patients, since these patients often attach profound meaning to the introduction and manipulation of drugs. For example, inpatient settings sometimes are a favorable opportunity for a safe, controlled trial of medication, but at other times, the inpatient unit may be the worst possible place and time: a patient may have come in after an overdose, the purpose of which was to express anger at the spouse for uncaring behavior. If the introduction of drug treatment is seen as the doctor's way of suggesting that the patient, not the spouse, must change, then the doctor may be in for trouble!

Impasses in the psychotherapy of difficult, borderline patients commonly stimulate requests for psychopharmacology consultations. Familiarity with key issues in psychotherapeutic care is most useful in handling these consultations (67,68). If the therapist has succumbed to guilty overinvolvement, countertransference hate, or emotional withdrawal, these can be provocative factors in the patient's distress. Utilizing utmost tact, some indirect exploration of the psychotherapy can be done in the context of thoughtful compliance with the (manifest) request for a psychopharmacology consultation.

Characterological Depression

This will ensure that the final recommendations have considered as many contributing variables as possible.

On the other hand, there is always the danger of patients being invested in idealizing the consultant and subsequently calling him or her at times when they are not satisfied with what their doctor is doing. To prevent this splitting, it is best to not discuss recommendations with the patient but only with the referring physician and to deal with any calls by indicating respectfully that you only respond to consultation requests that come directly from their physician.

Many borderline patients do want medication, and gratifying this desire may be a valuable part of the treatment plan, even if the direct pharmacological effects seem small (69). The patients often have an intense sense of empty aloneness and may have a defect in the ability to remember their positive experience of the therapist's comforting presence when they have left the office (70). Having a pill to take is like a transitional object that replaces the therapist for the time being. This becomes less necessary as they are able to feel more trust in the reliable availability and concern of the therapist over time.

Atypical Depression

Considerable effort has been devoted to identifying a group of patients for whom an MAOI would be the treatment of choice. Recent work suggests they are patients with the characterological syndrome as defined here, plus some of these additional features: high levels of anxiety, waves of lethargy, extreme sensitivity to rejection, and excessive eating and sleeping. Phenelzine seems highly effective in these patients, where imipramine is little better than placebo (71) when there is a history of panic attacks. It is unclear if other marketed MAOIs such as tranylcypromine and isocarboxazid would be as specifically effective. Recent work suggests that these three MAOIs do not have identical effects in atypical depressive syndromes (72).

Eating Disorders

Much attention has been focused recently on the use of drugs in bulimia and, to a lesser extent, anorexia nervosa. Although results are inconclusive and dropout rates seem very high (both initially and on even short term follow-up), there is evidence that pharmacotherapy may add something to the other aspects of treatment in this difficult group of patients (73). Cyclic antidepressants and MAOIs, sometimes enhanced by L-tryptophan, have been used in double-blind studies with bulimia. Lithium (74) and nomifensine (75), were also recently reported of value.* All of the drugs seem associated with high sensitivity to side effects in these patients.

Post-traumatic Stress Disorder

Researchers seem to be trying to separate this disorder from the larger group of characterological depression on the hypothesis that this syndrome develops in reaction to specific, often sustained traumata and then takes on a life of its own in that the patient becomes permanently overreactive to any stress that even slightly resembles the original trauma (76). Acute trauma and disasters can also have a profound, long-term impact to distort character, activate depressive or anxiety symptoms, and exacerbate psychosomatic responses (77). Drug treatment may be helpful in modifying the neurochemical substrates of the brain's adaption to the traumatic experience. Mainly anecdotal experience with drugs such as CAs, MAOIs, lithium, and propranolol have been reported so far (78), and the response pattern seems similar to that of the larger group of characterological depressives, namely that dramatic effectiveness is occasionally seen, but over the long run the role of the drugs is unclear.

There are numerous other diagnostic entities that have been proposed as potentially having relatively specific drug treatments associated with them, and there is no doubt that others will appear. However, empiricism will probably dictate the approach to most characterological patients for some time. The essence of the empirical approach may be summarized as follows: begin with guarded optimism and a cautionary attitude about the drugs. Then, the patient might be offered some of the following: a full trial of a CA, a trial of a nontypical antidepressant such as trazodone or alprazolam (*caution*: there are reports of disinhibition with the latter [79]), low-dose lithium, or an MAOI. The combination therapies and ECT have little support in the literature for their use in these patients and are rarely justified.

*Nomifensine was withdrawn from the market after a few cases of fatal hemolytic anemia were reported.

SCHIZOPHRENIA-RELATED DEPRESSION

Depressive symptoms occur commonly at various points in the course of schizophrenic disorders in up to 50% of patients. These symptoms also have been shown to be prominent in the early symptoms that occur as prelude to relapse, and in fact, are now considered appropriate target symptoms for reintroduction of antipsychotics (80). It seems unlikely that so much depressive symptomatology should reflect the chance of co-occurrence of depressive and schizophrenic disorders that can be treated concurrently on a symptom-focused basis. In most cases, the symptoms are probably secondary to the schizophrenia. In addition, virtually all the studies bearing on the treatment of depressive symptom complexes in the patients discussed so far made a point of excluding schizophrenic patients. Therefore, those drug studies have little application toward what should be done for schizophrenic patients with depression.

Diagnostic issues in schizophrenia-related depression are noted in Table 10-1. Evidence of schizophrenia is often overlooked in the young treatment-refractory depressed patient, who may have been diagnosed as psychotically depressed, but on careful history taking is revealed to have had a premorbid schizotypal personality, or 6 months of prodomal schizophrenia symptoms as listed in DSM-III. Similarly these same substrates may have preceded what looks like a nonpsychotic depression, and on interview with the consultant, the patient finally confesses that he has heard voices for years but did not tell anyone, including his therapist, for fear that they would think he was crazy.

The clinician and family often deny the implications of "crazy" material actually revealed by the patient out of understandable hope that it is not what it sounds like. However, the index of suspicion should be high in depressive presentations in young patients, among whom, on an epidemiological basis, one has a good chance of finding newly emerging cases of schizophrenia. Psychological testing reports, even when projective tests have been employed, often miss the diagnosis and should not be relied upon. The interpretation of the tests in subtle cases often depends on what the examiner considers "formal thought disorder" and other conceptions of schizophrenia that may not be those of DSM-III or the psychopharmacologist.

Other associated features, besides the early age of onset in these patients, include impairment in work and social functioning, substance abuse, and antisocial behavior of a less successful kind than their peers with only personality disorders. Regarding specific symptoms of depression, there have been efforts to subdivide these patients into those with a more anergic, anhedonic presentation (typically seen in the post-psychotic or neurasthenic phase) and those with intense dysphoria, demoralization, and suicidality. So far, no treatment differences have been demonstrated for the two subtypes (81).

Drug-treatment strategies for depression in schizophrenia have been disappointing. Controlled studies of adding antidepressants (CAs or MAOIs) or placebo to antipsychotics for depression in various phases of schizophrenia have overwhelmingly failed to demonstrate any positive effect of the active drug (82). On the other hand, most studies show little harm done in the form of worsening psychosis, although this has been frequently reported anecdotally. In the real world, it seems to be a widespread practice to employ CAs in schizophrenic patients. As newer agents are marketed, claims appear that they may be especially useful in these patients. Trazodone, for example, is undergoing investigation to try to substantiate an earlier report in this regard (83).

The following steps are recommended for the treatment-refractory patient with a schizophrenia-related depression.

1. If an antipsychotic has not been prescribed, a reasonable first step is the discontinuation of the current antidepressant treatments and substitution of an antipsychotic. This is particularly appropriate in the young patient presenting with a nonpsychotic depressive syndrome who has a clear history of a schizotypal personality. These patients should not be given an antidepressant alone because clinical experience suggests that extremely high rates of psychotic reactions have been reported to occur (as high as 40%) (84).

2. If the patient is already on antipsychotics, it is well to first look for akinesia or catatonic symptoms that could be secondary to drug treatment. Dosage reduction and/or treatment of these side effects with anticholinergic antiparkinson agents or amantadine may be effective in ameliorating the depressive picture (85,86).

3. If CAs are currently being employed and have been ineffective, they should probably be discontinued on the possibility that they are contributing to the depressive picture through

central anticholinergic toxicity or other nonspecific behavioral toxicity (87).

4. If the antipsychotic itself has not been demonstrably effective, the patient deserves a trial off it to at least minimize the risk of tardive dyskinesia. Some depressive symptoms may also be improved to the extent that they are the result of side effects from the antipsychotic.

5. There is no convincing evidence that drugs such as thiothixene, thioridazine, and loxapine have more antidepressant effects in schizophrenia than the other antipsychotics.

6. Empirically, a trial of lithium in addition to the antipsychotic may help some portion of the patient's symptoms. However, as with bipolar disorder, lithium has been reported to be less effective for the depressive compared to the excited phase of schizo-affective disorder (88).

7. If not previously tried, a CA or trazodone may be offered with minimal enthusiasm and with encouragement to discontinue the drug if a clear effect is not seen.

8. Some schizophrenic patients may become extremely suicidal, usually on a delusional basis. They may be totally preoccupied with the desire to kill themselves, and may require active restraint to prevent self-injury. Electroconvulsive therapy can be lifesaving in these instances. This does not definitively treat the depression or the schizophrenia, but usually resolves the acute crisis and enables the patient to return to his/her previous baseline (89).

9. For post-psychotic depressive patterns, it may be predicted that the affective symptoms will probably spontaneously improve in 3-6 months with or without antidepressant treatment, assuming adjustment has been made in dosage of the antipsychotic to minimize behavioral toxicity (90).

SCHIZO-AFFECTIVE DEPRESSION

For the purposes of this classification, schizo-affective disorder is defined as one in which DSM-III schizophrenic symptoms occur in the absence of a premorbid history of schizotypal personality features or DSM-III prodromal characteristics such as asocial, eccentric, or bizarre behavior (91). The psychotic symptoms may be episodic or chronic with exacerbations, but they are predominantly of the "positive" variety such as delusions and hallucinations (92). The clinician is often reluctant to diagnose these patients as schizophrenic because of their emotional warmth, capacity to relate to the examiner, and motivation for psychotherapy, even though they may have been hallucinating continuously for years. Their functioning in work, child care, and relationships is often surprisingly good despite their ongoing symptoms (see Table 10-1).

When the disorder is episodic, the characteristic course in the depressive episodes seems to be initial onset of psychotic symptoms followed by depressive symptoms as the patient becomes aware of impairment in concentration and functioning secondary to the thought disorder. This is in contrast to patients with delusional depression who most often initially experience depressive symptoms followed by psychotic ideation as the condition gets more and more severe. Another typical course in schizo-affective depression is to have simultaneous acute symptoms of depression and psychosis, and for the psychotic symptoms to dominate the clinical picture. Another distinguishing feature of this diagnosis is the generally much earlier average age of onset compared to delusional depression.

As with schizophrenic patients, there are highly variable patterns to the depressive symptoms, which, due to the lack of directly applicable research, so far cannot be broken down in a way that leads to specific drug treatment strategies. Thus, both unipolar and characterological symptoms may be present in various combinations. Delusions may be affect-consonant or nonconsonant; for the latter, a greater family history of schizophrenia has been found, and therefore the prognosis may be worse.

Despite the lack of data, there is reason to be more optimistic about the prognosis with schizo-affective depressives, compared with the schizophrenic group. Yet, there is a much more guarded prognosis compared to bipolar or unipolar patients (45,93). The current trend to apply the label "bipolar" to all patients who are not clearly chronic schizophrenic obscures the reality that there is this middle prognosis group for whom a more cautionary attitude is appropriate. This attitude enables the patient and family to begin the grief work and movement toward possible acceptance of the presence of a major disability that is an integral part of the rehabilitation process. Treatment resistance is experienced as doubly devastating in the context of excessive implied promises for the outcome of drug and/or psychotherapy treatment in these often engaging, rescue-fantasy-stimulating patients. Nevertheless, given the prognostic variability, the clinician is certainly justified in attempting an aggressive drug treatment approach in the refractory case. As might be expected, due to the lack of research on treatment of schizo-affective depressions as defined here, empiricism will again be the main guidepost. The following steps are suggested:

1. First, employ treatments appropriate to bipolar depression, with use of lithium and attempts to minimize or eliminate the antipsychotic (pages 279–280 and Table 10-2). These patients may be at above-average risk for tardive dyskinesia (94), so the necessity of the antipsychotic medication should be established. Sometimes chronic hallucinations and suicidal preoccupations are not influenced in any way by antipsychotics.

2. Electroconvulsive therapy is an option in refractory cases and usually is dramatically effective initially. Unfortunately, relapse can occur within weeks of the end of treatment. Recently, there has been renewed advocacy of ECT as a treatment that can work in schizophrenic psychoses (95). However, if no effective drug maintenance program has been found, the practical limits of ECT are soon reached, except for the occasional patient who can tolerate maintenance ECT treatments every 2–4 weeks.

3. Experience suggests that ultimately an antipsychotic is going to be a necessary component of treatment. In obtaining informed consent, it is appropriate to indicate that trials of treatments for affective disease pursuant to the first step described above carry sufficient risk of resulting in relapse or failure to respond. This should be weighed against the risks of neuroleptic therapy. It is important that the patient be brought into the center of the treatment cost–benefit deliberative process, rather than being directed toward a long list of treatments that have limited promise of effectiveness.

An approach to the clinical diagnosis and management of treatment-resistant cases of depression and dysphoria has been presented. The first step involves classifying the patient into one of five categories based on course, symptoms, and response patterns to drug treatment (if any are presently established). A treatment plan, including an impression of the likely benefits from further interventions, can then be formulated and shared with clinicians, patient, and family. This step in itself can be highly therapeutic. Then a course of treatment can be chosen that is in an appropriate context. As new data on course or symptoms arises, reformulation of the situation is readily accomplished.

Laboratory tests, such as the dexamethasone suppression test (DST), thyrotropin-releasing hormone (TRH) stimulation, urinary MHPG, platelet MAO, stimulant challenge, and other procedures are under active study to see if they can match or improve on the predictive power of the clinical measures described here. What seems most likely is that they will not substitute for comprehensive clinical assessment, but rather may help at certain points in the decision tree, for example, to make a final choice of what drug to try next. The ability of the tests to do this will probably advance in parallel with advances in our knowledge of how these drugs work in different kinds of depressed patients.

TREATMENT-RESISTANT PSYCHOSES: MANIC, SCHIZO-AFFECTIVE, AND ATYPICAL PRESENTATIONS

There is considerable sentiment toward a system of classification of psychotic disorders in the United States that attempts to define schizophrenia as a chronic, limited-treatment-response disorder, and lumps together most other patients of good or uncertain prognosis under the heading of bipolar disorder and variants (96). This spectrum concept of affective disorder and fixed notion of schizophrenia is interesting to contrast with the approach of Manfred Bleuler (97), whose nosology is much more popular in Europe. He uses a spectrum concept for schizophrenia, based on his father's pioneering work; only a small percent of Bleulerian schizophrenics have a chronic downhill course and many fully recover. Bipolar illness is defined with more limiting parameters.

Since the validity of neither approach has been established, it remains to be seen which is more useful to the practicing clinician. The spectrum concept of affective disease carries the implication that all these psychotic patients might respond to one of the growing list of drug treatments thought to be useful in bipolar illness. It suggests that antipsychotics may not be needed and so risk of tardive dyskinesia may be minimized. It avoids the discouraging connotations of the schizophrenic label. On the negative side, as discussed earlier (page 288–289), it sets up unrealistic rehabilitative therapeutic processes involving mourning the loss of normal functioning that the disease often causes and working toward family and patient acceptance of, and adaptation to, some degree of chronic disability.

A valuable first step is to discuss the benefits and risks of the various interventions with the patient and family in the light of a realistic prognostic assessment given past treatment response, family history of mental illness, and number of "negative" symptoms and schizotypal traits predictive of poor outcome. Then it is possible to embark on a reasonable treatment plan in a conducive atmosphere.

Here are some steps recommended in sorting out what to do with treatment-resistant psychotic individuals.

1. As with the depressive disorders, it is again assumed that the clinician has ruled out or dealt with the medical differential diagnosis, which involves various etiologies which have been recently reviewed (98). In recent years there has been a growing interest in neurological disorders that have psychiatric manifestations, such as temporal lobe epilepsy and other brain electrical disorders that may produce behavioral symptoms through a kindling-like process (99,100). Although electroencephalographic (EEG) and other laboratory evidence of such subictal mood or psychotic disorders (in the absence of evidence of clinical seizures) might have important treatment implications, such as suggesting the use of antiepileptic agents, clear support for this assertion is still lacking.

2. Often more fruitful is a close inquiry into potential sources of behavioral toxicity in the patient's current or recent drug regimen. Table 10–4 presents a list of common problems that should be eliminated before proceeding to more definitive

TABLE 10-4 Some Causes of Drug-Induced Behavioral Toxicity in Psychotic Patients

Examples	Possible Remedies	References
1. Akinesia	a. Lower dose of antipsychotic. b. Anticholinergic therapy a distant second choice remedy.	101
2. Akathisia	a. Lower dose of antipsychotic. b. Benzodiazepines and beta blockers are often better than anticholinergics.	102, 103
3. Catatonic (lead-pipe) rigidity from high potency neuroleptics	a. Discontinue neuroleptic if possible, restart later, if indicated, at much lower dose and be prepared to wait longer for desired effect. b. Amantadine and IV benzodiazepines may be useful. c. Observe for signs of neuroleptic malignant syndrome (elevated temp. and blood pressure, elevated serum CPK).	85, 104-107
4. Oversedation	a. Taper and discontinue high dose benzodiazepines. b. If lithium and neuroleptic are both being used, lower doses or elimination of one probably necessary, especially if partial clinical response has occurred. c. Sedating antidepressants may be contributing.	
5. Rapid irregular (metabolic) tremor	a. Look for lithium toxicity. May be present even if serum levels not elevated, especially if neuroleptic also being used. May also occur with excessive neuroleptic doses.	108
6. Confusional state from anticholinergic toxicity	a. Eliminate contributing causes such as antiparkinson drugs, cyclic antidepressants, thioridazine and chlorpromazine.	109

treatments (85, 101–108). Often considerable, if not complete, recovery will occur during this step.

3. In contrast to the depressive disorders, there seem at this time to be relatively few pharmacological treatment implications to diagnostic subdivisions of the affective psychoses. They are all at least potentially suitable for the drug treatments to be proposed, at least in the refractory case. The consultant may want to offer a prognostic estimate, however, and it is plausible that prominent negative symptoms, schizotypal premorbid personality traits, failure to return to normal functioning between episodes, and continuous illness for more than 6 months could be indicators of guarded prognosis. A patient who has just lost key social supports, and has not functioned independently in the past, is not expected to do well, particularly after discharge, without comparable replacements. Rapid cycling (three or more episodes per year) would be another negative predictor (109).

4. For pharmacotherapy, lithium salts are generally the first recommendation for this spectrum of illnesses. Blood levels up to 1.2 mEg/L or more may be necessary. These atypical cases are mistaken for schizophrenia or delusional depression because of obscure manic symptoms. For example, increased libido may have been missed because increased sexual interest and sensations in persons subjected to strict prohibitions in childhood may be dramatically denied or disguised. Projection of sexual impulses ("men are after me") may be prominent in these patients. Lithium can be dramatically effective in terminating these episodes, which have been termed "dysphoric mania."

5. For the patient whose psychosis has not responded to lithium, or who is not well maintained on this drug, the next drug of choice is probably carbamazepine. As Table 10–5 indicates (32,111–134), it is the most established newer treatment, although it has potential for toxicity and must be closely monitored, particularly for suppression of white cell and platelet counts. These should be checked every 2 weeks for 2 months, and every 3 months thereafter, and the patient should be instructed to report symptoms of infection

TABLE 10–5 Alternatives to Lithium in Manic Psychosis and its Variants

Drug	Type	Daily Dosage	Major Side Effects	Comment	References
Carbamazepine	Anticonvulsant	600–1600 mg/day	Suppression of white count, platelet count	Most established as effective. Blood levels 6–12 μg/ml. Have patient report any sign of infection	111–114
Valproic acid	Anticonvulsant	750–1500 mg/day	Hepatic toxicity: Must monitor SGOT, PT, bilirubin, alkaline phosphatase weekly for a month, then bimonthly	Considerable use in Europe. Blood levels 50–100 μg/ml. Causes nausea, tremor, weight gain, hair loss. Best effect may be when combined with lithium.	115–118
Verapamil	Calcium channel blocker	160–320 mg/day	Contraindicated in congestive heart failure due to negative inotropic effect	Promising because of low side effects. Limited use in refractory cases. Causes constipation, vertigo, headache.	121–125
Clonidine	Antihypertensive	0.4–2.0 mg/day	Lowered blood pressure	Must be increased very slowly	126
Thyroxine (T4)	Hormone	Up to 0.3–0.5 mg/day	Excess stimulation, cardiac toxicity	Dose started at 0.1 mg and increased or decreased by 0.1 mg/week. Give at least 0.1 if T4 less than 6 in rapid cyclers.	127
L-Tryptophan added to lithium	Amino acid	4–10 g/day	Weight gain, nausea, sedation	Must be taken between meals, at bedtime, or with carbohydrate snack	32, 128
Clonazepam	Anticonvulsant	0.5–16 mg/day	Sedation, ataxia	Few serious side effects. Long-term effectiveness questionable.	129–131
Methylene blue	Dye: affects electrolyte transport	200 mg/day		One case report: included here for heuristic interest.	134

promptly (114). Other common side effects include gastric irritation, sedation, and ataxia. Hepatic and renal toxicity are seen rarely. Clinicians not familiar with this drug should consult recent reviews as to the spectrum of problems encountered (111,114). Some neurologists have observed that the hazards of this drug have been exaggerated and that it causes less agranulocytosis than chlorpromazine (135). On the other hand, some advocate even more frequent monitoring than indicated above and suggest testing for serial serum iron as well (136).

Carbamazepine is most clearly effective in manic-depressive patients but is beneficial in a smaller percentage of schizo-affective and atypical cases. When it is effective, both manic and depressive phases seem to be reduced, though the effect on the manic phase may be somewhat greater. It may be especially useful in rapid cyclers who fail to respond to lithium (110). There is disagreement as to whether there is any correlation between benefits and the presence of EEG abnormalities. It may be combined with lithium salts, sometimes to advantage (137), although there are some reports of toxicity (138). A useful strategy when lithium seems to have been of at least some benefit is to add carbamazepine, see how the patient does, and later try to discontinue the lithium if the patient does well. Combining carbamazepine with an MAOI can lead to problems since the drug is structurally related to the CAs. We have seen hypertensive-neurotoxic reactions with phenelzine, although there is a report with tranylcypromine in which no problems occurred (139). It is unclear if any (as yet undemonstrated) benefit of that combination would be worth the risks.

Although no correlation between response and plasma level has been demonstrated, clinicians generally start slowly (200–400 mg/day) and gradually raise the dose until blood levels reach the antiepileptic range of 6–12 μg/ml. It is somewhat tricky to reach this range, since the drug tends to induce hepatic enzymes over the first several weeks of use, requiring gradually increased oral dose, often to well over 1,000 mg/day. However, other patients are highly sensitive to side effects and may only be able to tolerate 400 mg/day.

Patients who are known or likely good responders to lithium but have developed unacceptable side effects may not do well on carbamazepine (140). In these cases we often recommend considering one of the alternatives in step 6, below.

6. The rest of the pharmacological alternatives for treatment of refractory or lithium-intolerant affective psychoses are shown in Table 10-5. This is not necessarily the order in which they would be tried; that depends on the clinical presentation of the patient and individual side-effect sensitivities that might be predicted.

    Most of the work with valproate involves lithium nonresponders, while clonazepam has primarily been reported as an alternative to lithium in probable lithium responders. Verapamil has been studied both in lithium responders (121) and nonresponders (122). Valproate seems clearly effective independently (118), although perhaps even more effective (at least in prophylaxis) when combined with lithium (120). It seems to be useful in schizo-affective and overactive paranoid psychoses as well and may potentiate the effects of neuroleptics in those patients (118). Clonazepam, too, was useful in one report with atypical psychoses (132). There has been little reported experience with verapamil in nonbipolar patients.

    For maintenance treatment, carbamazepine and, to a lesser extent, valproate are fairly well-established as effective. Particularly good results have been reported with carbamazepine blood serum levels over 10 μg/ml (112), although it is not clear that levels had to be that high. A single case report of maintenance with verapamil has been described (123). Clonazepam has been used in more than 100 patients for maintenance according to one anecdotal report (133), but this needs to be documented with more systematic observations and replicated by others. Indeed, local experience with acute use of clonazepam in mania has been disappointing so far.

7. Electroconvulsive therapy is a very effective treatment for mania and other affective psychoses. It usually gets employed (subject to availability, which is often lacking in the public sector), when drugs are not working and the psychosis is extremely severe or prolonged to the point where the

patient and family are ready to ignore their biases against it. Patients who have been successfully treated with ECT often want it much earlier during a recurrence than they did originally. Some physicians use it quite early because of the high response rate and rapid effect. A recent report noted that nonresponders to unilateral ECT who subsequently responded to bilateral ECT showed many manic features (141). Accordingly, if no response is seen after 2 weeks of unilateral treatment, it would be reasonable to switch to bilateral treatment of affective psychoses. If the situation is urgent and severe, the physician may consider beginning with bilateral ECT administration.

The larger problem lies, once again, with the choice of maintenance for the patient with a history of recurrent episodes following successful ECT. If previous acute treatments have been ineffective, the clinician is left with two choices: (a) to try one of these ineffective treatments anyway to see if it will work as a maintenance regimen (frequently done but of questionable merit), or (b) to try some treatment that has not been offered in the past, including the alternatives in Table 10–5 (better, but still a guess).

8. The role of antipsychotics has not been stresssed here for the reasons stated earlier, namely that this group of disorders may include many patients who can do without a neuroleptic and be spared the risks of tardive dyskinesia. This does not imply that antipsychotics should always be withheld until every alternative listed here has been tried. It again is a difficult clinical judgment to make, taking into account the patient's symptoms, course, and response to treatment so far, as to when it is time to introduce them. There seems little doubt that for a large number of these patients, neuroleptics will be the most effective treatment available.

TREATMENT-RESISTANT SCHIZOPHRENIA

In this section, pharmacotherapeutic strategies employed with the chronic nonresponsive schizophrenic patient are outlined. The interface between these and the relevant psychosocial interventions that may be necessary are also described. The emphasis is on what to do when standard treatment is not working and the need for a consultation has arisen.

WHAT IS AN ADEQUATE TRIAL OF NEUROLEPTIC THERAPY?

In order to answer the question of what an adequate trial of neuroleptic therapy is, a working conception is needed of the usual pattern of response in chronic (as opposed to acute) patients. Extrapolation from the relatively rapid full response to these drugs (e.g., in 3–6 weeks) seen in many patients with mania, schizo-affective disorders, and so-called acute schizophrenia (from older literature) is clearly inappropriate. Extremely useful in this regard is the 2-year inpatient study of antipsychotics and psychotherapy in chronic schizophrenia from the late 1960s done at Massachusetts Mental Health Center (MMHC) (142). Unlike most contemporary studies, the milieu of the patient for the 2-year period was held quite constant while the primary treatments were being administered. We now know that changes in the environment and social network of these patients can have a potent effect on symptoms and relapse rate, and it is almost impossible to control for these variables in long-term drug treatment studies of contemporary patients who spend so much of their time in the community mental health system (143).

In looking closely at the course of response of the chronic patients on neuroleptic therapy in the MMHC study, it is striking that the improvement was gradual and took place over an extended time. Some were totally unresponsive, as has been confirmed repeatedly over the years in studies employing a variety of methodologies (144). For the responders, however, symptoms slowly improve over 8–12 weeks, reach a plateau, and then, further, small improvements were recorded over the next 3–9 months. Some patients made additional slight gains in the second year of treatment. Some of this gradual improvement may have been due to the concomitant psychotherapy, twice a week, with senior experienced psychodynamically oriented psychiatrists. On the other hand, no improvement, gradual or otherwise, was seen in the control chronic schizophrenics who had psychotherapy and no neuroleptic treatment. Therefore, at the least, the drug enabled the patient to gradually benefit from this particular psychosocial intervention.

The clinical implications of these findings are that chronic patients who are going to respond at standard constant doses do so slowly and steadily if the clinician can be patient and try to control the other variables that tend to obscure the evidence of this progressive drug effect. Examples of these variables would probably include some of the following: premature reduction in structure on the inpatient unit or discharge to a stressful living situation, overmedication producing behavioral toxicity and intolerable side effects, high-pressure "rehabilitation" efforts setting up performance failures, and concomitant physical illness causing pain or disability. Because of the inevitable occurrence of some of these factors, almost no patients seem to follow this smooth course of response. However, it may be reasonable to assume that constant medication has a gradually increasing positive input into the situation, and the physician should avoid the temptation to "treat" all the acute exacerbations and improvements with medication adjustments.

There is often considerable pressure from administrators of hospital units and community programs to medicate in these situations because they want to either get the patient out of some place where they are not wanted (e.g., the hospital) or keep them in some other place where they are not doing well (e.g., home, halfway house). It is no wonder that some people outside of the mental health field have the impression that neuroleptics are something used by psychiatrists to exercise social control over patients! Economic factors can be paramount here; if the busy prescribing physician can spare only 15 minutes to make a comprehensive assessment of a treatment-refractory case, the path of least resistance is to increase or change the medication. This becomes even more likely when the patients are brought to the clinic for evaluation without even a knowledgeable staff member accompanying them who could give the full story to the physician.

The dynamics of the relationship between the "medical backup" physician and the patient's therapist or case manager is also an interesting and powerful factor here (145). The non-medical clinicians are often invested in seeing the sociotherapy as the central influence in the patient's well-being and as their exclusive clinical domain. Psychiatrists and their medications are only on call to be triaged in if felt needed. Yet, the non-medical clinician's omnipotent fantasies about the doctor and the medication are revealed when it becomes clear that they (like the rebellious adolescent) expect that the doctor can solve any problem they have fallen into, with some medication change. If the physician refuses to medicate and tries to take the time to examine and alter elements of the patient's psychosocial regimen, there may be considerable resistance.

Despite the above difficulties, preliminary steps are strongly recommended in evaluating apparent treatment resistance in schizophrenic patients. That is, there should be an investigation for the presence of powerful stressors which drugs cannot be expected to override, combined with insufficient time having elapsed for previous drug therapy to exert its full effect.

Dosage Issues

How is the clinician to decide if the proper dose has been chosen to achieve this maximum effect as described above? In evaluating the treatment-refractory case, three issues that should be considered are: dose–response relationships, drug absorption, and clinical role of plasma levels.

Dose-Response Relationships. It is well documented that most patients get maximum effect from neuroleptic doses in the range of 300–600 mg/day of chlorpromazine or its equivalent (146). No studies have demonstrated any superiority of higher average doses. Yet, it seems to be widespread practice to employ higher doses, both acutely and for maintenance, particularly with high-potency drugs such as haloperidol and fluphenazine. Many physicians seem to feel that the usual doses of these drugs should be 20–40 mg/day (147), even though that is the equivalent of 1,000–3,400 mg/day of chlorpromazine (using conversion ratios of 50:1 to 85:1 suggested in standard texts) (148,149). The dosage adjustment range in which there seems to be a dose–response relationship (i.e., in which, as you raise the dose, you get an increased effect) is between 100 and 300 mg of Chlorpromazine or equivalent.

Although clinical evidence of behavioral toxicity at excessive doses has been frequently cited, recent confirmation of the idea that there may be problems with excessive dosaging has come from work with neuroleptic plasma levels. Evidence of inverted U-shaped curves, or therapeutic windows describing the relationship between response and plasma levels, has been found for the neuroleptics haloperidol, thiothixene, chlorpromazine, and possibly fluphenazine (150, 151). These findings are similar to the well-established plasma level–response curve found for the antidepressant nortriptyline (152). Not all plasma level studies show this pattern, but as larger numbers of patients are being studied, it is becoming possible to discern subpopulations of schizophrenics with different dose–response patterns (153). Thus not all, but some, patients may experience this toxicity at high dosage. To the clinician, this suggests that a justifiable early intervention with the refractory patient is lowering the antipsychotic dose back into a reasonable range (where it may never have been for long) or discontinuing it altogether for a period to allow for clearance of potential toxicity. The likelihood of this being helpful is increased if other obvious side effects, such as parkinsonism, are prominent. If indications for antipsychotic use persist, and particularly if there is a past history of at least some responsiveness to these drugs, then one may be restarted in a low to moderate dose (perhaps with an intermediate potency agent such as molindone or perphenazine), and a suitably long trial be allowed before additional manipulations are employed.

Absorption of Oral Neuroleptic. Another issue to address in approaching patients who are not improving is the question of whether the drugs are being absorbed adequately. Again from the plasma level work, we know there are patients who do not generate significant levels despite quite high oral doses (154). There can be many possible reasons: failure of the drug to be absorbed from the gastrointestinal tract (shown for some patients on chlorpromazine), extensive first-pass liver metabolism immediately after absorption, or breakdown by different metabolic pathways to inactive products (155). A clinical indicator of these patients is the complete absence of any side effects, even on careful examination for subtle degrees of cogwheeling (for example), as well as absence of antipsychotic efficacy. Experience suggests that these probable low plasma-level patients will often generate good levels on intramuscular administration of a neuroleptic (156). Therefore, if this situation is suspected, switching to fluphenazine decanoate would seem a reasonable suggestion if it has not already been tried.

Noncompliance, of course, is perhaps the more common cause of the triad of no side effects–no clinical effects–no blood level, even in the controlled setting of the inpatient unit. If, indeed, the patient has been successful for so long in secretly evading his/her oral medication, then it is certainly overdue to confront that deception. A liquid preparation might be offered, which will be effective in the noncompliance but not in the nonabsorption etiology (157). Alternatively, these patients as well may be offered parenteral medication.

Clinical Role of Plasma Levels. Are there occasions when it is justified to use high oral doses? Clinical experience says definitely yes, but the long-accepted standard approach of using high doses on everyone and then backing down as the patient improves is being replaced by an approach in which the physician begins with standard doses and goes up only if there is adequate justification to expose the patient to the increased risks of toxicity, including tardive dyskinesia (158). Although it is suggested that a neuroleptic plasma level obtained from an experienced commercial laboratory would sometimes aid in that justification, research on these plasma level determinations has clearly not progressed to the point where specific therapeutic ranges for the neuroleptics have been determined. Whether they are of any use at all to the clinician is still debated, with some prominent experts declaring that there is no place for levels in routine clinical use (155,159), and others stating that they do at present have value in helping reduce side effects and improving clinical response (160,161). Our experience supports the latter view. In the treatment-refractory case, an extremely low or zero neuroleptic level adds confidence to a clinical impression that a higher dose or switch to a parenteral preparation is appropriate. It also provides a way of monitoring the effect of these interventions. If the level is extremely high, lowering the dose may be justified, even if the patient has been on a high oral dose and it has seemed necessary.

Here is a frequent clinical situation: it will seem that every time the psychiatrist tries to lower the dose of, for example, haloperidol from 60 to 50 mg/day, the patient becomes more psychotic. Is this a true pharmacological effect, the result of unrelated environmental or internal stress, affective lability secondary to behavioral toxicity, or placebo effect? Patients like this are commonly seen in consultation because they are extremely vulnerable to relapse or severe symptomatology on a day-to-day basis. They may be discharged and then skip their medication for a day and suddenly become psychotic enough to need readmission. We know from clinical research that stable institutionalized patients who have had their antipsychotics suddenly discontinued do not have a relapse rate that significantly exceeds continuously medicated controls until 1 month has passed, and the maximum difference does not occur for 3 months (162). Measurable amounts of neuroleptic continue to be excreted in the urine of such patients for months (163). With fluphenazine decanoate, plasma levels may not decline significantly for 10 weeks or more in some patients following the last injection (164).

How then can these patients relapse so quickly? Some cases may be related to the phenomenon of withdrawal-emergent or "supersensitivity" psychosis, which may involve limbic kindling from repeated off-and-on exposure to the neuroleptic (165). Most, however, seem to be reacting to environmental stress, and the occurrence of this reaction is probably unmasking the ineffectiveness of the current drug regimen. It should not be blamed on missing the 1-day's dose! A serum level might help to determine if this apparent drug ineffectiveness is due to extremely low levels, or excessive levels with behavioral toxicity. Additionally, if the level is somewhere in-between, the interpretation could be that either the drug needs more time to work, or it has reached its maximum effectiveness for that patient, unsatisfactory though that might be (166).

In addition, a prolactin level may further clarify the excessive plasma level situation: if not elevated (as it should be in association with even minimal antipsychotic effect) (167), it could mean the patient is tolerant to the central nervous system effects of the drug even at these high plasma levels. In this event, perhaps a switch to a different neuroleptic would be appropriate with early monitoring of prolactin to see if levels were elevated on the new drug.

Switching to Other Antipsychotics

The preceding discussion of issues in dosaging and how to get the maximum benefit out of any single neuroleptic leads directly to the question of when to switch to a different neuroleptic. For decades, it has been considered axiomatic that for reasons no one has ever been able to specify, patients will sometimes fail to respond to one neuroleptic, but do very well on another. This provides justification for the existence of a large number of drugs with similar, in fact indistinguishable, clinical effects in psychosis, and with differences only in their side-effect profiles. The clinician has been encouraged to try these various options sequentially, in 4- to 6-week trials, in treatment-refractory cases (168). The newer information about drug response which has just been reviewed, however, seriously challenges this practice of switching antipsychotics. A strong clinical impression is developing that when a truly adequate trial of a neuroleptic has failed, the psychiatrist is unlikely to get a response from another. There has been some preliminary examination of this question with small numbers of patients using plasma levels which tends to confirm this idea. When several oral antipsychotics are given to the same patient, they all produce comparable levels of plasma activity, both in responders and nonresponders. Patients failing to respond to a drug despite a typical or average plasma level also fail to respond when tried on other neuroleptics (169).

Nevertheless, sometimes it is worth trying a different neuroleptic if (a) you suspect supersensitivity psychosis and the patient is on a high-potency drug, (b) prolactin levels are not elevated, or (c) side effects of the index neuroleptic have prevented a full therapeutic trial. Otherwise, the psychiatrist would probably be better advised to consider alternative, non-neuroleptic drug treatments.

The question of whether antipsychotics are fully interchangeable is a separate question. Switching medication in clinically stable, chronic schizophrenics may precipitate deterioration (170). However, this may be due to adverse reactions to drugs with different side-effect profiles, or supersensitivity psychosis, rather than differing primary (antischizophrenic) effects of the drugs.

Use of Adjunctive or "As Needed" Antipsychotics

The dosage of tranquilizer can be kept to a minimum by intensive use of the structure of the inpatient milieu. All efforts to reduce potentially stressful stimulation in the environment of the patient should be made through the use of quiet rooms and other sections of the ward into which other patients are not permitted to move freely. As the schizophrenic patient begins to respond to drug treatment, overly rapid restoration of "privileges" in the more stimulating patient areas should be avoided. All too often, the psychiatrist is called to add more medications when, 2 or 3 days after admission, the patient has had a major outburst just after being released to the general ward area after too short a time in the quiet room. Typically at this point, the patient will be given an emergency dose (p.r.n.), his/her standing dose of antipsychotic and/or benzodiazepine will be increased, and he/she will be escorted back to the restricted area. All this could have been avoided if his/her movement to a less restricted setting had been more gradual in keeping with the expected slow buildup of drug effects. Nevertheless, it still does not appear rational to increase medications at this point, p.r.n. or standing. All that is usually necessary is reinstitution of the one treatment that was working well before, namely, the increased structure and decreased stimulation of the quiet room. The original doses of medication, given a little more time, will soon be effective on the underlying condition.

The regular use of p.r.n. medication throughout the admission for the occurrence of agitation has another unfortunate side effect on the patient's understanding of the role of medications in the management of his illness. The message from the doctor and the nurse in the form of the p.r.n. is as follows: "If you feel agitated or about to be out of control, the answer is to take an extra pill." A better message would be: "If you feel agitated, try to identify what is stimulating or upsetting you, and avoid that stress, or talk to a staff member about how you can deal with it more directly and effectively." The latter approach is more likely to foster a sense of self-control and responsibility in the patient over the long run, whereas the former only reinforces inappropriate drug-taking behavior and externalization of responsibility for problem management.

In addition, the antipsychotics have little immediate effect in patients who have been taking them for awhile, and thus a p.r.n. and all medications are viewed as ineffective. When patients notice this and lose faith in the drug, the only option they can consider is more drugs or another drug, or ultimately no drug (which in their minds may require rejection of the entire mental health system). This unfortunate sequence can often be avoided by good patient education from the beginning about the relative roles of drugs and environmental factors in symptom formation. As patients improve, they can take larger roles in monitoring themselves and requesting appropriate assistance when needed.

Nursing staff often strongly believes in the effectiveness of p.r.n. medication, and they may push vigorously to have this management option available to them. At the heart of this pharmacologically irrational attitude may be a feeling that agitated patients are too impaired to respond to simple, direct, firm limits. When the nurse has just given the p.r.n. (especially if intramuscularly), he/she feels confident that the patient will be more docile and will comply with the limits (e.g., to go to and stay in the quiet room). The patient sees from the nurse's firm but relaxed attitude that he/she is expected to be in control and capable of cooperating with the demands made. Accordingly, the patient meets these expectations. Often staff do not see that it is their interpersonal communication and not the magic of the drug that enables the patient to comply with their directives. It is often useful to prove this assertion by demonstrating that for every difficult patient there are certain staff who are remarkably and consistently effective in getting the patient to do what they want done, and others who rarely get a positive response out of the patient. If the effective staff are asked how they do it, the answer invariably is something like, "Oh, that patient knows that when I ask him to do something, I mean business! But, he also knows I like him!"

Thus, inappropriate medication use can be sharply diminished if staff as a whole can be helped to set limits in a clear, firm, but kindly manner, and with a tone of expectation that they will be obeyed. Physical size, sex, age, or professional status of the staff member bears little relationship to effectiveness; sometimes the tiniest elderly mental health assistant can be a model for the entire hospital staff.

This is not meant to suggest that there are not some very violent patients, both acute and chronic, who can only be managed safely in a setting more secure than the usual inpatient facility, and/or who may temporarily at least need high doses of tranquilizers for purposes of chemical restraint.

ADDITIONAL DRUG TREATMENTS IN SCHIZOPHRENIA

Benzodiazepine drugs and lithium salts seem to have important roles in the management of some difficult cases of schizophrenia. When their benefits have been exhausted, the clinician is left with few good alternatives. Propranolol and carbamazepine may occasionally be of some benefit, and some of the newer treatments for affective psychosis reviewed earlier (Table 10–5) might have at least a remote chance of helping. We will review these alternatives in more detail.

Benzodiazepines in Schizophrenia

There are now over 60 published reports on the potential uses of the benzodiazepine tranquilizers in psychotic patients (171). This contrasts with earlier views that they had little role to play. It seems that when used in high oral doses or with parenteral administration, they do help treat the psychotic process, either by reducing the level of arousal and its psychosis-exacerbating effect, or by direct antipsychotic actions of their own. There is evidence that, through a complex mechanism involving facilitation of GABAergic neurons (gamma aminobutyric acid; a GABAergic neuron is a neuron that uses GABA as a neurotransmitter), benzodiazepines in high doses can produce dopamine blockade to a clinically significant degree (172).

As has been discussed, the evidence is beginning to mount that use of doses of antipsychotic larger than absolutely necessary for antipsychotic effect is unwise, both because there may be decreased efficacy at higher doses, and because there will be unnecessary additional exposure to the risk of side effects, including tardive dyskinesia. Management of agitation in the acute phase may be accomplished as well or better by the addition of benzodiazepines, than by the traditional approach of using higher-dose neuroleptics. Doses of, for example, 4-30 mg/day of lorazepam, given orally, intramuscularly, or intravenously in divided doses within the first few days of admission, have been successful in treating acutely manic patients (173). This can also be prescribed for the schizophrenic patient who is not adequately contained on a standard neuroleptic regimen.

Benzodiazepines have been used in extremely high doses (6 weeks of 200 mg of diazepam per day for example) for chronic treatment-refractory patients in a few studies (174). Possibly this treatment would only work in patients who have not had an adequate trial of dopamine blockade by a traditional neuroleptic. This would be the expected pattern if high-dose benzodiazepines work through dopaminergic mechanisms. Therefore, we have not been enthusiastic about this treatment alternative.

Lithium in Schizophrenia

Literature reviews have concluded that one-third to one-half of schizophrenic patients appear to benefit from treatment with lithium carbonate (88). This would seem to make it a reasonable, early option in approaching the neuroleptic-refractory case. The mechanism is unknown, though it seems to be more than just the raising of cellular levels of antipsychotic, as some have argued from animal studies. The improvement frequently involves affective symptoms and hyperactivity, but core schizophrenic symptoms may also improve, even with lithium alone (175). When lithium is going to be effective, significant improvement almost always begins in the first week (175). Sometimes the prominent lithium effect will be on impulse control, and it will seem that the primary benefit has been on concomitant (and often disabling) characterological difficulties.

When lithium is added to a neuroleptic, and significant benefit occurs, there is often a decreased need for the neuroleptic. The patient may become overly sedated, or show other signs of behavioral toxicity. This can be difficult to assess, but usually it is best to lower the dose of the neuroleptic and keep the lithium level moderate. Phenothiazines may raise intracellular lithium levels such that early signs of lithium toxicity may be seen despite apparently moderate plasma levels (176).

Carbamazepine and Propranolol in Schizophrenia

These two drugs, which are now being used in a growing list of psychiatric disorders, have been suggested as potentially beneficial in refractory schizophrenia.

Carbamazepine seems to be effective much less often in schizophrenia than in bipolar or even schizo-affective disorders. Nevertheless, case reports and anecdotal experience suggest that among chronic, hospitalized patients, there are a few who respond to this compound (115, 177). There so far seems to be no reliable correlation with presence or absence of EEG abnormalities, or with diagnosis of complex partial seizures. As with lithium, the symptoms that respond are unpredictable, and degrees of response range from slight to dramatic. Neuroleptic blood levels may be sharply lowered by concomitant use of carbamazepine. The clinical signficance is unclear, but the clinician should keep this in mind.

Propranolol generated some enthusiasm a few years ago as an adjunct in refractory schizophrenia (179), although recent experience has not supported this impression. It seems to raise neuroleptic plasma levels by up to several fold, which may be the mechanism of its action. However, several independent studies have shown that it helps control aggression in brain-damaged and mentally retarded individuals with conduct disorders; some schizophrenics were among those treated (180). Many patients were helped when propranolol was the only drug prescribed. Doses ranged from 20 mg/day up to 1,200 mg/day after gradual increases. Most patients seem to do well between 80 and 250 mg/day, and doses higher than that produce problems with hypotension. However, schizophrenic patients seem to tolerate, and eventually require, the higher doses. It is not unreasonable, when all else has failed, and with informed consent, to give propranolol or carbamazepine a cautious trial in the entrenched, treatment-resistant case of schizophrenia.

New Leads

Research offers hope for the future, although it has been estimated that it will be at least 5–10 years before any new drugs for the treatment of schizophrenia will be marketed (181). Remoxipride is a dopamine blocker which seems specific for the mesolimbic dopamine type 2 (D2) receptors and has little impact on the nigrostriatal dopamine pathway and consequently no parkinsonian side effects (and presumably no tardive dyskinesia). It has been reported to be effective in schizophrenic patients (182), but presumably it would work in the same spectrum of patients for which traditional neuroleptics are effective.

The search for drugs that work in an entirely different manner is more difficult, and there have been few promising leads. Vasopressin was recently reported helpful in improving symptoms in patients with schizophrenia (183). This is not a new idea, as the drug was first reported as useful in 1937, but the findings did not attract much interest. However, a long time also elapsed between the discovery of the effectiveness of lithium in mania and its adoption into widespread clinical use. Rubidium was in the news because of some promising studies a few years ago (184), but little has been reported about it since then. Naloxone seems to have small effects, at least temporarily, but more work is needed (185).

CRITICAL PSYCHOSOCIAL INTERVENTIONS

Valuable contributions to the understanding and management of treatment-resistant schizophrenic patients have come from new research on particular psychosocial treatments. These include the critical role of structure (already alluded to earlier), new methods of environmental management (in the family or the other residential arrangements), and the expansion of the social network of the patient. Basic to all these interventions is the effort to reduce the negative effect of environments and relationships that are too stressful for the patient and lead to failure, rejection, or criticism. It seems clear that stressful environments and relationships not only provoke more relapses and more severe symptomatology, but regularly override the positive effect of medication. Consequently, failure to evaluate the current status of the patient's psychosocial sphere will often result in his being sent on futile and unnecessary drug odysseys.

Structure—the Neglected Ingredient of Treatment

The current concern about patient rights to treatment in the least restrictive setting has been difficult to balance with the fact that unstructured settings are more stressful for many schizophrenic patients and may produce clinical deterioration. They may be overwhelmed by the requirements of more independent living or they may have concomitant characterological difficulties which lead them to use poor judgment (e.g., drug and alcohol abuse, sexual and violent acting out, and discontinuation of their medication). The outpatient physician often feels compelled to prescribe larger doses of medication in the hope of forestalling relapse, or to try to circumvent compliance problems with long-acting injectable medication. However, the allegedly enhanced efficacy of either approach has been seriously questioned (187-189).

A more recent development compounding the issues has been the widespread concern about the side effects of neuroleptics and the impression that they are often used in excessive doses and without the patient's fully informed consent. This situation, however, actually affords the psychiatrist an opportunity to give more balanced recommendations for treatment-refractory schizophrenic patients, involving increased structure and external controls (limit-setting) and less medication.

These issues apply especially to the young chronic patient, who has been receiving considerable attention in the community psychiatry literature (190,191). The majority of them are schizophrenic patients whose symptoms are masked by their more manifest antisocial, passive-aggressive, or narcissistic personality traits. They reject traditional sociotherapies and prefer to emulate peers who seem to be making a success of antisocial behavior. Their judgment is not as good, however, and they become psychotic, particularly when under the influence of drugs and alcohol. The physician is often puzzled as to whether the psychotic difficulties may be explained entirely by the drug use, but it is usually noted that the patient's companions who took the same drugs are not similarly affected. Ultimately, these young chronics are even rejected by their chosen peer group, and they become acutely suicidal; the death rate from suicide is remarkably high in this population (192).

This malignant interaction of psychotic and characterological difficulties needs to be managed in a firm manner because of the serious, disabling consequences of the problem. The primary intervention should be to work with community and hospital staff to set up structured, individual treatment programs for each patient. This can be done without new, locked, intensive treatment facilities by using available programs in a coordinated effort. For example, if the patient is in a community residence, an analysis is made of what kinds of activities are associated with the occurrence of potentially life-threatening incidents involving poor judgment. Given firm verbal limits, the patient is restricted from those activities. The activities are very gradually reintroduced as the patient demonstrates an ability to handle them. If the limit-setting in itself provokes rebellious uncooperativeness, the patient is further restricted, and if this escalates the situation into an unsafe clinical state, then brief hospitalization may be required for containment, adjustment of medication, and reinforcement of the outpatient treatment plan. Firm limits will be set there, as well, to discourage regression, and this must be coordinated so the inpatient staff knows exactly how to fit in with what the community programs are trying to accomplish.

After a while, the patient sees that the system as a whole takes his or her problems seriously, and intends to help him get a grip on them. He/she starts to have some hope, and after a few months a striking turnaround in the patient's attitude toward the treatment program often takes place, following which he/she becomes much more cooperative and motivated to progress (193).

Treatment plans like this have to be carefully planned in advance. It is useful, and well worth the time, to arrange a meeting with key individuals in the different agencies that will be involved in the program, including influential administrators as well as clinicians. Despite rivalries and past histories of not cooperating with one another, they will often come to the meeting because problem patients like this already occupy a lot of their time, and they welcome the opportunity to consider new ideas. After briefly reviewing the history and what has not worked in the past, the plan is presented, followed by consideration of details of how to respond to various contingencies. In this way, group consensus and commitment are reached. Someone then summarizes the treatment plan in writing and circulates it for amendment as a final step to help promote everyone's cooperation.

Family Management in Refractory Schizophrenia

Much has been written in recent years about the toxic role of expressed emotion (EE) in the family environments of schizophrenics and how, despite medication, this factor can induce relapse (194). There has been some demonstration, with respect to treatment, that a psychoeducational approach (195) (as opposed to traditional approaches) (196) with the families can reduce the level of criticism, rejection, and overinvolvement in the family environment and markedly improve the patient's symptoms. What seems less well recognized is that many typical nonfamily environments in which patients are found probably also have high EE levels and are potentially toxic. These are all suitable subjects for examination in the treatment resistant case.

Acute inpatient milieus are often very difficult for schizophrenic patients, especially in private hospitals, because high value is placed on expressing feelings openly to strangers, active participation in group, occupational, and recreational therapies, and self-restraint from inappropriate action. These are all areas of greatest impairment in many schizophrenics. Consequently, enormous pressure to perform and direct criticism of the patient's impairments often develop. Frustrated staff ask the physician to find medications that will get the patient to be more active in the milieu. A better approach is to educate the staff about the nature of this illness and to develop an individualized approach to the schizophrenic patient (197). As all inpatient units are under pressure to shorten length of stay, it is important to foster awareness that pressure past a critical point may produce regression and lengthen the total period in the hospital for these patients (198).

Similar observations pertain to intermediate-care community facilities. They are also becoming more oriented toward active treatment. Administrators are frustrated when patients seem to be bottlenecked in halfway houses, making it impossible to find placement for hospitalized patients ready for discharge. The solution has been to put more pressure on patients in community residences to pursue further rehabilitation programs so that they can leave for more independent living situations. Another strategy has been to suddenly impose a time limit on how long a patient may stay in a community residence. For many unfortunate patients, this becomes a prescription for relapse and readmission to the hospital, from which early return to the community may be barred because someone else has filled their place in the residence. This process of turning good patient environments into stressful ones should be taken into account before dealing with the situation in an exclusively pharmacological manner. Destructive, nonclinically motivated programmatic and management decisions and their impact on patients are regularly brought to the attention of the psychopharmacologist; this poses complex strategic as well as ethical dilemmas.

Reduction of EE level may reduce active symptoms and rehospitalization, but there is evidence that it is associated with decreased performance, negative symptoms, and chronicity (199). Reasonable pressure should be placed on patients, in a supportive and accepting environment, in order to determine what their maximum level of functioning can be. Then, it would seem humane to allow them the most comfortable environment consistent with their limitations. An interesting recent study (200) suggests that immediately following discharge, patients most appreciated factors such as material support, social approval, and opportunity to ventilate concerns. Least useful seemed to be reality testing, monitoring symptoms, and modeling of higher functioning behavior. Later, 6–12 months after discharge, needs for social approval and material support decreased, and there was an increase in the need for relationships in which there was equality in terms of giving and receiving. It would be worthwhile to monitor if these elements are going to be present in outpatient treatment plans.

Networking and Refractory Schizophrenia

Related to the final point in the last section is the need to assess the social network of the treatment-refractory patient. Is the social network "segmented" enough, or is there too much reliance on a few intense relationships? These concerns are the result of a decade of interest in the effects of these variables on relapse rate in psychotic patients (201–203). The results, in summary, are that schizophrenic patients do better with a large number of brief, low-intensity social contacts, each of which involves minimal demands and expectations, but in which there can be an opportunity for reciprocal interaction. Ideally, many of these contacts also talk to one another about the patient, which diffuses some of their anxiety about his/her abnormal behavior.

The most intense relationships are usually with relatives and administrators of their living situation, and if these are their only contacts, the patients tend to do poorly. There is better outcome when additional segments are added such as recreational activities, opportunities for social encounters, appropriate rehabilitation programs, and individual service providers (e.g., therapist, welfare worker, case manager, psychiatrist). These permit less intense and toxic dependency on the family and administrators. In a "network therapy" program, the explicit goal is to promote these more adaptive, segmented networks. The psychiatrist should expect that poor quality networks will be associated with drug treatment resistance, and pharmacological recommendations should be limited to what is rational in the context of an optimal comprehensive treatment plan.

Psychotherapy and Refractory Schizophrenia

As was indicated at the beginning of this section, there may be evidence that intensive psychodynamic (existential, Semradian, Sullivanian) psychotherapy may benefit chronic schizophrenic patients as long as neuroleptic therapy is being used concomitantly (142). A much more recent study from a prominent hospital specializing in this kind of therapy reached a similar conclusion (204). Distinguished senior clinicians continue to be persuasive in the view that individual psychotherapy can be helpful and should continue to be offered in selected cases (205–207), despite the confusing, equivocal results reported in recent sophisticated research paradigms (208).

It would be well if there were more documentation to support the encouragement of this inefficient and expensive modality. Nevertheless, experience suggests that many chronic, withdrawn, inactive, compensated schizophrenics on medication are more than shells of human beings organically impaired with enlarged cerebral ventricles. They are involved in massive defensive operations to protect their fragile self-esteem and avoid further failure and rejection. They can be reached by sitting with them, making a commitment to develop a relationship, trying to understand the what, how, and why of them as individuals and their withdrawal from trusting communication with others (207). Consistency, reliability, concern, and full acceptance of the patient's need to use these defenses at this time are essential. Over months, they will begin to trust enough to reveal more and more of their inner life, hidden wishes, and fears. Their ability to invest in the world can be reactivated through the catalyzing effect of the therapist's patient investment in them. This can move patients to try the next level of functioning and rehabilitation which they might have been avoiding for years, successfully resisting the more pushy approaches of the past. Therapists stick with patients through the inevitable regression and two-steps-foward, one-and-a-half-steps-back progression and try never to become critical or punitive when patients disappoint them. Experience suggests when all else has failed, this individual therapy strategy has been the critical factor in helping some schizophrenics to reach the maximum level of functioning of which they are capable.

It is unfortunate that many psychiatrists never have the opportunity in their training to experience this kind of long-term work with schizophrenics. This shapes the psychiatrist's subsequent attitude toward individual therapy; yet, how can one do, much less teach others, what one has never been taught?

This section presented an outline of pharmacological and psychosocial issues contributing to treatment-refractory cases of schizophrenia using a step-by-step approach to simulate how a psychopharmacology consultant might think through such cases. There are always unanswerable questions and unclear data that make it more difficult to proceed than might have been apparent in the foregoing discussion. In addition, new data are always appearing that contradict or challenge even the most accepted aphorisms. The clinicians' most valuable assets in approaching treatment-resistant problems are their ability to stay on top of the literature, question assumptions, ask for more data, and give the matter more thought and study.

Acknowledgement:

The author wishes to thank Chester Pearlman, M.D., for his thoughtful review of this chapter.

REFERENCES

1. Caplan, G. (1970). *The Theory and Practice of Mental Health Consultation*. New York: Basic Books.
2. Hall, R. C. W., Popkin, M. K., Devaul, R. A., Faillace, L. A., and Stickney, S. K. (1978). Physical illness presenting as psychiatric disease. *Archives of General Psychiatry* 35:1315–1320.
3. Gold, M. S., Pottash, A. C., Extein, L., Martin, D. M., Howard, E., Mueller, E. A., and Sweeney, D. R. (1981). The TRH test in the diagnosis of major and minor depression. *Psychoneuroendocrinology* 6:159–169.
4. Schildkraut, J. J., and Klein, D. F. (1975). The classification and treatment of depressive disorders. In *Manual of Psychiatric Therapeutics*, ed. R. I. Shader, pp. 39–62. Boston: Little, Brown.
5. Whybrow, P. C., Akiskal, H. S., and McKinney, W. T., Jr. (1984). Clinical and familial subtypes of mood disorders: Observation, opinion, and purpose. In *Mood Disorders*. New York: Plenum, 43–63.
6. Myers, J. K., Weissman, M. R., Tischler, G. L., Holzer, C. E. III, Leaf, P. J., Orvaschel, H., and Anthony, J. C. (1984). Six-month prevalence of psychiatric disorders in three communities. *Archives of General Psychiatry* 41:959–967.
7. Nelson, J. C., and Charney, D. S. (1981). The symptoms of major depressive illness. *American Journal of Psychiatry* 138:1–13.
8. Casper, R. C., Redmond, E., Jr., Katz, M. M., Schaffer, C. B., Davis, J. M., and Koslow, S. H. (1985). Somatic symptoms in primary affective disorder. *Archives of General Psychiatry* 42:1098–1104.
9. Glassman, A. H., and Carino, J. S. (1984). Use of antidepressants in the geriatric population. In *Guidelines for the Use of Psychotropic Drugs*, eds. H. C. Stancer, P. E. Garfinkel, and V. M. Rakoff, pp. 19–30. New York: Spectrum.
10. Flemenbaum, A. (1971). Methylphenidate: A catalyst for the tricyclic antidepressants. *American Journal of Psychiatry* 128:239.
11. Snyder, S. H., and Yamamura, H. I. (1977). Antidepressants and the muscarinic acetylcholine receptor. *Archives of General Psychiatry* 34:236–239.
12. Potter, W. Z., and Linnoila, M. (1984). Tricyclic antidepressant concentrations: Clinical and research implications. In *Neurobiology of Mood Disorders*, eds. R. M. Post and J. C. Ballenger, pp. 698–709. Baltimore: Williams and Wilkins.
13. Quitkin, F., Rabkin, J. G., Ross, D., and McGrath, P. J. (1984). Duration of antidepressant drug treatment. *Archives of General Psychiatry* 41:238–245.
14. Hirschowitz, J., Bennett, J. A., Zemlen, F., and Garver, D. L. (1985). Rapid dosing tricyclic antidepressant leads to early response. Presented at the American Psychiatric Association Annual Meeting, New Research, Dallas.

15. Lydiard, R. B. (1985). Tricyclic-resistant depressions: Treatment resistance or inadequate treatment? *Journal of Clinical Psychiatry* 46:412–417.
16. de Montigny, C., Cournoyer, G., Morissette, R., Langlois, R., and Caillé, G. (1983). Lithium carbonate addition to tricyclic antidepressant-resistant unipolar depression. *Archives of General Psychiatry* 40:1327–1334.
17. Heninger, G. R., Charney, D. S., and Sternberg, D. E. (1983). Lithium carbonate augmentation of antidepressant treatment. *Archives of General Psychiatry* 40:1335–1342.
18. Price, L. H., Charney, D. S., and Heninger, G. R. (1985). Efficacy of lithium-tranylcypromine treatment in refractory depression. *American Journal of Psychiatry* 142:619–623.
19. de Montigny, C. (1985). Using lithium to enhance the efficacy of antidepressants. *Currents in Affective Illness* 4:5–9.
20. Goodwin, F. K., Prange, A. J., Post, R. M., Muscettola, G., and Lipton, M. A. (1982). Potentiation of antidepressant effects by L-triiodothyronine in tricyclic nonresponders. *American Journal of Psychiatry* 139:34–38.
21. Schwarcz, G., Halaris, A., Baxter, L., Escobar, J., Thompson, M., and Young, M. (1984). Normal thyroid function in desipramine nonresponders converted to responders by the addition of L-triiodothyronine. *American Journal of Psychiatry* 141:1614–1616.
22. Cole, J. O., Schatzberg, A. F., Sniffin, C., Zolner, J., and Cole, J. P. (1981). Trazodone in treatment-resistant depression: An open study. *Journal of Clinical Psychopharmacology* 1(6, Suppl.): 49s–54s.
23. Stern, W. C., Harto-Truax, N., and Bauer, N. (1983). Efficacy of bupropion in tricyclic-resistant or intolerant patients. *Journal of Clinical Psychiatry* 44(Sect. 2):148–152.
24. White, K., and Simpson, G. (1985). Should the use of MAO inhibitors be abandoned? Commentary by D. V. Sheehan, D. Wheatley, T. A. Ban, E. S. Paykel, J. Davidson, and W. Z. Potter. *Integrative Psychiatry* 3:34–45.
25. Himmelhoch, J. M., Fuches, C. Z., and Symons, B. J. (1982). A double-blind study of tranylcypromine treatment of major anergic depression. *Journal of Nervous and Mental Disease* 170:628–634.
26. Gelenberg, A. J. (1984). Switching MAOIs. *Biological Therapies in Psychiatry* 7:33–36.
27. Jenike, M. A. (1984). Monoamine oxidase inhibitors in elderly depressed patients. *Journal of the American Geriatrics Society* 32:571.
28. Janicak, P. G., Davis, J. M., Ericksen, S., Chang, S., Gallagher, P., and Gibbons, R. D. (1985). Efficacy of ECT: A meta-analysis. *American Journal of Psychiatry* 142:297–302.
29. Crowe, R. R. (1984). Electro-convulsive therapy—a current perspective. *New England Journal of Medicine* 311:163–167.
30. White, K., and Simpson, G. (1981). Combined MAOI-tricyclic antidepressant treatment. A reevaluation. *Journal of Clinical Psychopharmacology* 1:264–282.
31. Baldessarini, R. J. (1984). Treatment of depression by altering monoamine metabolism: Precursors and metabolic inhibitors. *Psychopharmacology Bulletin* 20:238–244.

32. Hedaya, R. J. (1984). Pharmacokinetic factors in the clinical use of tryphophan. *Journal of Clinical Psychopharmacology* 4:347-349.
33. Fawcett, J., and Kravitz, H. M. (1985). Treatment refractory depression. In *Common Treatment Problems in Depression*, ed. A. F. Schatzberg, pp. 1-27. Washington, DC: American Psychiatric Press.
34. Feighner, J. P., Herbstein, J., and Damlouji, N. (1985). Combined MAOI, TCA, and direct stimulant therapy of treatment resistant depression. *Journal of Clinical Psychiatry* 46:206-209.
35. Feighner, J. P. (1983). Open label study of alprazolam in severely depressed inpatients. *Journal of Clinical Psychiatry* 44:332-334.
36. Mooney, J. J., Cole, J. O., Schatzberg, A. F., Gerson, B., and Schildkraut, J. J. (1985). Pretreatment urinary MHPG levels as predictors of antidepressants response to alprazolam. *American Journal of Psychiatry* 142:366-367.
37. Post, R. M., Uhde, T. W., Roy-Byrne, P. P., and Joffe, R. T. (1986). Antidepressant effects of carbamazepine. *American Journal of Psychiatry* 143:29-34.
38. Kocsis, J. H., Voss, C., Mason, B., Mann, J. J., Brown, R., Francis, A. J. (1985). Chronic depression: A study of clinical aspects. Paper presented at the Annual Meeting of the American Psychiatric Association, Dallas.
39. Nelson, W. H., Khan, A., and Orr, W. W., Jr. (1984). Delusional depression: Phenomenology, neuroendocrine function, and tricyclic antidepressant response. *Journal of Affective Disorders* 6:297-306.
40. Coryell, W., Tsuang, M. T., and McDaniel, J. (1982). Psychotic features in major depression: Is mood congruence important? *Journal of Affective Disorders* 4:227-236.
41. Spiker, D. G., Weiss, J. C., Dealy, R. S., Griffin, S. J., Hanin, I., Neil, J. F., and Perel, J. M. (1985). The pharmacological treatment of delusional depression. *American Journal of Psychiatry* 142:430-436.
42. Charney, D. S., and Nelson, J. C. (1981). Delusional and nondelusional unipolar depression: Further evidence for distinct subtypes. *American Journal of Psychiatry* 138:328-333.
43. Perry, P. J., Morgan, D. E., Smith, R. E., and Tsuang, M. T. (1982). Treatment of unipolar depression accompanied by delusions. *Journal of Affective Disorders* 4:195-200.
44. Wharton, R. N., Perel, J. M., Dayton, P. G., and Malitz, S. (1971). A potential clinical use for methylphenidate with tricyclic antidepressants. *American Journal of Psychiatry* 127:1619-1625.
45. Coryell, W., Lavon, P., Endicott, J., Keller, M., and Van Eerdewegh, M. (1984). Outcome in schizoaffective, psychotic, and nonpsychotic depression. *Archives of General Psychiatry* 41:787-791.
46. Coppen, A., Abou-Saleh, M. T., Milln, P., Bailey, J., Metcalfe, M., Burns, B. H., and Armond, A. (1981). Lithium continuation therapy following ECT. *British Journal of Psychiatry* 139:284-287.
47. Cole, J. O., and Schatzberg, A. F. (1983). Antidepressant drug therapy. In *Psychiatry Update II*, ed. L. Grinspoon, pp. 472-490. Washington, DC: American Psychiatric Press.
48. Price, L. H., Conwell, Y., and Nelson, J. C. (1983). Lithium augmentation of

combined neuroleptic-tricyclic treatment in delusional depression. *American Journal of Psychiatry* 140:318–322.
49. Mazure, C., and Nelson, J. C. (1985). Lithium in psychotic refractory depression. American Psychiatric Association Annual Meeting, New Research, Dallas.
50. Schaffer, C. B., Mungas, D., and Rockwell, E. (1985). Successful treatment of psychotic depression with carbamazepine. *Journal of Clinical Psychopharmacology* 5:233–235.
51. Schildkraut, J. J., Schatzberg, M. D., Mooney, J. J., and Orsulak, P. J. (1983). Depressive disorders and the emerging field of psychiatric chemistry. In *Psychiatry Update II*, ed. L. Grinspoon, pp. 457–471. Washington, DC: American Psychiatric Press.
52. Goodwin, F. K., and Wehr, T. A. (1980). Rapid cycling in manic depressives induced by tricyclic antidepressants. American Psychiatric Association Annual Meeting Symposium, San Francisco.
53. Jefferson, J. W., Greist, J. H., and Ackerman, D. L. (1983). Depression, acute. In *Lithium Encyclopedia for Clinical Practice*, pp. 99–100. Washington, DC: American Psychiatric Press.
54. Kukopulos, A., Reginaldi, D., Laddomada, P., Floris, G., Serra, G., and Tondo, L. (1980). Course of the manic-depressive cycle and changes caused by treatments. *Pharmacopsychiatria* 13:156–157.
55. Wright, G., Galloway, L., Kim, J., Dalton, M., Miller, L., and Stern, W. (1985). Bupropion in the long-term treatment of cyclic mood disorders: Mood stabilizing effects. *Journal of Clinical Psychiatry* 46:22–25.
56. Karliner, W., and Wehrheim, H. K. (1965). Maintenance convulsive treatments. *American Journal of Psychiatry* 121:1113–1115.
57. Jefferson, J. W., Greist, J. H., and Ackerman, D. L. (1983). *Lithium Encyclopedia for Clinical Practice*, pp. 115–116. Washington, DC: American Psychiatric Press.
58. Keller, M. B., and Shapiro, R. W. (1982). "Double depression": Superimposition of acute depressive episodes on chronic depressive disorders. *American Journal of Psychiatry* 139:438–442.
59. Sheehan, D. V. (1985). MAO inhibitors and alprazolam in the treatment of panic disorder and agoraphobia. *Psychiatric Clinics of North America* 8:49–52.
60. Liebowitz, M. R. (1985). Imipramine in the treatment of panic disorder and its complications. *Psychiatric Clinics of North America* 8:37–48.
61. Akiskal, H. S., Chen, S. E., Davis, G. C., Puzantian, V. R., Kashgarian, M., and Bulinger, J. M. (1985). Borderline: An adjective in search of a noun. *Journal of Clinical Psychiatry* 46:41–48.
62. Rifkin, A., Quitkin, F., Carillo, C., Blumberg, A. G., and Klein, D. F. (1972). Lithium carbonate in emotionally unstable character disorder. *Archives of General Psychiatry* 27:519–523.
63. Serban, G., and Siegel, S. (1982). Response of borderline and schizotypal patients to small doses of thiothixene and haloperidol. *American Journal of Psychiatry* 141:1455–1458.
64. Gunderson, J. G., and Kolb, J. E. (1978). Discriminating features of borderline patients. *American Journal of Psychiatry* 135:792–796.

65. Himmelhoch, J. M. (1984). Major mood disorders related to epileptic changes. In *Psychiatric Aspects of Epilepsy*, ed. D. Blumer, pp. 271-294. Washington, DC: American Psychiatric Press.
66. Griffith, J. L., and Murray, G. B. (1985). Clorazepate in the treatment of complex partial seizures with psychic symptomatology. *Journal of Nervous and Mental Disease* 173:185-186.
67. Adler, G. (1985). *Borderline Psychopathology and Its Treatment*. New York: Jason Aronson.
68. Kernberg, O. F. (1985). *Severe Personality Disorders: Psychotherapeutic Strategies*. New Haven: Yale University Press.
69. Havens, L. L. (1968). Some difficulties in giving schizophrenic and borderline patients medication. *Psychiatry* 31:44-50.
70. Adler, G., and Buie, D. H. (1979). Aloneness and borderline psychopathology: The possible relevance of child development issues. *International Journal of Psycho-Analysis* 60:83-96.
71. Liebowitz, M. R., Quitkin, F. M., Stewart, J. W., McGrath, P. J., Harrison, W., Rabkin, J., and Tricamo, E. (1984). Phenelzine versus imipramine in atypical depression. *Archives of General Psychiatry* 41:669-677.
72. Zisook, S., Braff, D. L., and Click, M. A. (1985). Monoamine oxidase inhibitors in the treatment of atypical depression. *Journal of Clinical Psychopharmacology* 5:131-137.
73. Pope, H. G., Jr., Hudson, J. I., and Jonas, J. M. (1983). Antidepressant treatment of bulimia: Preliminary experience and practical recommendations. *Journal of Clinical Psychopharmacology* 3:274-281.
74. Hsu, L. K. G. (1984). Treatment of bulimia with lithium. *American Journal of Psychiatry* 141:1260-1262.
75. Pope, H. G., Jr., Herridge, P. L., Hudson, J. I., Fontaine, R., and Yurgelun-Todd, D. (1985). Treatment of bulimia with nomifensine. American Psychiatric Association Annual Meeting, New Research, Dallas.
76. van der Kolk, B. A., Greenberg, M., Boyd, H., and Krystal, J. (1985). Inescapable shock, neurotransmitters and addiction to trauma: Toward a psychobiology of post-traumatic stress. *Biological Psychiatry* 20:314-325.
77. Horowitz, M. J. (1985). Disasters and psychological responses to stress. *Psychiatric Annals* 15:161-167.
78. Birkhimer, L. J., DeVane, C. L., and Muniz, C. E. (1985). Post-traumatic stress disorder: Characteristics and pharmacological response in the veteran population. *Comprehensive Psychiatry* 26:304-310.
79. Gardner, D. L., and Cowdry, R. W. (1985). Alprazolam-induced dyscontrol in borderline personality disorder. *American Journal of Psychiatry* 142:98-100.
80. Herz, M. I., and Melville, C. (1980). Relapse in schizophrenia. *American Journal of Psychiatry* 137:801-805.
81. Becker, R. E. (1985). Implications of the efficacy of thiothixene and a chlorpramazine-imipramine combination for depression in schizophrenia. *American Journal of Psychiatry* 140:208-211.
82. Johnson, D. A. W. (1985). Antipsychotic medication: Clinical guidelines for maintenance therapy. *Journal of Clinical Psychiatry* 46(5 Sect.2):6-15.
83. Singh, A. N., Saxena, B., and Nelson, H. L. (1978). A controlled clinical study

of trazodone in chronic schizophrenic patients with pronounced depressive symptomatology. *Current Therapeutic Research* 23:485–501.
84. Schildkraut, J. J., Orsulak, P. J., Gudeman, J. E., Schatzberg, A. F., Rohde, W. A., LaBrie, R. A., and Cahill, J. F. (1977). Norepinephrine metabolism in subtypes of depressive disorders. In *Psychopathology and Brain Dysfunction*, eds. C. Shagass, S. Gershon, and A. J. Friedhoff, pp. 125–138. New York: Raven Press.
85. Gelenberg, A. J., and Mandel, M. R. (1977). Catatonic reactions to high-potency neuroleptic drugs. *Archives of General Psychiatry* 34:947–950.
86. Van Putten, T., and May, P. R. A. (1978). Akinetic depression in schizophrenia. *Archives of General Psychiatry* 35:1101–1107.
87. DiMascio, A., and Shader, R. I. (1970). Behavioral toxicity. Part I: Definition. Part II: Psychomotor functions. In *Psychotropic Drug Side Effects*, eds. R. I. Shader and A. DiMascio. Baltimore, MD: Williams and Wilkins.
88. Delva, N. J., and Letemendia, F. J. J. (1982). Lithium treatment in schizophrenia and schizoaffective disorders. *British Journal of Psychiatry* 141:387–400.
89. Salzman, C. (1980). The use of ECT in the treatment of schizophrenia. *American Journal of Psychiatry* 137:1032–1041.
90. McGlashan, T. H., and Carpenter, W. T. (1976). An investigation of the postpsychotic depressive syndrome. *American Journal of Psychiatry* 133:14–19.
91. Schildkraut, J. J., Orsulak, P. J., Schatzberg, A. F., Gudeman, J. E., Cole, J. O., Rohde, W. A., and LaBrie, R. A. (1978). Toward a biochemical classification of depressive disorders I. *Archives of General Psychiatry* 35:1427–1433.
92. Andreasen, N. C., and Olsen, S. (1982). Negative versus positive schizophrenia: Definition and validation. *Archives of General Psychiatry* 39:789–794.
93. Welner, A., Croughan, J. L., and Robins, E. (1974). The group of schizoaffective and related psychoses—critique, record, follow-up, and family studies I and II. *Archives of General Psychiatry* 31:628–637.
94. Gelenberg, A. J. (1984). Patients with affective illness: Are they more prone to develop tardive dyskinesia? *Biological Therapies in Psychiatry* 7:6.
95. Van Valkenberg, C., and Clayton, P. (1985). Electroconvulsive therapy and schizophrenia. *Biological Psychiatry* 20:699–700.
96. Fenton, W. S., Mosher, L. R., and Matthews, S. M. (1981). Diagnosis of schizophrenia: A critical review of current diagnostic systems. *Schizophrenia Bulletin* 71:452–476.
97. Bleuler, M. E. (1978). The long term course of schizophrenia. In *The Nature of Schizophrenia*, ed. L. Wynne, R. L. Cromwell, and S. Matthysse, p. 631. New York: Wiley.
98. Stasiek, C., and Zetin, M. (1985). Organic manic disorders. *Psychosomatics* 26:394–446.
99. Adamec, R. E., and Stark-Adamec, C. (1983). Limbic kindling and animal behavior—implications for human psychopathology associated with complex partial seizures. *Biological Psychiatry* 18:269–293.
100. Trimble, M. R. (1982). The interictal psychoses of epilepsy. In *Psychiatric Aspects of Neurologic Disease*, Vol. 2, ed. D. F. Benson and D. Blumer, pp. 75–92. New York: Grune and Stratton.

101. Rifkin, A., Quitkin, F., and Klein, D. F. (1975). Akinesia. *Archives of General Psychiatry* 32:672–674.
102. Adler, L., Angrist, B., Peselow, E., Corwin, J., Rotrasen, J. (1985). Efficacy of propranolol in neuroleptic-induced akathisia. *Journal of Clinical Psychopharmacology* 5:164–170.
103. Ratey, J. J., Sorgi, P., and Polakoff, S., (1985). Nadolol as a treatment for akathisia. *American Journal of Psychiatry* 142:640–642.
104. Fricchione, G. L., Cassem, N. H., Hooberman, D., and Hobson, D. (1983). Intravenous lorazepam in neuroleptic-induced catatonia. *Journal of Clinical Psychopharmacology* 3:338–342.
105. McEvoy, J. P., and Lohr, J. B. (1984). Diazepam for catatonia. *American Journal of Psychiatry* 141:284–285.
106. Smego, R. A., Jr., and Durack, D. T. (1982). The neuroleptic malignant syndrome. *Archives of Internal Medicine* 142:1183–1185.
107. Kurlan, R., Hamill, R., and Shoulson, I. (1984). Neuroleptic malignant syndrome. *Clinical Neuropharmacology* 7:109–120.
108. Jefferson, J. W., Greist, J. H., and Ackerman, D. L. (1983). Neurological side effects. In *Lithium Encyclopedia for Clinical Practice*, pp. 186–192. Washington, DC: American Psychiatric Press.
109. Davies, R. K., Tucker, G. J., Harrow, M., Detre, T. P. (1971). Confusional episodes and antidepressant medication. *American Journal of Psychiatry* 128:95–99.
110. Roy-Byrne, P. P., Joffe, R. T., Uhde, T. W., and Post, R. M. (1984). Approaches to the evaluation and treatment of rapid-cycling affective illness. *British Journal of Psychiatry* 145:543–550.
111. Post, R. M. (1985). Clinical perspectives on the use of carbamazepine in manic-depressive illness. *Psychiatry Letter (Fair Oaks Hospital)* 3(4).
112. Post, R. M., Uhde, T. W., Ballenger, J. C., and Squillace, K. M. (1983). Prophylactic efficacy of carbamazepine in manic-depressive illness. *American Journal of Psychiatry* 140:1602–1604.
113. Klein, E., Bental, E., Lerer, B., and Belmaker, R. H. (1984). Carbamazepine and haloperidol versus placebo and haloperidol in excited psychoses. *Archives of General Psychiatry* 41:165–170.
114. Gelenberg, A. J. (1985). Carbamazepine for manic-depressive illness: An update. *Biological Therapies in Psychiatry* 8:21–24.
115. Puzynski, S., and Klosiewicz, L. (1984). Valproic acid amide in the treatment of affective and schizoaffective disorders. *Journal of Affective Disorders* 6:115–121.
116. Emrich, H. M., von Zerssen, D., Kissling, W., and Moller, H. J. (1981). Therapeutic effect of valproate in mania. *American Journal of Psychiatry* 138:256.
117. Ayd, F. J., Jr. (1984). Alternatives for lithium. *Psychiatric Annals* 14:7.
118. Brennan, M. J. W., Sandy, R., and Borsook, D. (1984). Use of sodium valproate in the management of affective disorders: Basic and clinical aspects. In *Anticonvulsants in Affective Disorders*, eds. H. M. Emrich, T. Okuma, and A. A. Muller, pp. 56–65. Amsterdam: Elsevier.
119. Puzynski, S., and Klosiewicz, L. (1984). Valproic acid amide as a prophylactic

agent in affective and schizoaffective disorders. In *Anticonvulsants in Affective Disorders*, ed. H. M. Emrich, M., T. Okuma, and A. A. Muller, pp. 68-75. Amsterdam: Elsevier.

120. Emrich, H. M., Altmann, H., and von Zerssen, D. (1982). Prophylactic action of sodium valproate in manic-depression: The GABA hypothesis of affective disorders. In *New Vistas in Depression*, ed. S. Z. Langer, R. Takahashi, T. Segawa, and M. Briley, pp. 81-85. New York: Pergamon Press.

121. Giannini, A. J., Houser, W. L., Jr., Loiselle, R. H., Giannini, M. C., and Price, W. A. (1984). Antimanic effects of verapamil. *American Journal of Psychiatry* 141:1602-1603.

122. Giannini, A. J., Loiselle, R. H., Price, W. A., and Giannini, M. C. (1985). Comparison of antimanic efficacy of clonidine and verapamil. *Journal of Clinical Pharmacology* 15:307-308.

123. Gitlin, M. J., and Weiss, J. (1984). Verapamil as maintenance treatment in bipolar illness: A case report. *Journal of Clinical Psychopharmacology* 4:341-343.

124. Stone, P. H., and Braunwald, E. (1985). Calcium channel blocking agents: mechanisms of action, clinical pharmacology, and clinical application. In Update VI: *Harrison's Principles of Internal Medicine*, ed. R. G. Petersdorf, R. D. Adams, E. Braunwald, K. J. Isselbacher, J. B. Martin, and J. D. Wilson, pp. 109-131. New York: McGraw Hill.

125. Doran, A. R., Narang, P. K., Meigs, C. Y., Wolkowitz, O. M., Roy, A., Breier, A., and Pickar, D. (1985). Verapamil concentrations in cerebrospinal fluid after oral administration. *New England Journal of Medicine* 312:1261.

126. Zubenko, G. S., Cohen, B. M., Lipinski, J. F., and Jonas, J. M. (1984). Clonidine in the treatment of mania and mixed bipolar disorder. *American Journal of Psychiatry* 141:1617-1618.

127. Stancer, H. C., and Persad, E. (1982). Treatment of intractable rapid-cycling manic-depressive disorder with levothyroxine. *Archives of General Psychiatry* 39:311-312.

128. Brewerton, T. D., and Reus, V. I. (1983). Lithium carbonate and L-tryptophan in the treatment of bipolar and schizoaffective disorders. *American Journal of Psychiatry* 140:757-760.

129. Chouinard, G., Young, S. N., and Annable, L. (1983). Antimanic effects of clonazepam. *Biological Psychiatry* 18:451-466.

130. Victor, B. S., Link, N. A., Binder, R. L., and Bell, I. R. (1984). Use of clonazepam in manic and schizoaffective disorder. *American Journal of Psychiatry* 141:1111-1112.

131. Freinhar, J. P., and Alvarez, W. H. (1985). Use of clonazepam in two cases of acute mania. *Journal of Clinical Psychiatry* 46:29-30.

132. Frykholm, B. (1985). Clonazepam—antipsychotic effect in a case of schizophrenia-like psychosis with epilepsy and in three cases of atypical psychosis. *Acta Psychiatrica Scandinavica* 71:539-542.

133. Chouinard, G. (1985). Antimanic effects of clonazepam. *Psychosomatics* 26(Suppl.):7-12.

134. Thomas, R. D., and Callender, K. (1985). Methylene blue in treatment of bipolar illness. *Biological Psychiatry* 10:120.

135. Trimble, M. R. (1985). Recent advances in epilepsy and the relevance for psychiatry. Paper presented at the Annual Meeting of American Psychiatric Association, Dallas.
136. Goldensohn, E. S., Glaser, G. H., and Goldberg, M. (1984). Epilepsy. In *Merritt's Textbook of Neurology*, ed. L. P. Rowland, p. 647. Philadelphia: Lea and Febiger.
137. Lipinski, J. F., and Pope, H. G. (1982). Possible synergistic action between carbamazepine and lithium carbonate in the treatment of three acutely manic patients. *American Journal of Psychiatry* 139:948-949.
138. Shulka, S., Godwin, C. D., Long, L. E. B., and Miller, M. G. (1984). Lithium-carbamazepine neurotoxicity and risk factors. *American Journal of Psychiatry* 141:1604-1606.
139. Joffe, T. W., Post, R. M., and Uhde, T. W. (1985). Lack of pharmacokinetic interaction of carbamazepine with tranylcypromine (letter). *Archives of General Psychiatry* 42:738.
140. Lerer, B., Moore, N., Meyendorff, E., Cho, S. R., and Gershon, S. (1985). Carbamazepine and lithium: Different profiles in affective disorder? *Psychopharmacology Bulletin* 21:18-22.
141. Small, J. G., Small, I. F., Milstein, V., Kellams, J. J., and Klapper, M. H. (1985). Manic symptoms: An indication for bilateral ECT. *Biological Psychiatry* 20:125.
142. Grinspoon, L., Ewalt, J. R., and Shader, R. I. (1972). *Schizophrenia: Pharmacotherapy and Psychotherapy*. Baltimore, MD: Williams and Wilkins.
143. Hogarty, G. E., Schooler, N. R., Ulrich, R., Mussare, F., Peregrino, F., and Herron, E. (1979). Fluphenazine and social therapy in the aftercare of schizophrenic patients. *Archives of General Psychiatry* 36:1283-1294.
144. Csernansky, J. G., Kaplan, J., and Hollister, L. E. (1985). Problems in classification of schizophrenics as neuroleptic responders and nonresponders. *Journal of Nervous Mental Disorders* 173:325-331.
145. Chiles, J. A., Carlin, A. S., and Beitman, B. D. (1984). A physician, a nonmedical psychotherapist, and a patient: The pharmacotherapy-psychotherapy triangle. In *Combining Psychotherapy and Drug Therapy in Clinical Practice*, ed. B. D. Beitman and G. L. Klerman. New York: Spectrum.
146. Linden, R., David, J. M., and Rubinstein, J. (1982). High versus low dose treatment with antipsychotic agents. *Psychiatric Annals* 12:769-781.
147. Baldessarini, R. J., Katz, B., and Cotton, P. (1984). Dissimilar dosing with high potency and low potency neuroleptics. *American Journal of Psychiatry* 141:748-752.
148. Davis, J. M. (1976). Comparative doses and costs of antipsychotic medication. *Archives of General Psychiatry* 33:858-861.
149. Mason, A. S., and Granacher, R. P. (1980). *Clinical Handbook of Antipsychotic Drug Therapy*, p. 33. New York: Brunner/Mazel.
150. McIntyre, I. M., and Gershon, S. (1985). Interpatient variations in antipsychotic therapy. *Journal of Clinical Psychiatry* 46(5, Sect. 2):3-5.
151. Mavroidis, M., Kanter, D. R., Hirschowitz, J., and Garver, D. L. (1984). Fluphenazine plasma levels and clinical response. *Journal of Clinical Psychiatry* 45:370-373.

References

152. Kragh-Sorensen, P., Hansen, C. E., Baastrup, P. C., and Hvidberg, E. G. (1976). Self-inhibiting action of nortriptyline's antidepressive effect at high plasma levels: A randomized double-blind study controlled by plasma concentrations in patients with endogenous depression. *Psychopharmacologia* 45:305-312.
153. Garver, D. L., Hitzemann, R. M., Mavroidis, M. V., and Hirschowitz, J. (1985). Plasma antipsychotic sigmoidal response curves. American Psychiatric Association Annual Meeting, New Research, Dallas.
154. Smith, R. C., Crayton, J., Dekirmenjian, H., Klass, D., and Davis, J. M. (1979). Blood levels of neuroleptic drugs in nonresponding chronic schizophrenic patients. *Archives of General Psychiatry* 36:579-584.
155. Cohen, B. M. (1984). The clinical utility of plasma neuroleptic levels. In *Guidelines for the Use of Psychotropic Drugs*, pp. 245-260, eds. H. C. Stancer, P. E. Garfinkel, and V. M. Rakoff. New York: Spectrum.
156. Adamsen, L. (1973). Fluphenazine decanoate trial in chronic inpatient schizophrenics failing to absorb chlorpromazine. *Diseases of the Nervous System* 34:181-191.
157. Fann, W. E., and Moreira, A. F. (1985). Neuroleptic bioequivalency: Tablet versus concentrate. *Journal of Clinical Pharmacology* 25:305-306.
158. Teicher, M. H., and Baldessarini, R. J. (1985). Selection of neuroleptic dosage. *Archives of General Psychiatry* 42:636.
159. Ko, G. N., Korpi, E. R., and Linnoila, M. (1985). On the clinical relevance and methods of quantification of plasma concentrations of neuroleptics. *Journal of Clinical Psychopharmacology* 5:153-262.
160. Simpson, G. M., and Yadalam, K. (1985). Blood levels of neuroleptics: State of the art. *Journal of Clinical Psychiatry* 46(5, Sect. 2):22-28.
161. Curry, H. (1985). Commentary: The strategy and value of neuroleptic drug monitoring. *Journal of Clinical Psychopharmacology* 5:263-271.
162. Davis, J. M. (1975). Maintenance therapy in psychiatry: I. Schizophrenia. *American Journal of Psychiatry* 132:1237-1245.
163. Forrest, I. S., Carr, C. J., and Usden, eds. (1973). *Advances in Biochemical Pharmacology.* Volume 9: *Phenothiazines and Structurally Related Drugs.* New York: Raven Press.
164. Harris, P. Q., Friedman, M. J., Cohen, B. M., and Cooper, T. B. (1982). Fluphenazine blood levels and clinical response. *Biological Psychiatry* 17:1123-1130.
165. Chouinard, G., and Steinberg, S. (1984). New clinical concepts on neuroleptic-induced supersensitivity disorders: Tardive dyskinesia and supersensitivity psychosis. In *Guidelines for the Use of Psychotropic Drugs*, ed. H. Stancer, P. E. Garfinkel, and V. M. Rakoff. New York: Spectrum.
166. Brown, W. A., and Silver, M. A. (1985). Serum neuroleptic levels and clinical outcome in schizophrenic patients treated with fluphenazine decanoate. *Journal of Clinical Psychopharmacology* 5:143-147.
167. Gruen, P. H., Sachar, E. J., and Langer, G. (1978). Prolactin responses to neuroleptics in normal and schizophrenic subjects. *Archives of General Psychiatry* 35:108-116.
168. Ayd, F. J., Jr. (1975). Treatment resistant patients: A moral, legal, and thera-

peutic challenge. In *Rational Psychopharmacotherapy and the Right to Treatment*, ed. F. J. Ayd. Baltimore, MD: Ayd Medical Communications.
169. Osser, D. N. Unpublished observations.
170. Gardos, G. (1974). Are antipsychotic drugs interchangeable? *Journal of Nervous and Mental Diseases* 159:343–348.
171. Donaldson, S. R., Gelenberg, A. J., and Baldessarini, R. J. (1983). The pharmacologic treatment of schizophrenia: A progress report. *Schizophrenia Bulletin* 9:504–527.
172. Suranyi-Cadotte, B. E., Nestoros, J. N., Naer, N. P. V., Lal, S., and Gauthier, S. (1985). Parkinsonism induced by high doses of diazepam. *Biological Psychiatry* 20:455–457.
173. Modell, J. G., Lenox, R. H., and Weiner, S. (1985). Inpatient clinical trial of lorazepam for the management of manic agitation. *Journal of Clinical Psychopharmacology* 5:109–113.
174. Jimerson, D. C., van Kammen, D. P., Post, R. M., Docherty, J. P., and Bunney, W. E., Jr. (1982). Diazepam in schizophrenia: A preliminary double-blind study. *American Journal of Psychiatry* 139:489–491.
175. Zemlan, F. P., Hirschowitz, J., Sautter, F. J., and Garver, D. L. (1984). Impact of lithium therapy on core psychotic symptoms of schizophrenia. *British Journal of Psychiatry* 144:64–69.
176. Gelenberg, A. J. (1984). Serious toxicity from lithium. *Biological Therapies in Psychiatry* 7:21–22.
177. Roy-Byrne, P. P., Uhde, T. W., and Post, R. M. (1984). Carbamazepine for aggression, schizophrenia, and nonaffective syndromes. *International Drug Therapy Newsletter* 19:9–12.
178. Jann, M. W., Ereshefsky, L., Saklad, S. R., Seidel, D. R., Davis, C. M., Burch, N. R., and Bowden, C. L. (1985). Effects of carbamazepine on plasma haloperidol levels. *Journal of Clinical Psychopharmacology* 5:106–109.
179. Hansse, T., Heyden, T., Sundberg, I., Alfredsson, G., Nybäck, H., and Wetterberg, L. (1980). Propranolol in schizophrenia. *Archives of General Psychiatry* 37:685–690.
180. Silver, J. M., and Yudofsky, S. (1985). Propranolol for aggression: Literature review and clinical guidelines. *International Drug Therapy Newsletter* 20:9–12.
181. Cole, J. O. (1985). Tardive dyskinesia: A review and recommendations. APA Task Force on Tardive Dyskinesia. American Psychiatric Association Annual Meeting Workshop, Dallas.
182. Chouinard, G., and Turnier, L. (1985). Phase II: Clinical trial of remoxipride in schizophrenia. American Psychiatric Association Annual Meeting, New Research, Dallas.
183. Iager, A-C, Kirch, D. G., Pliskin, N., Bigelow, L. B., Wyatt, R. J., and Karson, C. N. (1985). Vasopressin treatment of schizophrenia. American Psychiatric Association Annual Meeting, New Research, Dallas.
184. Chouinard, G., and Annable, L. (1983). Rubidium chloride in the treatment of schizophrenia: A double-blind study. American Psychiatric Association, New Research, New York.
185. Mueser, K. T., and Dysken, M. W. (1983). Narcotic antagonists in schizophrenia: A methodological review. *Schizophrenia Bulletin* 9:213–225.

186. Lamb, H. R. (1980). Structure: The neglected ingredient of community treatment. *Archives of General Psychiatry* 37:1224-1228.
187. Rifkin, A., Quitkin, F., Rabiner, C. J., and Klein, D. F. (1977). Fluphenazine decanoate, fluphenazine hydrochloride given orally, and placebo in remitted schizophrenia. *Archives of General Psychiatry* 34:43-47.
188. Kane, J. M. (1985). Compliance issues in outpatient treatment. *Journal of Clinical Psychopharmacology* 5(3, Suppl.):225-275.
189. Schooler, N. R., and Levine, J. (1983). Strategies for enhancing drug therapy of schizophrenia. *American Journal of Psychotherapy* 37:521-532.
190. Pepper, B., and Ryglewicz, H., eds. (1982). The young adult chronic patient. In *New Directions for Mental Health Services*, ed. H. R. Lamb. Washington, DC: Jossey-Bass.
191. Pepper, B., Ryglewicz, H., eds. (1984). Advances in treating the young adult chronic patient. In *New Directions for Mental Health Services*, ed. H. R. Lamb. Washington, DC: Jossey-Bass.
192. Pepper, B., Kirshner, M. C., Ryglewicz, H. (1981). The young adult chronic patient: Overview of a population. *Hospital and Community Psychiatry* 12:463-469.
193. Masterson, J. F. (1972). *Treatment of the Borderline Adolescent: A Developmental Approach.* New York: Wiley.
194. Vaughn, C. E., Snyder, K. S., Jones, S., Freeman, W. B., and Falloon, I. R. H. (1984). Family factors in schizophrenic relapse. *Archives of General Psychiatry* 41:1169-1177.
195. Leff, J., Kuipers, L., Berkowitz, R., and Sturgeon, D. (1985). A controlled trial of social intervention in the families of schizophrenic patients: Two year follow-up. *British Journal of Psychiatry* 146:594-600.
196. Terkelsen, K. G. (1983). Schizophrenia and the family: II. Adverse effects of family therapy. *Family Process* 22:191-200.
197. Barter, J. T. (1984). Psychoeducation: Its role in the treatment of the chronic patient. In *The Chronic Mental Patient Five Years Later*, ed. J. A. Talbott. New York: Grune and Stratton.
198. Brown, G. W., Birley, J. L. T., and Wing, J. K. (1972). The influence of family life on the course of schizophrenia. *British Journal of Psychiatry* 121:241-258.
199. Wing, J. K., and Brown, G. W. (1970). *Institutionalism and Schizophrenia.* Cambridge, England: Cambridge University Press.
200. Breier, A., and Strauss, J. S. (1984). The role of social relationships in the recovery from psychotic disorders. *American Journal of Psychiatry* 141:949-955.
201. Cutler, D. L., and Madore, E. (1980). Community-family network therapy in a rural setting. *Community Mental Health Journal* 16:144-155.
202. Greenblatt, M., Becerra, R. M., and Serafetinides, E. A. (1982). Social networks and mental health: An overview. *American Journal of Psychiatry* 139:977-984.
203. Cutler, D. L. (1984). Networks. In *The Chronic Mental Patient Five Years Later*, ed. J. A. Talbott. New York: Grune and Stratton.
204. Feinsilver, D. B., and Yates, B. T. (1984). Combined use of psychotherapy and drugs in chronic, treatment-resistant schizophrenic patients: A retrospective study. *Journal of Nervous and Mental Diseases* 172:133-139.

205. Fromm-Reichmann, F. (1950). *Principles of Intensive Psychotherapy*. Chicago: University of Chicago Press.
206. Will, O. A., Jr. (1983). The relationship of psychopharmacology and schizophrenia. In *Psychopharmacology and Psychotherapy*, ed. M. H. Greenhill and A. Gralnick. New York: The Free Press.
207. Semrad, E. V. (1969). Comments in psychotherapy of the psychoses. In *Teaching Psychotherapy of Psychotic Patients*, ed. D. W. Buskirk and E. V. Semrad, pp. 31–44. New York: Grune and Stratton.
208. Gunderson, J. G., Frank, A. F., Katz, H. M., Vannicelli, M. L., Frosch, J. P., and Knapp, P. H. (1984). Effects of psychotherapy in schizophrenia: II. Comparative outcome of two forms of treatment. *Schizophrenia Bulletin* 19(4):564–584.

11

Atypical Depression

Ronald W. Pies, M.D.

How atypical is "atypical" depression? The impression of some clinicians is that atypical forms of depression—variously defined—are quite common in everyday practice. Thus, Nies (1) has commented:

> . . . patients whose depressive symptoms are more typical of the classical textbook descriptions of melancholia probably represent no more than ten percent of patients with significant depressive symptoms . . . [p. 75].

Indeed, features of atypical depression (AD) seem so common in depressed populations as to impugn the diagnostic validity of the concept (2,3). Nevertheless, many clinicians find the concept of AD helpful both in understanding and in treating certain patients. Evidence continues to grow that specific drugs are especially beneficial in at least some subtypes of AD. Moreover, the notion of AD has considerable heuristic value, since it overlaps several important conditions: panic disorder (4), agoraphobia (5), and borderline personality disorder (6). An improved understanding of AD may lead to refined understanding and treatment of these other disorders. In short, whatever its ambiguity, AD seems destined to shape both our concept and treatment of depressive illness.

Before pursuing AD further, it behooves us to ask an obvious question: What is "typical" depression? Since the concept may not evolve from the frequency with which typical depression is encountered, what sense can we give this term? It is surely not to be found in DSM-III, at least not in any obvious form. Nevertheless, most clinicians would call "typical" those cases of depression meeting DSM-III criteria for major depressive episode with melancholia. As we shall see, AD, in its many guises, generally approximates a "non-melancholic" form of depression (7). A variety of associated features are then elaborated to define AD more precisely. These notions of AD differ fundamentally from the residual category of "atypical affective disorder" in DSM-III.

HISTORICAL DEVELOPMENT OF THE AD CONCEPT

One sometimes feels that there are as many concepts of AD as there are articles on the subject. The notion of AD, in some form or another, dates back to at least 1948, when Huston and Locker described a group of depressed inpatients characterized by agitation, paranoid features, and responsivity to electroconvulsive therapy (ECT) (8). Shortly thereafter, Jarvie described a similar depressed population characterized by agitation, persecutory ideas, hallucinations, marked neuroticism, psychopathy, inadequacy, and poor adjustment to life (9). Electroconvulsive treatment was again effective in this group. Although the Huston-Locker-Jarvie populations seem quite unlike many patients now called atypically depressed, they do overlap with our modern notions of borderline personality (10), delusional depression (11), and anxious depression (12), of which only the first is represented in DSM-III.

It was not until around 1959 that our current notion of AD began to coalesce, mostly as a result of clinical observations by English workers. Thus, West and Dally (13) described a group of depressed patients characterized by anxiety, hysterical features, phobic complaints, emotional overreactivity, psychophysiological symptoms, fatigue, reversed diurnal mood variation (i.e., mood worse in the evening), poor response to ECT, and generally good premorbid personality. (This last feature proves to be an important differentiating factor, with respect to other types of AD.) The West and Dally population showed a good response to the monoamine oxidase inhibitor (MAOI) iproniazid, except in patients with life-long inadequate personalities.

Sargant (14), also in England, described a similar group of depressed patients characterized by a precipitating stressor, emotional instability, a tendency to blame others, hysterical exaggeration of symptoms, and (once again) good premorbid personality. Some of Sargant's patients also had premenstrual symptoms, and—contrary to the usual pattern in AD—weight loss. Sargant's patients, like those of West and Dally, responded to MAOI (phenelzine or isocarboxazid). In neither population were quantitative or controlled measures of drug response described.

Roth (15), roughly at the same time, drew attention to a small minority of agoraphobic patients in whom acute, benign, and short-lived schizophreniform illness developed under severe stress. Premorbidly, these patients had been anxious, oversensitive, self-conscious, lacking in self-esteem, and phobic, though generally able to function. This symptom cluster came to be known as the "phobic-anxiety-depersonalization" syndrome. As we shall see, it overlaps significantly with more recent concepts such as borderline personality disorder, hysteroid dysphoria (16), and a symptom profile described by Shader (17).

In 1978, Robinson and colleagues described a group of nonendogenous depressives, who scored high on measures of anxiety, weight gain, long-standing phobia, and hysterical personality (18). The MAOI phenelzine was effective in this population. The patients of Robinson and colleagues approximate those studied by the British workers, and it is convenient to group these patients and their symptoms together as the "British atypical depressives" (AD-B).

Recently, Beeber and Pies (7) have extracted those features of AD seen in at least two of the three aforementioned studies by West and Dally, Sargant, and Robinson and colleagues. Allowing for difficulties in direct comparisons of patients' traits, the following extracted factors for atypical depression (EFAD) emerge: (a) prominent anxiety, (b) histrionic features, (c) phobic features, (d) fatigue, (e) usually initial (rather than midcycle or terminal) insomnia, (f) adequate premorbid personality, and (g) psychosomatic complaints. We have developed a questionnaire based on these putative "core" features of AD.

In a review of the literature, Davidson and colleagues (19) discerned two broad types of atypical depression. The "A" type is depression accompanied by severe anxiety. The "V" type shows atypical or reversed vegetative features; for example, increased weight, appetite, or sleep. Both types have in common early age at onset, female predominance, outpatient status, mild intensity, rarity of attempted suicide, nonbipolarity, nonendogenicity, and minimal psychomotor changes.

Liebowitz and Klein have delineated another (presumed) subtype of AD, termed hysteroid dysphoria (HD) (16). They define HD as "a chronic, nonpsychotic disturbance involving repeated episodes of abruptly depressed mood in response to feeling rejected." These patients are "attention junkies," with an exquisitely fragile sense of self-esteem. Depressive bouts are usually characterized by overeating (especially chocolate or other sweets), oversleeping, extreme fatigue, and responsivity to attention and applause (nonautonomy of mood). In their nondepressed periods these HD patients tend to be histrionic, flamboyant, seductive, self-centered, and demanding. They also tend to abuse sedatives or stimulants, indulge in chronic dieting to maintain normal weight, make suicidal gestures or threats, and show poor social judgment, often with idealization of love objects. Klein has posited abnormal regulation of phenylethylamine (PEA) in HD patients (20), and speculated that the HD patient's chocolate–craving may stem from this defect. As yet, however, no direct empirical evidence has been adduced to support this hypothesis. Moreover, at least two studies (2, 3) have impugned the diagnostic validity of HD. Thus, the symptomatic overlap between HD and DSM-III Borderline Personality Disorder is evident and was borne out in a study by Beeber and colleagues (3).

Despite these uncertainties, recent pharmacological data (discussed below) lend some support to the concept of HD. In my experience, particularly with depressed female college students, HD has been a useful diagnostic category.

Beeber and Pies (7) have reviewed the plethora of syndromes that overlap with AD, which include:

- subaffective dysthymia;
- atypical depression, British (AD-B);
- anorexia nervosa, bulimia;

- episodic dyscontrol;
- minimal brain damage;
- borderline personality disorder;
- hysteroid dysphoria;
- character spectrum disorder;
- depression spectrum disorder.

It is evident that the pharmacological treatment of AD may differ markedly from subgroup to subgroup. Moreover, even the syndromes just listed do not cover the range of conditions sometimes considered atypical forms of depression. Depression in the elderly (21) or in children (22) sometimes takes "atypical" or "masked" forms, though recent evidence supports the utility of conventional DSM-III criteria for major depression in these age groups (23). Patients with chronic pain syndromes are sometimes viewed as atypically depressed (24). However, recent data showing divergent dexamethasone suppression test responses in chronic pain patients with or without depression cast doubt on this assumption (24). Pope and others have called attention to eating disorders as possible variant forms of depression (25). Numerous "neurotic" states, including obsessive-compulsive (26), hysterical conversion (27), and hypochondriacal disorders (28), have been viewed as atypical forms of depression. However, it is often difficult to know whether such conditions are manifestations of depression or whether depression is merely secondary to the underlying neurosis.

Since so-called treatment-resistant depressions are often treated with monoamine oxidase inhibitors (MAOIs) (alone or in combination with trycyclics), it is tempting to view these as atypical forms of depression. Generally, however, such resistant cases are merely the result of inadequate treatment for an inadequate period of time (29).

Finally, the work of Rosenthal and others (30) has pointed out the symptomatic overlap between atypical depression and the light-sensitive, seasonal energy syndrome (31). Thus, patients with fall-winter symptoms often complain of anergia, hypersomnia, sugar craving, increased appetite, and weight gain. Interestingly, these patients often show Raynaud's phenomenon, a finding also seen in one case of panic disorder associated with bipolar mood swings (32). Clearly, the relationship between AD, on the one hand, and anxiety states, vasomotor disturbance, and major affective disorder, on the other, remains quite unclear. I consider the following to be core features of atypical depression (EFAD):

- prominent anxiety;
- histrionic features;
- phobic features;
- fatigue
- initial insomnia, usually;
- adequate premorbid personality;
- psychosomatic complaints.

Subsequent references to AD will refer to these features, unless otherwise specified.

These extracted factors are primarily of clinical and heuristic value. Their validity will need to be confirmed by means of large-scale, controlled studies, utilizing demographic, biochemical (33), and prognostic variables.

CONCEPTUAL AND METHODOLOGICAL PROBLEMS IN STUDYING DRUG RESPONSE OF AD

Carroll (34) has pointed out a number of problems with current diagnostic criteria for depression. For example, several patients may end up with the same DSM-III diagnosis of major depression and yet have none of the twenty or more possible symptoms in common. Moreover, the diagnostic criteria do not in themselves ensure that groups of patients will be homogeneous. Finally (34),

> DSM-III merely provides a set of nonstatistical algorithms which . . . have never been validated by . . . response to specific treatments, studies of natural history or family history, or use of biological markers [p. 15].

Approaching the problem of classification from a statistical standpoint, Andreasen (35) has noted some pitfalls in the use of cluster analysis, a method by which similar patients are grouped together so as to generate subtypes of depression. Because there is no way of knowing the "correct" number of clusters inherent in a set of data, cluster analysis never assures us that the correct number of depressive subtypes has been determined.

Such general problems of classification pervade the literature on drug response in AD. For example, depending on the criteria used to select an AD population, a particular drug may or may not be effective. Thus, "atypical" patients with high, generalized anxiety may not do well on deprenyl (a selective MAO-B inhibitor described later) (36), but do quite well on phenelzine (37). Similarly, if one systematically excludes panic disorder patients from one's AD population, MAOIs may prove no more effective than tricyclics (37).

Essentially technical factors also complicate the drug response studies of AD. First, there is wide variation in the dosage of medication used. Thirty milligrams of phenelzine may be ineffective in treating AD, whereas 60 mg may be quite effective (38). Dosage also appears critical in isocarboxazid therapy (39).

Nies has pointed out that comparisons between drugs may be somewhat misleading in studies of AD (1). Thus, "the non-specific effect of each drug is large enough to weigh down and obscure their specific differences." Drug–placebo comparisons may obviate this problem but leaves us ignorant of differential pharmacotherapeutic effects. Finally, the literature on drug treatment of AD seems to have spawned a number of misconceptions. In this regard, let us consider these three superficially related propositions:

1. MAOIs are better than tricyclics in the treatment of AD (however defined).

2. "Typically" depressed patients (e.g., melancholic type) should not be treated with MAOIs.

3. MAOI responders do poorly on tricyclics or other agents.

As we shall see, proposition 1 is gaining modest experimental support. Clinicians may reason intuitively from this proposition to 2 and 3. However, there is little evidence to support these other notions, and some data to the contrary, as we shall see below.

REVIEW OF SELECTED RECENT LITERATURE

With the foregoing complexities in mind, can we extract, nevertheless, some useful conclusions from the literature on atypical depression? The earlier studies of drug response in AD (e.g., 1959–1981) have been reviewed exhaustively by Quitkin and colleagues (40), Davidson and colleagues (19), and Nies and Robinson (41). I shall focus, in some detail, on some of the better controlled studies completed within the past 3 years.

Monoamine Oxidase Inhibitor (MAOI) Studies

Paykel and colleagues (42) studied 131 outpatients with mixed anxiety and depression, who were treated for 6 weeks with phenelzine (60–75 mg/day), amitriptyline (150–190 mg/day), or placebo in a double-blind study. Patients were assessed according to three definitions of "atypical" depression: (a) the presence of marked anxiety, (including phobic and panic symptoms), (b) reversed neurovegetative signs (e.g., hypersomnia or increased weight), or (c) absence of endogenous features (using several measures of endogenicity). There proved to be only "a tendency" for phenelzine to have stronger effects in patients with marked anxiety. Consistent with the report of West and Dally (13), patients with characterological depression tended to do worse with phenelzine than with amitriptyline. Generally, however, the authors found little evidence to support a differential response to either active drug, based on any of the concepts of AD. Specifically (42),

> The two classes of antidepressants show many more similar effects in clinically defined subgroups than has been believed, with some probable differences, but relatively weak ones . . . [p. 1048].

This conclusion was later questioned by Nies (1), who suggests (as noted in the previous section) that the nonspecific effects of each drug are large enough "to weigh down and obscure" their specific differences. Reanalyzing Paykel's data along a drug–placebo dimension, Nies (1) concludes that:

> . . . in comparison with placebo, phenelzine outcome shows a pattern of response to predictors which are associated with atypical depression [p. 74].

Specifically, patients with high overall levels of anxiety and absence of characterological depression show this response to phenelzine.

Nies himself has provided modest support for the specificity of phenelzine, as compared with amitriptyline, in a heterogeneous group of depressed outpatients (1). Phenelzine (60 mg/day) showed no significant advantage over amitriptyline (150 mg/day) in patients whose atypical features included somatic anxiety and hypochondriasis. However, there was a weak trend for phenelzine to be superior in treating psychic anxiety and in energizing patients. Predictors of better response to phenelzine included high pretreatment anxiety, panic-type symptoms, hysteroid dysphoria, and secondary depression with primary phobic symptoms.

Liebowitz and colleagues (37) in an especially well-designed study, looked at the effects of imipramine, phenelzine, or placebo in a group of atypical depressives. AD was defined operationally as follows:

1. Patients met Research Diagnostic Criteria (RDC) criteria for major, minor, or intermittent depression.
2. Patients showed "mood reactivity" when depressed (non-autonomy of mood).
3. Patients showed two or more of the following features:
   - increased appetite or weight gain while depressed;
   - oversleeping;
   - severe fatigue or heaviness in the limbs while depressed;
   - rejection sensitivity.

Anxiety was not required for a diagnosis of AD. The patients so selected were further divided as follows:

1. AD patients (including hysteroid dysphorics) with a history of panic attacks,
2. AD patients without panic attacks, who also met criteria for hysteroid dysphoria,
3. AD patients with neither panic attacks nor HD ("plain" AD).

Excluded were patients with psychotic, sociopathic, obsessive-compulsive, anorexic, or bulimic features, as well as patients with recent drug abuse. (These exclusion criteria would probably eliminate many patients with DSM-III Borderline Personality Disorder.)

The procedure involved a 10-day, single-blind placebo trial for all patients. Those not significantly improved were randomized to 6-week treatment on imipramine, phenelzine, or placebo. Double-blind conditions were maintained. Imipramine dosage eventually exceeded 200 mg, p.o., q.h.s., while phenelzine dosage was in the range of 60–90 mg/day—both considered adequate for clinical purposes. Treatment response was measured via psychiatrists' ratings on the CGI (Clinical Global Impression) Change Scale.

Broadly speaking, phenelzine, but not imipramine, proved markedly superior to placebo. Interestingly, phenelzine was superior to imipramine on two self-rated measures of interpersonal vulnerability and discomfort—a trait commonly seen in borderline and HD patients. Comparison among subgroups showed that in the "plain" AD group (lacking HD and panic attacks), patients showed a 50% response to all treatments, including placebo. However, the panic attack subgroup showed a greater response to phenelzine than to placebo or imipramine. This was also true in the HD subgroup, though the phenelzine–imipramine difference was not statistically significant.

Liebowitz and colleagues concluded that AD patients with panic attacks, and possibly those with HD, appear specifically responsive to phenelzine. So-called plain AD patients (by the criteria used) appear equally responsive to MAOIs, imipramine, or placebo. One confounding factor, noted by the authors, was the high baseline anxiety and phobia scores in the panic-attack subgroup, in comparison to the "plain" ADs. These features might have contributed to the observed MAOI response in the panic attack group. (Of course, even if this were so, it would support the traditional "anxious-phobic" category of AD, long viewed as specifically responsive to MAOIs.) With respect to the very high placebo response of the plain ADs, it must be remembered that the criteria for AD used by Liebowitz and colleagues are only one of the many possible sets of criteria. As shown in Table 11–1, there is only partial overlap with the "core" features (EFAD) utilized by Beeber and Pies (7). It is conceivable that a different set of entrance criteria for AD would have produced a more phenelzine-responsive population.

TABLE 11-1 Comparison of Liebowitz and Colleagues Criteria for Atypical Depression with Beeber and Pies (EFAD)

Liebowitz and Colleagues (37)	Beeber and Pies (EFAD) (7)
Patients meet RDC criteria for major, minor, or intermittent depression. Patients show "mood reactivity" when depressed. Patients show two or more of the following: • increased appetite or weight gain while depressed, • oversleeping, • severe fatigue or heaviness in the limbs while depressed, • rejection sensitivity.	Prominent anxiety. Histrionic features. Phobic features. Fatigue. Usually initial insomnia. Adequate premorbid personality. Psychosomatic complaints.

Quitkin and colleagues (43), in a companion study to the criteria in Table 11-1 examined drug response in depressed patients (a) meeting RDC criteria for major, minor, or intermittent depression; and (b) showing reactivity of mood while depressed, but showing only one or none of the associated features described above (essentially, hypersomnia, hyperphagia, lethargy, and rejection sensitivity). In a sense, these subatypical patients were chosen so as to reveal the core features of phenelzine responsivity. A 10-day placebo period was initiated (single blind) for all patients. Placebo responders were excluded, and the rest entered into a 6-week active treatment period on either imipramine (up to at least 200 mg/day) or phenelzine (at least 60 mg/day).

In the group ($n = 41$) with mood reactivity and one associated atypical feature, 35% responded to placebo, 38% to imipramine, and 73% to phenelzine. No single associated feature was clearly associated with response to either active treatment (owing to insufficient sample size).

In the patients with mood reactivity but no associated atypical features ($n = 27$), 30% responded to placebo, 75% to imipramine, and 77% to phenelzine. Because there were only four patients in the imipramine group, no conclusion vis-à-vis imipramine versus phenelzine was possible.

Quitkin and colleagues concluded that patients with reactive mood and only one associated atypical feature may respond preferentially to phenelzine, compared to imipramine or placebo. There were insufficient data on patients with mood reactivity alone to permit any conclusions. However, the study generally supports the utility of phenelzine in at least one type of nonmelancholic depression.

If the pattern of response in the Quitkin study were to hold in studies of larger cohorts—in particular, the marked drop in efficacy of imipramine (from 75% to 38%) when even one atypical feature is "added"—one might postulate actual resistance to tricyclics in atypically depressed patients, as defined by the Quitkin criteria. At present, it is by no means clear which associated feature (hypersomnia, hyperphagia, etc.) is critical in conferring phenelzine responsiveness or a putative tricyclic resistance. Moreover, other studies (using different concepts of AD) do not support the notion of tricyclic resistance in atypical depression (42, 44). Kayser and colleagues (44) looked at phenelzine versus amitriptyline response in a group of fifty-one depressed outpatients evaluated for HD. Of the forty-seven patients completing the study, fourteen were considered to be high scorers on the HD questionnaire, and thirty-three, low scorers. Significantly more of the high HD scorers had moderate to marked improvement on phenelzine (60 mg/day) than on amitriptyline (100% vs. 60%). Low HD scorers responded equally well to the two drugs (79%).

These data generally bolster the Klein-Liebowitz hypothesis that HD is a discrete diagnostic and pharmacological subtype. However, it is clear from the Kayser study that 60% of the high HD score group had a good response to amitriptyline. Though the number of patients (five) was very small in this subgroup, the finding lends no support to the notion that atypically depressed patients generally do poorly on standard antidepressants. Conversely, many depressed patients with a low HD score did well on phenelzine (79%), thus impugning the notion that MAOIs are useful only in atypically depressed patients (assuming that HD is a form of atypical depression). Nevertheless, the Kayser study does support the use of phenelzine as the drug of first choice in HD.

Thus far, we have focused exclusively on phenelzine, in contrast to other MAOIs. Indeed, phenelzine is the most widely used and studied MAOI, but an overreliance on phenelzine as a model of MAOI pharmacodynamics may lead to unwarranted generalizations.

The MAOIs may be classified in a variety of ways (41,45); as hydrazine or nonhydrazine, reversible or irreversible, selective or nonselective. Thus, phenelzine is a hydrazine-type, irreversible, nonselective MAOI. Unfortunately, the precise clinical significance of these pharmacological distinctions is not clear. The hydrazines may be more effective than the nonhydrazines but appear to have greater hepatotoxicity (40,41). The possible clinical significance of reversible and selective MAOIs will be discussed below, in relation to specific drugs.

Suffice it to say, at this point, that reversibility refers to how "tightly" the MAOI is bound to its respective MAO enzyme. Selectivity refers to the preference of the MAOI for one or the other type of MAO enzyme, termed A and B. These subtypes (A and B) differ in their substrates and in their main site of action. Thus, MAO-A acts primarily upon serotonin and norepinephrine and predominates in the gut and liver. MAO-B acts primarily on phenylethylamine and benzylamine and predominates in the brain. The commonly used MAOIs (phenelzine, tranylcypromine, isocarboxazid) are termed nonselective, since they act on both MAO-A and MAO-B.

However, this simplified discussion (41,45) omits the many complexities of MAO and MAOIs, as detailed by Murphy and colleagues (46). For example, although tranylcypromine is usually considered an irreversible MAOI, its bonding properties actually place it in an intermediate position of reversibility; it may be more reversible than phenelzine, but less so than the investigational MAOI meclobemide (see p. 344). From the clinician's perspective, reversibility has implications for the drug's potential toxicity. Selectivity of the MAOI may have implications for both drug toxicity and site of action; in theory, for example, one might expect a selective MAO-B inhibitor to act primarily on the brain. By acting minimally on gut and liver MAO, such a drug might spare the individual from the harmful effects of tyramine overload (41,45).

Isocarboxazid (Marplan) is an irreversible, nonselective, hydrazine MAOI. There appear to be no controlled studies comparing isocarboxazid with either standard antidepressants or other MAOIs, in a strictly defined population with AD. Giller and colleagues (47) studied the characteristics of patients who responded to isocarboxazid, using discriminant function analysis. The patients ($n = 60$) were mainly middle-aged, male outpatients meeting DSM-III criteria for Major Depressive Episode and, in seven cases, melancholia. Other inclusion criteria were dysphoric mood, anxiety, somatic symptoms of anxiety, and a Hamilton Depression Rating Scale (HAM-D) score of 20 or higher. The first phase of the study was double blind and placebo controlled. The second phase was an open, active-drug trial for patients not improved on placebo. In phase 1, the dose of isocarboxazid was adjusted to yield 90% platelet MAO inhibition. The mean daily dose at 6 weeks was roughly 58 mg. Forty-three patients had a trial on active medication. Ratings on HAM-D and clinical global impression (CGI) showed that 60% of those on active treatment improved significantly. Only 18% on placebo did. Interestingly, all seven patients with DSM-III melancholia had a good response to isocarboxazid. Response was associated with higher pretreatment platelet MAO, higher diastolic blood pressure at entry into the study, and the presence of psychomotor agitation or retardation. The authors concluded that the MAOI showed little specificity for atypical depression in that it improved the melancholic subgroup. However, the results were consistent with other data on MAOIs, insofar as this population showed high levels of anxiety and somatization. Nonetheless, the Giller study calls into question the notion, discussed in the previous section, that MAOIs should not be used in typically depressed patients.

Zisook and colleagues (48) studied a group of sixty-nine anxious, somatizing AD outpatients who did not meet DSM-III criteria for melancholia. In a 6-week, double-blind study using either isocarboxazid (up to 80 mg/day) or placebo, isocarboxazid was clearly superior to placebo for the total group. However, no subgroups could be identified as specifically responsive to isocarboxazid. The single item associated with a statistically significant advantage of isocarboxazid over placebo was loss of anticipatory pleasure.

Neither typical nor atypical vegetative symptoms, presence or absence of phobias, fatigue, anergia, or endogenous features predicted outcome. Hypersomnia and rejection-sensitivity were not studied. That the loss of anticipatory pleasure—as opposed to consummatory or experiential pleasure—was correlated with isocarboxazid response is of some theoretical interest, since this symptom is characteristic of HD (16).

Tranylcypromine (Parnate) is an irreversible, nonselective, nonhydrazine MAOI. There have been relatively few controlled studies of tranylcypromine in well-defined AD populations, and it is not prescribed as widely as phenelzine (40). Early studies did provide evidence of tranylcypromine's superiority to placebo, and its roughly equal efficacy in comparison to tricyclics, in heterogeneous depressed populations (49). Recently, McGrath and colleagues (50) studied the effect of tranylcypromine in twelve outpatients meeting DSM-III criteria for melancholia. All patients went through a 10-day placebo trial, after which placebo-responders were eliminated. Of the twelve patients who went on to tranylcypromine treatment, nine (75%) responded. Responders, though melancholic, were rated as less depressed at baseline than were nonresponders. Again, the specificity of MAOI for AD patients was impugned. Interestingly, one of the responders was delusionally depressed.

l-Deprenyl (Selegiline) is a selective MAO-B inhibitor not now marketed for routine use which has received little study in the treatment of AD. Quitkin and colleagues (36), in a 6-week open trial of seventeen patients with AD (using the criteria of Liebowitz and colleagues [37]), found that 59% of patients responded to l-deprenyl. When compared with a six-week placebo treatment, administered in a separate double-blind study, l-deprenyl responders had lower baseline anxiety rates. A history of absence of panic attacks had no effect on response to l-deprenyl—again in contrast to phenelzine. Interestingly, patients who had a dysphoric response to a single intravenous dose of d-amphetamine tended to have a good response to l-deprenyl. This study points out the probable heterogeneity of MAOI effects and the difficulty of drawing conclusions about what type of depression responds to MAOIs. The amphetamine-challenge data are of some theoretical interest, since response to ordinary antidepressants may be correlated with good response to amphetamine (51). The reversed outcome with respect to l-deprenyl may reflect a biochemically distant type of depression. Indeed, one wonders if a subset of AD patients might be, as it were, "wired backward," and became euphoric on depressant-type drugs.

In reviewing their own and other studies of l-deprenyl, Mann and colleagues (52) concluded that this drug is probably most effective in nonendogenous depression and for those (endogenous or nonendogenous) who present with certain "reverse" neurovegetative signs—particularly hyperphagia. l-Deprenyl appears ineffective in depressed patients with associated panic attacks and phobic symptoms, suggesting that MAO-A inhibition is critical to treatment of these symptoms. Because *l*-deprenyl does not significantly alter tyramine sensitivity (52), it may have a safety advantage over currently marketed MAOIs. Pargyline (Eutonyl), like *l*-deprenyl, is a (partially) selective MAO-B inhibitor, marketed as an antihypertensive agent. Quitkin and colleagues (40) have reviewed most of the earlier studies demonstrating pargyline's efficacy in a variety of depressed populations. More recently, Pickar and colleagues (53) reported on the use of pargyline in thirteen patients meeting RDC criteria for major depression. Mania and hypomania were noted as complications in somewhat less that 15% of cases. At present, the specific advantages and indications of pargyline, if any, are unclear.

Clorgyline is an investigational MAO-A inhibitor that is no longer manufactured. Several controlled studies have demonstrated its antidepressant effects, but it appears to have no special advantages over other MAOIs (52).

Thus far, we have discussed the irreversible MAOIs. Several investigative compounds are reversible MAOIs, for example, meclobemide (Roche), MD 780515 (Delande), and FLA 336 (+) (Astra) are all reversible MAO-B inhibitors (52). Recently, Norman and colleagues (54) compared meclobemide with amitriptyline in twenty-five depressed inpatients. Sixty percent responded to meclobemide, versus 55% to amitriptyline. Vague generalized headaches, but no hypertensive reactions, were reported with meclobemide. Since the reversible MAOIs may actually be displaced from MAO by tyramine, these drugs may prove safer for patients who depart from a tyramine-free diet. The utility of these reversible MAOIs has yet to be established in well-defined AD populations.

Depending on one's definition of atypical depression, a variety of non-MAOI medications may be useful in selected cases. Sovner (55) found the relatively nonsedating secondary amine tricyclic desipramine useful in anxious patients with atypical vegetative signs. The use of nonsedating tricyclics makes intuitive sense for lethargic, hypersomnic patients, and I have had success (in one case of AD with hypersomnia and lethargy) using protriptyline. However, I know of no controlled studies comparing MAOIs to secondary amine tricyclics in rigorously defined AD populations.

Other non-MAOI antidepressants have acquired a reputation for anxiolytic properties, for example, imipramine, doxepin, and trazodone. Crook (56) concluded that "tricyclic antidepressants, particularly imipramine and doxepin, are superior to the benzodiazepines chlordiazepoxide and diazepam in alleviating both anxiety and depression in mixed anxious-depressed adults." However, few studies have compared imipramine and doxepin with other tricyclics, vis-à-vis anxiolytic properties. It seems likely that the sedative and/or anticholinergic properties of imipramine and doxepin may account for at least some of their reputed anxiolytic effects. In contrast, in one study (57), trazodone, which lacks anticholinergic properties, appears to be superior to both desipramine and imipramine in relieving psychic and somatic anxiety associated with depression. Trazodone also proved as effective in relieving anxiety as chlordiazepoxide in one controlled study (58).

On the whole, the benzodiazepines are not useful in primary depressive illness and may occasionally exacerbate depression (59). However, controlled studies in rigorously defined AD populations are lacking. Certainly, the new "triazolo" benzodiazepine, alprazolam (Xanax) merits consideration in anxious depressives, since it has anxiolytic (generalized or panic-type anxiety) and antidepressant properties (60). The author has reported two cases of mixed depression and panic attacks successfully treated with alprazolam (doses ranging from 1.5 to 2.0 mg orally per day), accompanied by normalization of the DST in both cases (61). Recently, concern has arisen over the possible disinhibiting (62) and habituating (63) properties of alprazolam, though I have not been impressed with these problems in more than fifty cases of alprazolam use.

The use of antipsychotic agents in well-defined AD populations has not been studied systematically. If one considers Borderline Personality Disorder (BPD) a variant of affective illness, or a form of atypical depression, it might make intuitive sense to treat BPD with antidepressants; indeed, this has been suggested, using both conventional antidepressants or MAOIs (64). However, low-dose antipsychotics have also been suggested for BPD patients, especially those with thought process disorder or schizophrenic psychopathology (64).

Klein and colleagues (65) have also used antipsychotics (notably thioridazine) in so-called emotionally unstable character disorder, a syndrome with marked similiarity to BPD. Similarly, Brinkley and colleagues (66) found neuroleptics with "activating properties" (more accurately, less sedating properties) such as thiothixene or trifluoperazine useful in BPD, over a wide spectrum of symptoms.

Klein and Shader (67) and Cole and Sunderland (64) have offered useful typologies of BPD with guidelines for pharmacotherapy. However, the whole issue is fraught with diagnostic uncertainty and a paucity of well-controlled studies. Moreover, the precise relationship between BPD and AD remains unclear, despite significant symptomatic overlap. A similar picture, unfortunately, also prevails with respect to use of lithium carbonate in AD. Once again, "emotionally unstable character disorder" may respond to lithium (65), as may a cyclothymic subgroup of Akiskal's "subaffective dysthymic" patients (68). Both types of patient overlap with HD and other concepts of AD. I have found no controlled comparisons of antipsychotics or lithium versus MAOIs in the treatment of well-defined AD populations.

Andrulonis and colleagues (69) described a possible organic subgroup of BPD, characterized by "episodic dyscontrol," that is, spontaneous and uncontrolled attacks of rage or violence. These patients often have depression and free-floating anxiety as part of their syndrome and thus overlap with several types of AD. Anticonvulsants (such as carbamazepine) might be useful in such episodic dyscontrol syndromes, particularly when temporal lobe abnormalities are seen on electroencephalogram (EEG).

So-called minimal brain dysfunction (MBD) may also present with affective and borderline features, such as depression, anxiety, mood swings, impulsivity, aggressive outbursts, drug abuse, and suicide gestures (69). To this extent, MBD, like episodic dyscontrol syndrome, has affinities with atypical depression. Minimal brain dysfunction in adults may respond to stimulants, as it does in children (69). However, the use of stimulants (such as methylphenidate) in most AD patients would be risky, owing to the potential for both abuse and drug-induced hypomania.

Finally, a number of newer (and as yet unreleased) agents show some promise in the treatment of AD. Bupropion (Wellbutrin), a nontricyclic antidepressant, showed better anxiolytic properties than did imipramine, in one double-blind, controlled study (70). However, imipramine dosage reached only 150 mg/day. Patients with psychosomatic complaints also appear responsive to bupropion (71) but not those with panic-phobic type symptoms (72). Should bupropion prove useful in AD, it may do so in those patients with generalized anxiety and somatic complaints. (It has been removed from the market by the U.S. FDA but continues to have research programs associated with it.) Buspirone (Buspar) is an anxiolytic agent chemically unrelated to any other psychotropic drug (73). Some preliminary evidence suggests that buspirone is better than clorazepate

(Tranxene) in relieving depression and "interpersonal sensitivity" (74). Feighner and colleagues (75), in a double-blind study comparing buspirone with diazepam, concluded that "buspirone may be particularly indicated for anxious patients who have a strong depressive component" (p. 107).

Polypharmacy

Virtually unexplored is the efficacy of combination treatments in well-defined AD populations. In principle, one could consider (among other possibilities) MAOI/tricyclic, lithium/tricyclic, lithium/MAOI, or a benzodiazepine plus any of the above in the treatment of AD. I know of no controlled studies of AD utilizing such regimens, much less studies comparing polypharmacy to MAOI.

White and Simpson (76) have reviewed the use of MAOI-tricyclic therapy in refractory depression, but it is by no means clear that this entity, even it is valid, overlaps significantly with any concept of AD.

Monoamine oxidase inhibitors can be safely combined with lithium and with neuroleptics, though there may be some potentiation of extrapyramidal effects with the latter (77). While MAOIs and benzodiazepines are often used in combination, Davidson and colleagues (77) caution that behavioral disinhibition may occur with this regimen.

In short, the use of MAOIs in combination with other drugs has not been studied systematically in this very diverse population. I urge caution in adding polypharmacy to polymorphism.

Electroconvulsive Therapy (ECT)

The use of ECT has not been studied systematically in AD. It will be recalled that West and Dally's (13) AD patients had a poor response to ECT. In contrast, van Valkenburg and Winokur's (78) "depression spectrum" patients were "overwhelmingly" responders to ECT.

These ECT responders were selected from a depressed population on the basis of alcoholic, rather than depressed, first-degree relatives. This depression-spectrum group appears to have affinities with BPD. However, psychotic features were common in van Valkenburg and Winokur's cohort and it may be that this psychotic subgroup, primarily, had a good response to ECT. In general, response to ECT appears correlated with signs and symptoms of typical, endogenous, psychotic, or melancholic types of depression (79). However, Mandel's suggestion (80) that ECT may be effective in chronic pain associated with depression is of interest, since some regard chronic pain as a form of masked depression (24).

PRACTICAL CONSIDERATIONS

It is too early to speak of a "definitive" pharmacological treatment for AD, however defined. Nevertheless, the research to date does permit some tentative, and largely pragmatic, recommendations. What follows is essentially a "what I would do" approach to AD, rather than a scientifically established set of guidelines.

Let us return to the putative core features of AD (EFAD) listed earlier in this chapter, that is, prominent anxiety, histrionic features, initial insomnia, psychosomatic complaints, phobic complaints, marked fatigue, and good premorbid adjustment. What should the clinician prescribe for the patient with most, or all, of these features? Figure 11-1 attempts to diagram a tentative pragmatic approach to such a patient.

It must first be said that, within this group of AD patients, individuals will differ as to the relative intensity of specific symptoms. Thus, some patients may have severe, incapacitating anxiety, but only moderate fatigue or hypersomnia. Others may have only moderate anxiety, but severe fatigue and hypersomnia, such that the patient spends 18–20 hours per day in bed. As we shall see, these quantitative differences have implications for pharmacological treatment. However, the first clinical decision, as shown in Figure 11-1, is qualitative, that is, deciding whether the patient may be lithium-responsive. Although Nelson and Charney (81) concluded that "the unipolar-bipolar distinction depends on a history of mania rather than the character of the depressive syndrome," and though DSM-III does not distinguish between unipolar and bipolar depressive states, some clinicians maintain that the two differ phenomenologically (82). Thus, hypersomnia and psychomotor retardation are said to be more common in bipolar depression (82). If this is true, it follows that some AD patients (without known history of manic episodes) may be "covert" bipolar patients. Certainly, the clinician should attempt to elicit a history of marked cyclothymia, drug-induced mania (53) or

Practical Considerations

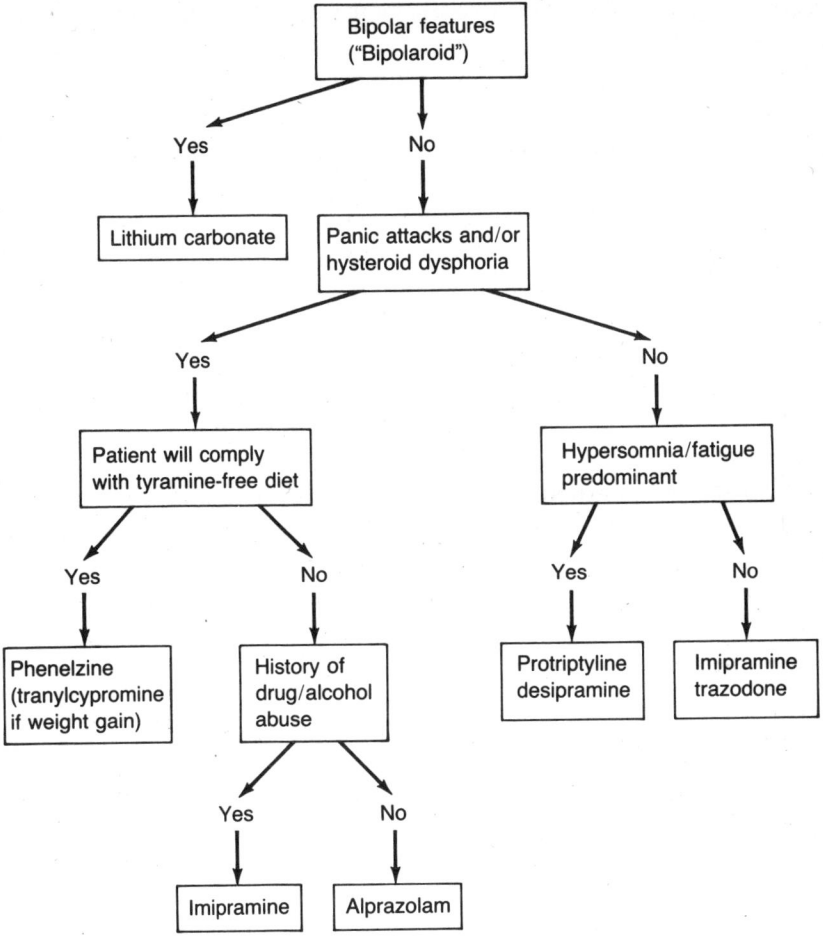

FIGURE 11-1. Tentative approach to the treatment of atypical depression (EFAD criteria).

family history of bipolar disorder from every AD patient, but particularly from those with hypersomnia and psychomotor retardation. If the patient has two or more of these features—patients I call "bipolaroid"—I would begin treatment with lithium. This is motivated less by the conviction that lithium will be spectacularly effective than by the concern that MAOIs or tricyclics will induce mania in such patients (53). I recently saw an AD patient with a history of phenelzine-induced mania who spent $3,000 (most of her savings) in a matter of days. She subsequently had a psychotic episode following use of imipramine.

Using the data of Liebowitz and colleagues (37) we must then deal with the next issue, the presence or absence of panic attacks and/or hysteroid dysphoria. If either or both of these are present, a trial on phenelzine is probably the treatment of first choice. If weight gain becomes a problem, tranylcypromine may be used (83). However, some patients will not agree to a tyramine-free diet, and some will not comply with it (84). Furthermore, some borderline patients will use the diet as a suicide threat (84).

In such unwilling or unreliable patients, a trial of imipramine or alprazolam may be preferable to an MAOI. If the patient has a history of alcohol or sedative abuse, imipramine may be safer than alprazolam.

If the AD patient lacks both panic attacks and/or criteria for HD, the treatment of first choice is less clear cut. I believe it is helpful to subdivide such patients into those with hypersomnia and fatigue as the predominant complaint, and those in whom other EFAD symptoms predominate (i.e., anxiety, histrionic features, initial insomnia, psychosomatic complaints, or phobias).

In the fatigued, hypersomnic group, I would initiate treatment with either protriptyline or desipramine. Both drugs are nonsedating, and protriptyline may be especially useful in treating hypersomnia (85). [Caution is warranted, however, in patients prone to overdosing, since protriptyline has a very long half-life, approaching 80 hours (86). On the other hand, some animal data suggest that protriptyline is less cardiotoxic than desipramine or nortriptyline (87).] In patients without marked fatigue and hypersomnia, I would initiate treatment with imipramine or trazodone. These relatively sedating (and perhaps anxiolytic) drugs can be prescribed at bedtime for patients with initial insomnia. If response is poor in either subgroup, treatment may be initiated with phenelzine or alprazolam, as diagrammed for patients with panic attacks or HD. Clearly, large-scale, controlled trials are sorely needed to establish the validity of this algorithm.

The question of combined medication and psychotherapy is covered in Chapter 14. With respect to AD, the data are quite scanty. Liebowitz and Klein (16) used a primarily supportive (nonpsychoanalytic) type of therapy in a small group of HD patients concomitantly treated with phenelzine. Though the combination seemed to be effective, psychotherapy was quite "stormy," characterized by intense transference reactions and acting out. Moreover, the relative contribution of medication versus psychotherapy was not clear.

In my experience, many AD patients—particularly those with hysteroid dysphoric or borderline features—do poorly in unstructured, "time-unlimited," "uncovering" types of therapy. This is not to say that psychoanalytic principles should be ignored; on the contrary, confronting and interpreting negative transference and understanding countertransference reactions is a practical necessity with such patients. However, a structured (88), time-limited (89), supportive approach (in which mature defenses are bolstered) is most useful in the hysteroid-borderline type of AD patient. As with most pharmacological approaches, this claim stands in need of large-scale controlled studies.

Atypical depression remains an elusive concept, despite more rigorous definition in recent years. AD undoubtedly overlaps with a variety of conditions, including DSM-III BPD and such non-DSM-III categories as Akiskal's character-spectrum disorder. The pharmacological treatment of AD may depend, in part, on how the category is defined and on the presence of specific symptoms such as panic attacks. In general, an MAOI is probably the drug of choice. Imipramine, alprazolam, and a variety of other agents may also be useful. Of critical importance in this field is the need for further, well-designed studies.

REFERENCES

1. Nies, A. (1984). Differential response patterns to MAO inhibitors and tricyclics. *Journal of Clinical Psychiatry* 45:70-77.
2. Spitzer, R. L., and Williams, J. B. W. (1982). Hysteroid dysphoria: An unsuccessful attempt to demonstrate its syndromal validity. *American Journal of Psychiatry* 139:1286-1291.
3. Beeber, A. R., Kline, M. D., and Pies, R. W. (1984). Hysteroid dysphoria in depressed inpatients. *Journal of Clinical Psychiatry* 45:164-166.
4. Sheehan, D. V., Ballenger, J., and Jacobsen, G. (1980). Treatment of endogenous anxiety with phobic, hysterical, and hypochondriacal symptoms. *Archives of General Psychiatry* 37:51-59.
5. Whiteford, H. A., and Evans, L. (1984). Agoraphobia and the dexamethasone suppression test: Atypical depression? *Australian and New Zealand Journal of Psychiatry* 18:374-377.
6. Stone, M. H. (1979). Contemporary shift of the borderline concept from a subschizophrenic disorder to a subaffective disorder. *Psychiatric Clinics of North America* 2:577-594.

7. Beeber, A. R., and Pies, R. W. (1983). The nonmelancholic depressive syndromes: An alternative approach to classification. *Journal of Nervous and Mental Disease* 171:3–9.
8. Huston, P. E., and Locker, L. M. (1948). Manic-depressive psychosis. *Archives of Neurology and Psychiatry* 60:37–48.
9. Jarvie, H. F. (1950). On atypicality and the depressive state. *Journal of Nervous and Mental Sciences* 96:208–225.
10. Kernberg, O. (1975). *Borderline Conditions and the Pathological Narcissism.* New York: Jason Aronson.
11. Charney, D. S., and Nelson, J. C. (1981). Delusional and nondelusional unipolar depression: Further evidence for distinct subtypes. *American Journal of Psychiatry* 138:328–333.
12. Roth, M. (1978). The classification of affective disorders. *Pharmakopsychiatrie* 11:27–42.
13. West, E. D., and Dally, P. J. (1959). Effect of iproniazid in depressive syndromes. *British Medical Journal* 1:1491–1494.
14. Sargant, W. (1961). Drugs in the treatment of depression. *British Medical Journal* 1:225–227.
15. Roth, M. (1959). Phobic-anxiety-depersonalization syndrome. *Proceedings of the Royal Society of Medicine* 52:587–595.
16. Liebowitz, M. R., and Klein, D. F. (1979). Hysteroid dysphoria. *Psychiatric Clinics of North America* 2:555–575.
17. Shader, R. I. (1984). A new axis II diagnosis: Troubles (editorial). *Journal of Clinical Psychopharmacology* 4:241.
18. Robinson, D. S., Nies, A., Ravaris, C. L., Ives, J. O., and Bartlett, D. (1978). Clinical pharmacology of phenelzine. *Archives of General Psychiatry* 35:629–635.
19. Davidson, J. R., Miller, R. D., Turnbull, C. D., and Sullivan, J. L. (1982). Atypical depression. *Archives of General Psychiatry* 39:527–534.
20. Klein, D. (1974). Pathophysiology of depressive syndromes (letter). *Biological Psychiatry* 8:119–120.
21. Gurland, B. J. (1976). The comparative frequency of depression in various adult age groups. *Journal of Gerontology* 31:283–292.
22. Kovacs, M., and Beck, A. T. (1977). An empirical-clinical approach toward a definition of childhood depression. In *Depression in Childhood*, J. G. Schulterbrand and A. Raskin, ed. pp. 1–25. New York: Raven Press.
23. Poznanski, E. O. (1982). Clinical phenomenology of childhood depression. *American Journal of Orthopsychiatry* 52:308–313.
24. France, R. D., Krishnan, K. R., Houpt, J. L., and Maltbie, A. A. (1984). Differentiation of depression from chronic pain with the dexamethasone suppression test and DSM-III. *American Journal of Psychiatry* 141:1577–1579.
25. Pope, H. G., Jr., Hudson, J. I., Jonas, J. M., and Yurgelun-Todd, D. (1983). Bulimia treated with imipramine: A placebo-controlled, double-blind study. *American Journal of Psychiatry* 140:554–558.
26. Insel, T. R., Kalin, N. H., Guttmacher, L. B., Cohen, R. M., and Murphy, D. L. (1982). Dexamethasone suppression test in patients with primary obsessive-compulsive disorder. *Psychiatry Research* 6:153–160.

References

27. Bick, P. A. (1982). Hypnosis (letter). *British Journal of Psychiatry* 140:207-213.
28. Dorfman, W. (1968). Hypochondriasis as a defense against depression. *Psychosomatics* 9:248-251.
29. Keller, M. B., Klerman, G. L., Lavori, P. W., Fawcett, J. A., Coryell, W., and Endicott, J. (1982). Treatment received by depressed patients. *Journal of the American Medical Association* 248:1848-1855.
30. Rosenthal, N. E., Sack, D. A., Gillen, J. C., Lewy, A. J., Goodwin, F. K., and Davenport, Y. (1984) Seasonal affective disorder. *Archives of General Psychiatry* 41:72-80.
31. Mueller, P. S., and Allen, N. G. (1984). Diagnosis and treatment of severe light-sensitive seasonal energy syndrome (SES) and its relationship to melatonin anabolism. *Fair Oaks Hospital Psychiatry Letter* 2 (9).
32. Pies, R. (1985). Raynaud's syndrome, panic disorder, and mood changes. *Journal of the American Medical Association* 253:28-33.
33. Davidson, J. R., McLeod, M. N., Turnbull, C. D., White, H. L., and Feuer, E. J. (1980). Platelet monoamine oxidase activity and classification of depression. *Archives of General Psychiatry* 37:771-773.
34. Carroll, B. J. (1984). Problems with diagnostic criteria for depression. *Journal of Clinical Psychiatry* 45:14-18.
35. Andreasen, N. C. (1982). Concepts, diagnosis and classification. In *Handbook of Affective Disorders*, ed. E. S. Paykel, pp. 24-44. New York: Guilford Press.
36. Quitkin, R. M., Liebowitz, M. R., Stewart, J. W., McGrath, P. J., Harrison, W., Rabkin, J. G., and Markowitz, J. (1984). *l*-Deprenyl in atypical depressives. *Archives of General Psychiatry* 41:777-781.
37. Liebowitz, M. R., Quitkin, F. M., Stewart, J. W., McGrath, P. J., Harrison, W., Rabkin, J. G., and Tricamo, E. (1984). Psychopharmacologic validation of atypical depression. *Journal of Clinical Psychiatry* 45:22-25.
38. Ravaris, C. L., Nies, A., Robinson, D. S., Ives, J. O., Lamborn, K. R., and Korson, L. (1976). A multiple-dose controlled study of phenelzine in depressive-anxiety states. *Archives of General Psychiatry* 33:347-350.
39. Davidson, J., and Turnbull, C. (1984). The importance of dose in isocarboxazid therapy. *Journal of Clinical Psychiatry* 45:49-52.
40. Quitkin, F., Rifkin, A., and Klein, D. F. (1979). Monoamine oxidase inhibitors. *Archives of Psychiatry* 36:749-764.
41. Nies, A., and Robinson, D. S. (1982). Monoamine oxidase inhibitors. In *Handbook of Affective Disorders*, ed. E. S. Paykel, pp. 246-261. New York: Guilford Press.
42. Paykel, E. S., Rowan, P. R., Parker, R. R., and Bhat, A. V. (1982). Response to phenelzine and amitriptyline in subtypes of outpatient depression. *Archives of General Psychiatry* 39:1041-1049.
43. Quitkin, F. M., Harrison, W., Liebowitz, M., McGrath, P., Rabkin, J. G., Stewart, J., and Markowitz, J. (1984). Defining the boundaries of atypical depression. *Journal of Clinical Psychiatry* 45:19-21.
44. Kayser, A., Robinson, D. S., Nies, A., and Howard, D. (1985). Response to phenelzine among depressed patients with features of hysteroid dysphoria. *American Journal of Psychiatry* 142:486-488.

45. Murphy, D. L., Garrick, N. A., and Aulakh, G. S. (1984). New contributions from basic science to understanding the effects of monoamine oxidase inhibiting antidepressants. *Journal of Clinical Psychiatry* 45:37–43.
46. Murphy, D. L., Garrick, N. A., and Cohen, R. M. (1983). Monoamine oxidase inhibitors and monoamine oxidase: Biochemical and physiological aspects relevant to human psychopharmacology. In *Drugs in Psychiatry: Antidepressants,* ed. D. Burrows, T. R. Norman, and B. Davies, pp. 209–227 (vol 1). Amsterdam: Elsevier/North Holland Biomedical Press.
47. Giller, E., Jr., Bialos, D., Harkness, L., and Riddle, M. (1984). Assessing treatment response to the monoamine oxidase inhibitor isocarboxazid. *Journal of Clinical Psychiatry* 45:44–48.
48. Zisook, S., Braff, D. L., and Glick, M. A. (1985). Monoamine oxidase inhibitors in the treatment of atypical depression. *Journal of Clinical Psychopharmacology* 5:131–137.
49. Lieb, J., and Collins, C. (1978). Treatment of delusional depression with tranylcypromine. *Journal of Nervous and Mental Disease* 166:805–808.
50. McGrath, P. J., Quitkin, F. M., Harrison, W., and Stewart, J. W. (1984). Treatment of melancholia with tranylcypromine. *American Journal of Psychiatry* 141:288–289.
51. van Kammen, D. P., and Murphy, D. L. (1978). Prediction of imipramine antidepressant response by a one-day *d*-amphetamine trial. *American Journal of Psychiatry* 135:1179–1184.
52. Mann, J. J., Aarons, S. F., Frances, A. J., and Brown, R. D. (1984). Studies of selective and reversible monoamine oxidase inhibitors. *Journal of Clinical Psychiatry* 45:62–66.
53. Pickar, D., Murphy, D. L., Cohen, R. M., Campbell, I. C., and Lipper, S. (1982). Selective and nonselective monoamine oxidase inhibitors. *Archives of General Psychiatry* 39:535–548.
54. Norman, T. R., Ames, D., and Burrows, G. D. (1985). A controlled study of a specific MAO-A reversible inhibitor (RO 11-1163) and amitriptyline in depressive illness. *Journal of Affective Disorders* 8:29–35.
55. Sovner, R. (1981). The clinical characteristics and treatment of atypical depression. *Journal of Clinical Psychiatry* 46:285–289.
56. Crook, T. (1982). Diagnosis and treatment of mixed anxiety-depression in the elderly. *Journal of Clinical Psychiatry* 43:35–52.
57. Kellams, J. J., Klapper, M. H., and Small, J. G. (1979). Trazodone, a new antidepressant: Efficacy and safety in endogenous depression. *Journal of Clinical Psychiatry* 40:390–395.
58. Wheatley, D. (1976). Evaluation of trazodone in the treatment of anxiety. *Current Therapeutic Research* 20:74–83.
59. Ryan, H. F., Merrill, B. F., Scott, G. E., Krebs, R., and Thompson, B. L. (1968). Increase in suicidal thoughts and tendencies associated with diazepam therapy. *Journal of the American Medical Association* 203:1137–1139.
60. Feighner, J. P., Aden, G. C., Fabre, L. F., Rickels, K., and Smith, W. T. (1983). Comparison of alprazolam, imipramine, and placebo in the treatment of depression. *Journal of the American Medical Association* 249:3057–3064.

References

61. Pies, R. (1983). Alprazolam for panic disorder and depression. *American Journal of Psychiatry* 140:640.
62. Strahan, A., Rosenthal, J., Kaswan, M., and Winston, A. (1985). Three case reports of acute paroxysmal excitement associated with alprazolam treatment. *American Journal of Psychiatry* 142:859-861.
63. Breier, A., Charney, D. S., and Nelson, J. C. (1984). Seizures induced by abrupt discontinuation of alprazolam. *American Journal of Psychiatry* 141:1606-1607.
64. Cole, J. O., and Sunderland, P. (1982). The drug treatment of borderline patients. In *Psychiatry 1982 Annual Review*, ed. L. Grinspoon, pp. 456-469. Washington, DC: American Psychiatric Association.
65. Klein, D. F., Gittleman, R., Quitkin, F., and Rifkin, A. (1980). *Diagnosis and Drug Treatment of Psychiatric Disorders*. Baltimore, MD: Williams and Wilkins.
66. Brinkley, J. R., Beitman, B. D., and Friedel, R. O. (1979). Low-dose neuroleptic regimens in the treatment of borderline patients. *Archives of General Psychiatry* 36:319-326.
67. Klein, D. F., and Shader, R. I. (1975). The borderline state: Psychopharmacologic treatment approaches to the undiagnosed case. In *Manual of Psychiatric Therapeutics*, ed. R. I. Shader, pp. 281-293. Boston: Little, Brown.
68. Akiskal, H. S. (1981). Subaffective disorders: Dysthymic, cyclothymic, and bipolar II disorders in the "borderline" realm. *Psychiatric Clinics of North America* 4:25-46.
69. Andrulonis, P. A., Glueck, B. C., Stroebel, C. F., Vogel, N. G., Shapiro, A. L., and Aldridge, D. M. (1981). Organic brain dysfunction and the borderline syndrome. *Psychiatric Clinics of North America* 4:47-66.
70. Branconnier, R. J., Cole, J. O., Ghazvinian, S., Spera, K. F., Oxenkrug, G. F., and Bass, J. L. (1983). Clinical pharmacology of bupropion and imipramine in elderly depressives. *Journal of Clinical Psychiatry* 44:130-133.
71. Shopsin, B. (1983). Bupropion: A new clinical profile in the psychobiology of depression. *Journal of Clinical Psychiatry* 44:140-142.
72. Sheehan, D. V., Davidson, J., Manschreck, T., and Van Wyck Fleet, J. (1983). Lack of efficacy of a new antidepressant (bupropion) in the treatment of panic disorder with phobias. *Journal of Clinical Psychopharmacology* 3:28-31.
73. Temple, D. L., Yevich, J. P., and New, J. S. (1982). Buspirone: Chemical profile of a new class of anxioselective agents. *Journal of Clinical Psychiatry* 43:4-9.
74. Goldberg, H. L., and Finnerty, R. (1982). Comparison of buspirone in two separate studies. *Journal of Clinical Psychiatry* 43:87-91.
75. Feighner, J. P., Merideth, C. H., and Hendrickson, G. A. (1982). A double-blind comparison of buspirone and diazepam in outpatients with generalized anxiety disorder. *Journal of Clinical Psychiatry* 43:103-107.
76. White, K., and Simpson, G. (1984). The combined use of MAOI's and tricyclics. *Journal of Clinical Psychiatry* 45:67-69.
77. Davidson, J., Zung, W. W. K., and Walker, J. I. (1984). Practical aspects of MAO inhibitor therapy. *Journal of Clinical Psychiatry* 45:81-84.
78. van Valkenburg, C., and Winokur, G. (1979). Depression spectrum disease. *Psychiatric Clinics of North America* 2:469-482.

79. Kiloh, L. G. (1982). Electroconvulsive therapy. In *Handbook of Affective Disorders*, ed. E. S. Paykel, pp. 262–275. New York: Guilford Press.
80. Mandel, M. (1975). Electroconvulsive therapy for chronic pain associated with depression. *American Journal of Psychiatry* 132:632–636.
81. Nelson, J. G., and Charney, D. S. (1981). The symptoms of major depressive illness. *American Journal of Psychiatry* 138:1–13.
82. Whybrow, P. C., Akiskal, H. S., and McKinney, W. T. (1984). *Mood Disorders: Toward a New Psychobiology*. New York: Plenum.
83. Rabkin, J., Quitkin, F., Harrison, W., Tricamo, E., and McGrath, P. (1984). Adverse reactions to monoamine oxidase inhibitors. Part I. A comparative study. *Journal of Clinical Psychopharmacology* 4:270–278.
84. Walker, J. I., Davidson, J., and Zung, W. W. K. (1984). Patient compliance with MAO inhibitor therapy. *Journal of Clinical Psychiatry* 45:78–80.
85. Schmidt, H. S., Clark, R. W., and Hyman, P. R. (1977). Protriptyline: An effective agent in the treatment of the narcolepsy-cataplexy syndrome and hypersomnia. *American Journal of Psychiatry* 134:183–185.
86. Baldessarini, R. (1980). Drugs used in the treatment of disorders of mood. In *The Pharmacological Basis of Therapeutics*, ed. L. S. Goodman, A. Gillman, p. 423. New York: MacMillan.
87. Bonaccorsi, A., Dejana, E., Franco, R., and Garattini, S. (1977). Plasma levels and cardiotoxic effects of some antidepressant drugs in the rat. In *Depressive Disorders* (symposia medica Hoechst 13), pp. 367–375. New York: FK Schattauer Verlag.
88. Zetzel, E. R. (1971). A developmental approach to the borderline patient. *American Journal of Psychiatry* 127:867–871.
89. Mann, J. (1973). *Time-limited Psychotherapy*. Cambridge, MA: Harvard University Press.

12

Attention-Deficit Disorder, Residual Type (ADD, RT) or Adult Hyperactivity

Paul H. Wender, M.D.

Attention-Deficit Disorder, Residual Type (ADD, RT) is the new DSM-III designation for the residual (persisting) form of the common syndrome of childhood formerly designated as the hyperactive child syndrome, hyperkinesis, minimal brain dysfunction, or minimal brain damage. The childhood form is designated attention-deficit disorder—hyperactivity (ADDH) or just ADD, depending on whether or not hyperactivity is present. The new name obviously designates one symptom—an attention deficit—as pathognomic. It avoids any allusions to etiology (damage, dysfunction) or motoric hyperactivity (which is thought not to be an essential component of the syndrome in childhood).

PREVALENCE

Attention-deficit disorder is the most common chronic psychiatric disorder of childhood, occurring in 3–10% of the childhood population. Significant symptoms of the disorder probably persist into adult life in one- to two-thirds of instances.

Diagnosis

The correct recognition of ADD, RT is the critical issue in its management. Although the pharmacological treatment frequently employs drugs not routinely used in adult psychiatry, namely, the stimulants, it is relatively straightforward.

The DSM-III diagnostic criteria state that: (a) the individual once met the criteria for ADDH; (b) "signs of hyperactivity are no longer present, but other signs of the illness have persisted to the present without periods of remission, as evidenced by signs of both attentional deficits and impulsivity (e. g., difficulty organizing work and completing tasks, difficulty concentrating, being easily distracted, making sudden decisions without thought of the consequences)" (p. 45); (c) that the symptoms of inattention and impulsivity result in some impairment of social-occupational functioning; and (d) that the symptoms are not due to schizophrenia, affective disorder, severe or profound mental retardation, or schizotypal or borderline personality disorders.

This definition poses two problems: (a) How can one be sure of the necessary pre-existing diagnosis of childhood ADDH? (b) Are inattentiveness and impulsivity sufficient symptoms? That is, does hyperactivity usually disappear?

THE UTAH APPROACH FOR THE DIAGNOSIS OF ADD, RT

Diagnosis of Childhood ADDH

The diagnosis of the adult patient's childhood psychiatric status is the most critical—and from a practical standpoint often the most difficult—part of the diagnosis. One way would be to obtain information from an earlier psychiatric evaluation, but obviously few individuals have been psychiatrically evaluated in childhood. Parental informants may not be available or the patient may not wish to involve them.

The Utah criteria suggest that the childhood diagnosis may be made in either of two ways: (a) Query the patient directly about the signs and symptoms of childhood ADD as listed in DSM-III. Patients are frequently unable to remember if they had the behavioral attributes whose presence is necessary for a DSM-III diagnosis of ADDH. If they cannot, the Utah criteria employ a broad diagnostic approach; (b) Query the patient in a general clinical manner about the presence of hyperactivity and inattention in childhood as well as certain other characteristics (see the Appendix to this chapter). Many patients are often unable to remember even these less-specific clinical cues.

When information about the patient is inconclusive, or if—as in studies—we want more certain diagnostic ascertainment, we employ a third method. We request that the patient's mother or father (only if the mother is not available) fill out a rating scale describing the now adult patient's behavior when he or she was between the ages of 6 and 10. This rating scale, which is a slight modification of the Connors' Rating Scale, has been normed. The parents' rating scale and the scoring are given in the Appendix. A score of 12 or greater places an individual in the 95th or higher percentile of childhood hyperactivity. From a practical standpoint, the form should be sent to the parents directly with a return envelope, following notification by the patient that they will be receiving it. Otherwise, some patients may fill out the form themselves. Obviously, mothers and fathers may be unavailable or dead. Much older siblings may be employed, and their records taken as approximate. A patient self-rating scale is currently under development.

It should be strongly emphasized that the presence of childhood ADDH (hyperactivity) as determined by these methods does not constitute a specific retrospective diagnosis of the child. Symptoms of inattentiveness, hyperactivity, and impulsivity are often seen in conjunction with other childhood psychiatric disorders, such as conduct disorder and specific developmental disorders. These other disorders are frequently associated in childhood with ADDH as well as with psychiatric syndromes that are not generally associated with ADDH. These psychiatric syndromes include developing (pre-)schizophrenia (not a DSM-III diagnosis but an important diagnosis nonetheless), overanxious disorder (perhaps without the impulsivity), and major mood disorders of childhood. In other words, a childhood diagnosis of ADDH is a necessary but not a sufficient condition for the diagnosis of ADD, RT.

Adult Criteria

These are listed in the Appendix, in part II of the Utah criteria for the diagnosis of ADD, RT. There are several important points to be made about these adult criteria:

1. The Utah criteria specify the continuing presence of both hyperactivity and inattentiveness, while the DSM-III criteria state that motoric hyperactivity may disappear.

2. These adult symptoms are not specific to ADD, RT. Many individuals with major depressions are not only depressed (moody) but also are agitated (motor hyperactivity), inattentive (distractable, forgetful, unable to concentrate), manifest affective lability, lack stick-to-itiveness to complete tasks (are disorganized), and are irritable and hot tempered. So again, the presence of these symptoms is a necessary but not sufficient condition. The diagnosis of ADD, RT excludes the diagnoses listed in the Appendix, part II, B of the Utah criteria.

3. The criteria not only exclude the presence of full-fledged schizotypal and borderline personality disorders (BPDs) but also exclude individuals who manifest any of the specific attributes of these disorders as listed in the Appendix, part II, C of the Utah criteria. We state specific, because there are attributes shared by ADD, RT and BPD. These would include such attributes as impulsivity or unpredictability with regard to gambling, spending, and so forth. One characteristic seemingly shared between ADD, RT and BPD is anger. However, clinically the differences are marked. It is characteristic for patients with ADD, RT to anger quickly; they explode rapidly and cool down rapidly. In this regard their anger is very different from the lingering intense anger seen in many individuals with BPD.

It is important to emphasize that the Utah criteria are provisional and are meant to be restrictive. Homogeneity is particularly important at this stage of syndromal definition and data collection. If criteria are too broad and wide, medication will be used with heterogeneous populations, and studies of drug response and other associated features will be difficult. In that case, it would not be the diagnostic entity that was at fault but the breadth of the criteria employed.

PHARMACOLOGICAL MANAGEMENT OF ADD, RT

The drugs useful in the management of ADD, RT are the same ones that are useful in the management of ADDH in childhood as well as some agents which have to date been used only in adults (see Table 12–1). The principal issues in the treatment of ADD, RT are correct diagnosis, measuring the severity of the symptoms, and measuring the change in the symptoms in response to drug therapy.

ASSESSMENT OF PATIENT SYMPTOMATOLOGY AND ITS CHANGE DURING TREATMENT

What is true of children with ADDH is also true of adults with ADD, RT. They are very often unaware of their behavior (as opposed to their symptoms) or its effect on others. They will tell the physician how they are treated; they do not perceive their role in engendering such treatment. Therefore, as with children, it is necessary, or at least very desirable, that a close other be used as an informant. People interested in and living with the patient (parents, spouses, etc.) are usually far more sensitive to quantitative and qualitative aspects of symptom and behavior change than the patient himself (1–4).

STANDARDIZED RATING SCALES

Because many patients are imperceptive and because most standardized self-rating scales (such as the SCL-90) have few specific ADD items, standardized rating scales are generally not helpful, either as measures of initial psychopathology or of changes in symptoms. We have found a Physician's Target Symptoms scale (PTS) and Physician's Global Rating (PGR) (see Appendix) to be useful. On the basis of information supplied by the patient and others during the interview, the physician rates six target areas: hyperactivity, inattentive-

TABLE 12-1 Drugs Useful in Treatment of ADD, RT

Drug	Usual Dose Range (mg/day)	Starting Single Dose (mg)	Usual No. of Doses Per Day	Duration of Action of Tablets (hours)	Long-Acting Forms (mg)	Comments
d-Amphetamine (e.g., Dexedrine) Methamphetamine (Desoxyn)	10–40	2.5	b.i.d. or t.i.d.	3–6	5, 10, 15	Afternoon dose (3–4 P.M.) may be associated with insomnia
Methylphenidate (Ritalin)	10–60	5	t.i.d. or q.i.d.	2–4	20	Long acting form (Ritalin S-R) may have to be given b.i.d.
Pemoline (Cylert)	18.75–150	18.75	Usually every A.M.; may have to give b.i.d.[a]	6–24	"Intrinsic"	Must titrate slowly upward in some patients. In others can begin with full dose. Must obtain LFT[b]
Pargyline (Eutonyl)	10–100	5–10	If arousing A.M. only; otherwise A.M. and noon in divided doses	24+	Similar to MAOIs	Watch for orthostatic hypotension

[a] Manufacturer's recommendation, but efficacy wears off in some patients by early afternoon.
[b] LFT-liver function test. Optimal frequency for obtaining laboratory tests are not known. Manufacturer states that "liver function tests should be obtained prior to and 'periodically' during treatment with Cylert."

ness, instability of mood and depression, temper, disorganization, and impaired social relationships. An alternative scale with specified anchor points is under development.

PHARMACOLOGICAL MANAGEMENT

Stimulant Drugs

The drugs we and most others have employed in the treatment of ADD, RT are the stimulant drugs, *d*-amphetamine (e. g., Dexedrine), methamphetamine (Desoxyn), methylphenidate (Ritalin), and pemoline (Cylert). When the drugs are effective, the following symptomatic and behavioral changes are seen: decreased fidgetiness and restlessness, decreased inattentiveness and distractability, decreased affective lability, with an elimination of ups as well as downs, decreased loss of temper, increased organization, and better relationships with others. In the doses we have employed with the patients described above, we have not seen euphoria.

SPECIFIC FEATURES

Amphetamines (d-Amphetamine and Methamphetamine)

The usual dose range is between 5 and 40 mg. We begin with 2.5 mg morning and noon and increase the amount by 2.5 mg per dose every 2 days. An afternoon dose (3–4 P.M.) may be necessary. The anti-ADD, RT effect of amphetamine tablets appears to last between 3 and 6 hours. Arousing effects may last for longer periods of time and if the medication is given after 3 or 4 P.M., insomnia may result.

d-Amphetamine is available in scored, 5-mg tablets and in slow-release forms which last from 8 to 12 hours and which may be given once a day. These are (conveniently) available in 5-, 10-, and 15-mg doses so that doses may be titrated to the nearest 5 mg/day. These are satisfactory only for some patients. This is because some formulations seem to release a very large bolus initially, and the patient initially experiences the effects (usually unpleasant) of too much medication. Unlike methylphenidate (MP), amphetamines rarely produce sedation. As the dose is increased, some patients complain of irritability.

Some clinicians use both *d*-amphetamine and methamphetamine in children; the doses are said to be equivalent. There are no experimental data documenting a difference, and we have no experience with methamphetamine.

Methylphenidate (MP)

Methylphenidate produces an effect similar to that of amphetamines. It appears to be approximately one-half as potent as amphetamines, and the dose is accordingly usually twice that of amphetamines. MP is available in scored 5-, 10-, and 15-mg tablets and as a proprietary 20-mg, long-acting form (slow release), Ritalin-SR. The usual dose range is between 10 and 60 mg/day. Our procedure is to begin with 5 mg morning and noon and increase the dose by 2.5 mg every 2 days. The duration of action of MP tablets is briefer than that of the amphetamines, and medication must frequently be given three or four times a day. Some patients find that MP produces tiredness and grogginess when the dose is excessive. (This is probably an adult description of a subjective response corresponding to the zombie-like behavior seen in some ADDH children who have received too much MP.) We have no experience with the use of Ritalin-SR in adults. Experience with the slow-release form in children is limited. Clinicians report that Ritalin-SR usually does not last throughout the day and either it must be given b.i.d. or supplemented with tablets late in the day. Absorption may be less adequate, larger doses of Ritalin-SR may be necessary, and some idiosyncratic responses may occur (presumably due to the vehicles). The availability of one long-acting dosage form is a disadvantage (as described for amphetamines, above).

Pemoline

This is the most recently introduced of the stimulant drugs. There are several respects in which it is different from amphetamines and MP. Pemoline is effective at a lower percentage of ADD, RT patients than amphetamines and MP, although there are some who respond best to this drug. Whereas amphetamines and MP are classified as schedule II drugs, pemoline is a schedule IV drug. It is apparently not a popular recreational drug and is relatively insoluble and cannot be injected intravenously. Pemoline is available as scored 18.75-, 37.5- and 75-mg tablets. In treating patients, we begin at a low dose (e. g., one-half of the 18.75-mg tablet) and increase the dose as tolerated every few days. The average optimum dose of pemoline for good responders in our controlled study was 65 mg; doses ranged from 18.75 to 150 mg/day. Side effects, to which tolerance may develop, include anorexia, abdominal discomfort, headaches, and insomnia.

Whether or not the drug has a delayed onset is uncertain since increases of dose often must take place over a period of days to 2–3 weeks. However, there are some patients in whom the drug may be begun immediately at the dose that proves to be therapeutic and in whom the onset of action may be immediate. Duration of action varies. The *Physicians' Desk Reference* (PDR) states that once-daily dosage is usual, but some patients require a b.i.d. schedule. An additional respect in which pemoline differs from amphetamines and MP is that periodic laboratory screening is necessary (at uncertain intervals), since elevated liver enzymes and jaundice have been reported. The manufacturer's package insert states that "liver function tests should be performed prior to and periodically during therapy."

Monoamine Oxidase Inhibitors (MAOIs)

We have conducted systematic, uncontrolled trials of both pargyline and *l*-deprenyl. In low doses, both are specific MAOI-B inhibitors. Monoamine oxidase–B inhibits the oxidation of phenethylamine and dopamine, and these drugs have been employed because of a hypothesized decrease in phenethylaminergic and dopaminergic activity in individuals with ADD.

Pargyline was developed in the 1960s as an antidepressant and is now marketed as an antihypertensive (Eutonyl). *l*-Deprenyl is currently not commercially available in the United States. Its distinctive feature is that in low doses it does not produce a cheese reaction (tyramine induced hypertension). Pargyline is available in 10 and 25 mg tablets and is begun at a level of 5 mg/day. The 10-mg tablet must be cut in two and thereafter administered on a morning-and-noon basis. Blood pressure must be followed in nonhypertensive individuals. Twenty to thirty milligrams is generally the most that is initially tolerated. Over a period of weeks to months, some patients develop some degree of tolerance to pargyline. In our experience this has never been absolute (e. g., patients have gone from 20 mg/day to 100 mg/day over a period of 2 years and then remained at the upper dose with no increasing tolerance).

The latency until onset of action with pargyline is similar to that seen with other MAOIs. The precautions and side effects are likewise similar to those of other MAOIs. Its particular advantage is that, when effective, it provides pharmacological suppression of symptoms 24 hours/day. Stimulants are not ideal in those patients with interpersonal difficulties who may have troubles with others (generally their spouses) prior to taking their medication in the morning or following its wearing off in the evening. Pargyline has been an excellent drug in two patients who were both hypertensive and had ADD.

Amphetamines, MP, pemoline, pargyline, and deprenyl are the only drugs that have been systematically explored in the treatment of ADD, RT. None is ideal. The requirements for an ideal ADD, RT drug are as follows:

1. It would be nonabusable, like the MAOIs.
2. It would have a rapid onset of action, like A and MP.
3. It would be continuously active, without daily troughs and peaks, like MAOIs.
4. It would not require laboratory monitoring, unlike pemoline.
5. It would be safe to use with impulsive individuals (including impulsive alcoholics). Since impulsive people are liable, at least when drunk, to violate the food and drug restrictions, the use of MAOIs may be dangerous.
6. It could be used with ADD, RT alcoholics. There is no good drug for use in ADD, RT alcoholics. The MAOIs are ruled out for the reason specified, amphetamines and MP are potentially abusable (an undesirable attribute for someone who is already a substance abuser), and pemoline is associated with possible hepatotoxicity.

Clinical hints about the use of drugs:

1. With stimulants, gradually increase the dose until benefits plateau out or side effects become annoying. Do not fail to raise the dose because the patient has shown a positive response. He or she may respond more with a further increase in dose.

2. With short-acting stimulants, try to space them through the day so their effect is relatively constant.

3. Determine the latest time in the afternoon that a stimulant can be administered without producing insomnia. Unfortunately, the arousing effect seems to last longer than the anti-ADD effects, and a dose of amphetamine at 3 P.M. may provide behavioral coverage to 7 P.M. but keep the patient awake until midnight.

4. In patients for whom late afternoon doses are necessary and in whom they produce insomnia, consider the use of small amounts of sedative neuroleptics, for example, thioridazine, 10–50 mg. Obviously, one is concerned about cumulative neurological toxicity, although the risks are low in this dose range. The risks of neuroleptics should be discussed with the patient as should the risks and benefits of using benzodiazepines (BZPs) for sleep (tolerance and dependence). BZPs are obviously unsatisfactory on a long-term basis.

5. If a patient's response to one stimulant is not optimal, try another stimulant. Overall, amphetamines and MP seem equally efficacious, but some patients seem to do better on one, some on another. A smaller percentage of patients seem to respond to pemoline, but there are some for whom it is the best drug.

6. Long-acting forms of amphetamines and MP can sometimes be substituted for the tablets. As mentioned, long-acting preparations of amphetamines sometimes produce an unpleasant spiking in dose, and the long-acting preparation of MP is variable in duration and usually must be given twice a day. Pemoline may be given once per day in some instances but may need to be given twice a day for others.

7. Pargyline is an excellent treatment for teetotalers and individuals who are anxious about the use of possible abusable drugs.

THE PROBLEM OF DRUG ABUSE

It is uncertain whether ADD patients will experience a "high" on large doses of intravenously administered stimulants (i. e., will experience the same effect as a non-ADD individual). Even if the patients themselves do not abuse the drugs, the drugs can be sold and have a high street value. Accordingly, we use amphetamines and MP only in responsible individuals and preferably in responsible individuals with partners. In high-risk patients, we use pemoline and sometimes pargyline. We do not employ amphetamines or MP, even if patients fail to respond to the former agents.

Depending on local concerns about the prescription of schedule II drugs, prescribing physicians are well advised to support their position legally and medically. From a practical standpoint, it is a good idea to get an independent confirmation of the diagnosis of ADD, RT patients from another physician. Administrative safeguards will vary from state to state, but the physician who treats many of these patients should take appropriate precautions to avoid being labeled a "speed doctor."

PATIENTS WHO FAIL TO RESPOND TO STIMULANTS OR MAOIs

There are no systematic studies of other drugs in the treatment of ADD, RT. In our experience, an occasional patient responds to tricyclics, benzodiazepines, or low doses of high-potency neuroleptics (e. g., 1–5 mg of trifluoperazine per day).

Since only 60–70% of patients with ADD, RT show a favorable response to stimulant medications or MAOIs, there is ample room for pharmacological experimentation.

APPENDIX *

Utah Criteria for the Diagnosis of ADD, RT

I. CHILDHOOD history consistent with ADD of childhood. Diagnostic criteria for ADD in childhood:
   A. DSM-III ("NARROW") CRITERIA
      The child displays, for his or her mental and chronological age, signs of developmentally inappropriate inattention, impulsivity, and hyperactivity. The signs must be reported by

* Reprinted with permission from the *Diagnostic and Statistical Manual of Mental Disorders, Third Edition, Revised,* Copyright 1987 American Psychiatric Association.

adults in the child's environment, such as parents and teachers. Because the symptoms are typically variable, they may not be observed directly by the clinician. When the reports of teachers and parents conflict, primary consideration should be given to the teacher's reports because of greater familiarity with age-appropriate norms. Symptoms typically worsen in situations that require self-application, as in the classroom. Signs of the disorder may be absent when the child is in a new or a one-to-one situation.

The number of symptoms specified (below) is for children between the ages of eight and ten, the peak age range for referral. In younger children, more severe forms of the symptoms and a greater number of symptoms are usually present. *The opposite is true of older children.*

1. INATTENTION (at least *three* of the following):
   a. often fails to finish things he or she starts,
   b. often doesn't seem to listen,
   c. easily distracted,
   d. difficulty concentrating on school-work or other tasks requiring sustained attention,
   e. difficulty sticking to a play activity.

2. IMPULSIVITY (at least *three* of the following):
   a. often acts before thinking,
   b. shifts excessively from one activity to another,
   c. difficulty organizing work (unrelated to cognitive impairment),
   d. needs a great deal of supervision,
   e. often calls out in class,
   f. difficulty awaiting turn in games or group situations.

3. HYPERACTIVITY (at least *two* of the following):
   a. runs about or climbs on things excessively,
   b. difficulty sitting still or fidgets excessively,
   c. difficulty staying seated,
   d. moves about excessively during sleep,
   e. is always "on the go" or acts as if "driven by a motor."

4. ONSET before age of 7

5. DURATION of at least 6 months

6. NOT DUE TO schizophrenia, affective disorder, or mental retardation (DSM-III criteria)

B. "BROAD" CRITERIA

Presence in childhood of both characteristics 1 and 2, and one characteristic of 3 through 6.
1. more active than other children, unable to sit still, fidgetiness, restlessness, always on the go, talking excessively;
2. attention deficits, sometimes described as "short attention span," characterized by inattentiveness, distractibility, inability to finish school work;
3. behavior problems in school;
4. impulsivity;
5. overexcitability;
6. temper outbursts.

II. ADULT CRITERIA

A. Presence in adulthood of both characteristics 1 and 2 (below)—which the patient observes or says others observe about him—together with two of characteristics 3 through 7.
1. PERSISTENT MOTOR HYPERACTIVITY, as manifested by restlessness, inability to relax, "nervousness" (inability to settle down rather than anticipatory anxiety), inability to persist in sedentary activities (e.g., watching movies, TV, reading newspaper), always on the go, dysphoria when inactive.
2. ATTENTION DEFICITS, as manifested by inability to keep mind on conversation, distractibility (aware of other stimuli when trying to filter them out), inability to keep mind on reading materials, difficulty keeping mind on job, frequent "forgetfulness" (often losing or misplacing things, forgetting plans, etc.), "mind frequently somewhere else."
3. AFFECTIVE LABILITY (usually described as antedating adolescence and in some instances as far back as the patient can remember), as manifested by definite shifts from a normal mood to depression or mild euphoria or excitement; depression described as "down," "bored" or "discontented"; mood shifts usually last hours to (at most) a few days and are present without significant physiological concomitants; mood shifts may occur spontaneously or be reactive.
4. INABILITY TO COMPLETE TASKS: lack of organization in job, running household or performing school work;

tasks frequently uncompleted; switches from one task to another in haphazard fashion; disorganization in activities, problem solving, organizing time.

5. HOT TEMPER: explosive, short-lived outbursts. Loss of control, sometimes frightened by his own behavior; easily provoked; constant irritability. Temper problems interfere with personal relationships.

6. IMPULSIVITY: makes decisions quickly and easily without reflection, often on the basis of insufficient information (to his disadvantage); inability to delay acting without experiencing discomfort. Manifestations include: poor occupational performance; abrupt initiation or termination of relationships (e.g., multiple marriages, separations, divorces); antisocial behavior (e.g., joy-riding, shop-lifting); excessive involvement in pleasurable activities without recognizing risks or painful consequences (e.g., buying sprees, foolish business investments, reckless driving).

7. STRESS INTOLERANCE: cannot take ordinary stresses in stride and reacts excessively or inappropriately with depression, confusion, uncertainty, anxiety or anger. Emotional responses interfere with appropriate problem solving; repeated crises in dealing with routine life stresses.

B. Absence of signs and symptoms of the following diseases:
   1. schizophrenia,
   2. schizo-affective disorder,
   3. primary affective disorder.

C. Absence of the following characteristics of schizotypal or borderline personality disorders:
   1. magical thinking,
   2. ideas of reference,
   3. recurrent delusions,
   4. odd communications,
   5. inadequate rapport in face-to-face interactions,
   6. suspiciousness or paranoid ideation.

Parents' Rating Scale

Name _____ Number _____ Date _____

This form is to be completed by your *mother* (or father only if mother is not available).

Listed below are items concerning children's behavior and the problems they sometimes have. Read each item carefully and decide how much you think your child was bothered by these problems when he/she was between six and ten years old. Rate the amount of the problem by putting a check in the column that describes your child at that time.

	Score	0 Not at all	1 Just a little	2 Pretty much	3 Very much
1.	Restless, overactive				
2.	Excitable, impulsive				
3.	Disturbs other children				
4.	Fails to finish things (short attention span)				
5.	Fidgeting				
6.	Inattentive, distractible				
7.	Demands must be met immediately (gets frustrated)				
8.	Cries				
9.	Mood changes quickly				
10.	Temper outbursts (explosive and unpredictable behavior)				

Each item is scored 0 to 3 as indicated above. The PRS score is simply their sum.

Physician's Target Symptoms (PTS)

Name _____ Week and Drug _____
Date _____ Physician _____

TARGET AREAS	NONE 0	MILD 1	MODERATE 2	MARKED 3
Concentration difficulties	___	___	___	___
Hyperactivity	___	___	___	___
Mood instability and depression	___	___	___	___
Temper	___	___	___	___
Disorganization	___	___	___	___
Social difficulties	___	___	___	___

Physician's Global Rating (PGR)

GLOBAL RATING OF IMPROVEMENT (CIRCLE ONE)

___ +3   very much improved

___ +2   moderately improved

___ +1   mildly improved

___ 0   no change

___ −1   mildly worse

___ −2   moderately worse

___ −3   very much worse

Note: Whenever possible, evaluations should be based both on the reports of the patient and the spouse or "significant other."

REFERENCES

1. Wood, D. R., Reimherr, F. W., and Wender, P. H. (1976). Diagnosis and treatment of minimal brain dysfunction in adults. *Archives of General Psychiatry* 33:1453–1461.
2. Wender, P. H., Reimherr, F. W., and Wood, D. R. (1981). Attention deficit disorder (minimal brain dysfunction) in adults: A replication study of diagnosis and drug treatment. *Archives of General Psychiatry* 38:449–456.
3. Wender, P. H., Wood, D. R., Reimherr, F. W., and Ward, M. (1983). An open trial of pargyline in the treatment of attention deficit disorder, residual type. *Psychiatry Research* 9:329–336.
4. Wender, P. H., Reimherr, F. W., Wood, D., and Ward, M. (1985). A controlled study of methylphenidate in the treatment of attention deficit disorder, residual type. *American Journal of Psychiatry* 142:547–552.

13

Drug Combinations and Interactions

Charles B. Schaffer, M.D.
Patrick T. Donlon, M.D.
Linda C. Schaffer, M.D.

Clinical psychiatrists have become increasingly aware of the importance of the drug interactions that occur when psychiatric medications are combined with other psychiatric or nonpsychiatric agents. Several factors have established these drug combinations and interactions as important topics in psychopharmacology. The first is simply the burgeoning numbers of clinically significant interactions. In 1972, the Boston Collaborative Drug Surveillance Program was the first large-scale study to report a significant incidence of adverse effects resulting from drug interactions, an incidence of approximately 7% (1).

Further, in the last decade the use of psychiatric medications has increased, especially in the treatment of affective disorders. This increase has lead to greater use of psychiatric medications by both psychiatrists and nonpsychiatric primary-care physicians and, thus, to a greater frequency of drug combinations and potential interactions. An additional factor is the growing number of geriatric patients, a population at high risk for significant drug interactions both because of the increasing number of medications usually prescribed with advancing age and because of the increased sensitivity to the adverse effects of medications seen in the elderly.

Recent advances in laboratory technology which now allow identification and serum-level determination of numerous medications have also contributed to the importance of this topic in psychopharmacology. With this newly available data, physicians can more effectively and accurately monitor drug combinations and document aspects of significant interactions. More sophisticated research in these areas, both in the laboratory and clinical setting, continues to provide useful clinical information and to stimulate theoretical hypotheses for continued investigation. Expansion of pharmacological, neurotransmitter, receptor physiology, and metabolism information has also facilitated recognition of interactions. Lastly, and unfortunately, the increase in litigation involving adverse drug interactions has been an additional factor in establishing the importance of drug combinations and interactions in psychopharmacology.

DETERMINANTS OF DRUG INTERACTIONS

There are several determinants of the effects of drug combinations. These include pharmacological and pharmacokinetic interactions, age of the patient, individual sensitivities to medication mixtures, individual doses of combined drugs, duration of drug treatment, and medical condition of the patient.

Pharmacological Interactions

The pharmacological interactions are those which occur at the receptor site, central or peripheral. These interactions may result in one of four effects: additive, synergistic, antagonistic, or no effect. A common example of the additive (or potentiation) effect is the increased sedation caused by the combination of two or more agents that possess central nervous system (CNS) depressant qualities. A synergistic effect is seen in the increased efficacy of antipsychotics and antidepressants when combined in the treatment of patients suffering from major depression with psychotic features. Patients treated with antipsychotics (dopamine antagonists) who also require the administration of L-dopa (a dopamine agonist), demonstrate an antagonist effect. The combination of lithium and a benzodiazepine anxiolytic agent has no interactional effects, though each agent has its own adverse effect profile.

Pharmacokinetic Interactions

Pharmacokinetic processes are those involved in the transport of medications to and from the receptor site. They consist of four stages: absorption, distribution, metabolism, and excretion. Pharmacokinetic interactions can be quite complex and occur when one agent alters any of the four transport stages of another.

Absorption. The availability of a drug to the body after absorption from the gastrointestinal (GI) tract is known as bioavailability. Bioavailability is a function of both the completeness and the rate of absorption of a given dose. Drug interactions in the GI tract can enhance or inhibit absorption in several ways. Generally, medications are better absorbed in the non-ionized form; some drug interactions promote ionization, thus inhibiting absorption. The pH level influences the rate of absorption, and some drug interactions change the pH of the absorption site. Other medications alter GI motility, which affects both speed and completeness of absorption. Lastly, some medications combine with other medications or foods to decrease the rate of absorption into the body.

Distribution. The rate of distribution of medications is a function of four variables: (a) regional flow of blood to various tissues and organs in the body, (b) lipid solubility of the medication, (c) degree of binding of a drug to plasma proteins (primarily albumin), and (d) active transport of medications across cell membranes. In psychopharmacology, drug interactions most commonly exert their influence on the distribution of medication by the degree to which one drug displaces another from bound plasma protein. Even small changes in shifting bound to unbound drug, and vice versa, can significantly alter the availability of free or active medication to target organs or tissues.

Metabolism. An important and frequent result of drug interactions in the body is the ability of one drug to alter the metabolism of another drug. This can occur by several mechanisms. Enzymes in the liver degrade most medications. As many of these metabolizing enzymes are nonspecific, they can be inhibited or induced (enhanced) by drugs that are pharmacologically unrelated.

The rate of hepatic drug metabolism is also influenced by the amount of hepatic blood flow and degree of protein binding of a drug. The delivery of medications which undergo a rapid and significant hepatic clearance, "a first-pass effect," is particularly vulnerable to agents that can decrease hepatic circulation. Lastly, some drugs can compete for enzyme reactive sites in the liver, thus decreasing metabolism of the competitive drug.

Excretion. Renal excretion or clearance is an important mechanism by which many drugs are eliminated from the body. Drugs are excreted by the kidneys in three ways: (a) glomerular filtration, (b) tubular reabsorption, and (c) active tubular secretion. Some drugs can alter the renal excretion of others by modifying one of these three pathways. Of the psychiatric medications, lithium is most influenced by the renal environment and its effects on speed of elimination.

ASSESSING CLINICAL RELEVANCE

In recent years, many publications have reported adverse reactions from drug combinations. Unfortunately, some warnings about adverse drug interactions in the literature are inflated. There are authors who base their warnings on one or two rare case reports. Others rely on clinical folklore, beliefs that have never been substantiated by scientific data or that are only theoretical in origin. And lastly, some reported adverse reactions are documented only in select populations (for example, studies limited to normal subjects or aged psychiatric patients) and may not apply to all patients. Thus, assessing the clinical relevance of a report involves attention to scientific method, frequency of the adverse effects, and the study population.

STEPS TO REDUCE ADVERSE EFFECTS

There are several steps the practicing psychiatrist can take in order to avoid or, at least minimize, adverse drug reactions. Before starting medications, a careful medical and drug history must be obtained from every patient. In addition, every effort should be made to make the correct diagnosis in order to avoid "shotgun" polypharmacy. Clinicians should also keep abreast of the current literature and remain familiar with the pharmacology of commonly used psychiatric medications and nonpsychiatric medications frequently used by psychiatric patients. Patients should be well educated about the potential adverse effects of drug combinations so that they are prepared and can contact their physicians early and appropriately with any problem.

When treatment begins, clinicians should start with conservative doses, increase dosage slowly, and assess the patient frequently. In some instances, serum levels of medications can be useful in determining proper dosage. Patients at known risk for adverse medication interaction should be monitored particularly carefully at the onset. Psychiatrists should not hesitate to consult other specialists when treating difficult patients or those who are on nonpsychiatric medications. This is especially relevant in patients on cardiovascular medications, for these agents often interact with psychiatric drugs. Lastly, the treating psychiatrist should be readily accessible to patients, especially early in the course of therapy when more than one medication is involved. This allows quick intervention when unpleasant and/or adverse effects occur, thus alleviating patient anxiety, increasing patient compliance, and in the end, facilitating treatment.

DRUG-DRUG INTERACTIONS

Drug–drug interactions for each major family of psychiatric medications are listed in table form. Comment is provided on reported possible adverse effects, underlying biological mechanism, and clinical importance. The interested reader is referred to several general articles and texts on drug–drug interactions which provide specific references to supplement the information presented in the tables (2-18). The following narrative provides additional clarification.

Tricyclic Antidepressants

Knowledge of the pharmacological actions of the tricyclic antidepressants (TCAs) helps explain their therapeutic, adverse, and interactional effects. All of the currently marketed TCAs have some anticholinergic effect. They also potentiate synaptic activity which may result from the blockage of norepinephrine and serotonin reuptake into the presynaptic neurons. As all marketed TCAs have similar efficacy, agent selection is guided primarily by the desire to have or omit select adverse effects.

The common adverse effects occur in the following systems: cardiovascular (orthostatic hypotension, hypertension, tachycardia, etc.), CNS and neuromuscular (sedation, confusion, agitation, disturbed sleep, tremor, etc.), autonomic nervous system (dry mouth, blurred vision, constipation, etc.), GI (nausea, epigastric distress, etc.), and others (weight gain or loss, urinary frequency, alopecia, etc.). Other than monoamine oxidase inhibitors (MAOIs), only trazodone and alprazolam are antidepressants that are significantly different from the TCAs. The former is sedating and acts with other CNS depressants to increase sedation. Alprazolam is a benzodiazepine and has comparable interactions.

TCAs are one of the psychiatric medications most frequently prescribed by both psychiatrists and nonpsychiatric physicians; they are also probably the most common psychiatric agents prescribed for the elderly. Thus, they are frequently used in combination with other nonpsychiatric medications. There are many studies and case reports documenting significant drug interactions with TCAs. These interactions can alter the pharmacokinetics or pharmacological action of either the TCAs, the drug being combined, or both. They can cause a significant change in the blood levels of TCAs, increase the risk of adverse or toxic effects, or enhance or negate the therapeutic effects (Table 13-1).

The kinetics of the TCAs can be affected by other medications at any of the four stages: absorption, distribution, metabolism, and excretion. The most common and important interactions, however, occur during distribution (e. g., protein binding) and metabolism (many drugs impair or induce enzyme activity in the liver). At the receptor site, significant pharmacological effects occur when TCAs are combined with other medications. These effects are the most common and clinically important results of drug combinations with these agents.

Several populations are at particular risk for significant interactions when TCAs are combined with other agents. The elderly are vulnerable, first, because they are often prescribed multiple medications; as the number of medications increases, the risk of clinically significant drug interactions also increases. In addition, they often take medications that interact with TCAs: cardiac drugs, antiparkinson agents and medications with CNS depressant effects. Further, the elderly have both decreased serum albumin and hepatic enzyme activity. They are more sensitive to the CNS effects of any medica-

TABLE 13-1 Tricyclic Antidepressants

Drug	Effect	Mechanism	Clinical Significance
Anticholinergic drugs	[a]↑ Anticholinergic effects/toxicity	Additive anticholinergic at receptor sites	Yes
Antipsychotics	↑ Plasma TCA levels ↑ Plasma antipsychotic levels ↑ Clinical efficacy in psychotic depression	[b]↓ Metabolism ? ?	Yes Yes Yes
MAOIs	↑ Plasma TCA levels, risk of toxicity	↓ Metabolism	Yes
Antihypertensives (Guanethedine, Bethanidine, Debrisoquine, Clonidine)	↓ Antihypertensive effect	Antagonism at receptor site	Yes
Thiazide diuretics	↑ Hypotensive effect from ↑ plasma levels diuretic	↑ Kidney reabsorption of diuretic	Yes
Coumarin anticoagulants	↑ anticoagulant effect coumarin	↓ Metabolism	Yes
Barbiturates	↓ Plasma TCA levels	↑ Metabolism	Yes
Sympathomimetics	↑ Pressor response to sympathomimetics	Potentiate at peripheral receptor sites	Yes
Amphetamines	↑ Stimulant effects	Potentiate at central receptor sites	Yes

TABLE 13-1 (*continued*)

Drug	Effect	Mechanism	Clinical Significance
Alpha-adrenergic agonists (Levophed, Norepinephrine)	↑ Pressor response to alpha-adrenergic agonists	Potentiate action at peripheral receptor sites	Yes
Methylphenidate	↑ Plasma TCA levels ? Enhanced antidepressant response	↓ Metabolism ? Potentiate at central receptor sites	Yes Yes
Cimetidine	↑ Plasma TCA levels	↓ Clearance and ↑ bioavailability	?
Ethchlorvynol	↑ Delirium risk	?	Yes
Acetaminophen	↑ Plasma TCA levels	↓ Metabolism	?
Disulfirum	↑ Plasma TCA levels	↓ Metabolism	?
Phenytoin, Mysoline	↓ Plasma TCA levels	↑ Metabolism	?
Nonbarbiturate hypnotics	↓ Plasma TCA levels	↑ Metabolism	?
Griseofulvin	↓ Plasma TCA levels	↑ Metabolism	?
Carbamazepine	↓ Plasma TCA levels	↑ Metabolism	?
Levodopa	↑ Levodopa antiparkinson effects	Potentiate anticholinergic effects	Yes
Rauwolfia alkaloids	↓ Rauwolfia alkaloid hypotensive effects	Antagonism at receptor site	Yes
Fenflurane	? Risk of seizures (2 cases)	?	?

Baclofen	↑ Muscle weakness	Potentiate antispastic effect of baclofen	Yes
Beta-adrenergic blockers	↓ Beta-blocker antihypertensive effects	Antagonize at receptor site	?
Quinidine procainamide	Cardiac conduction prolonged	Potentiate antiarrhythmic effects	?
Beta-adrenergic agonists (Epinephrine, etc.)	↑ Pressor effect	Potentiate at receptor site	Yes
Anesthetics (Halothane, Flurane)	Tachycardia with imipramine	?	?
CNS depressants	↑ Depressant effect	Potentiate at central receptor site	Yes
Oral contraceptives	↓ Plasma TCA levels	↑ Metabolism	?
Phenylbutazone	↓ Phenylbutazone clinical effect	↓ GI absorption	?
Meperidine	↑ Meperidine respiratory depression	Potentiate at central receptor sites	Yes
Smoking	↓ Plasma TCA levels	↑ Metabolism	?
Chloramphenicol	↑ Plasma TCA levels	↓ Metabolism	?
Thyroid (T4)	↑ Antidepressant TCA effects	? Potentiate at central receptor sites	?
Lithium	↑ Antidepressant TCA effects	? Potentiate at central receptor sites	?

^{a}↑ = increased
^{b}↓ = diminished/decreased/reversed

tions and especially those of the psychotropics. The elderly are also more vulnerable to anticholinergic, CNS depressant, and cardiovascular effects; and all of these are present when TCAs are given either alone or in combination with agents that potentiate these adverse effects at the receptor site.

Cardiac patients of any age are another group at greater risk for drug-drug interactions, as TCAs are often given in addition to their cardiac medications. Commonly prescribed cardiac agents that may interact with TCAs include beta blockers, antihypertensives, and antiarrhythmic agents.

Patients who abuse or drink alcohol in excess are also candidates for adverse interactions with TCAs. The most common problem is the additive CNS depressant effect when alcohol and TCAs are combined. In addition, chronic alcohol abusers with impaired liver function may experience increased blood levels of TCA, thus creating a greater risk for adverse effects or toxicity. In contrast, alcohol induces liver enzymes and if there is no serious liver pathology, TCA blood levels will be depressed.

Demented patients have a greater incidence of adverse interactions when TCAs are used in addition to other medications. Potential adverse effects include greater sensitivity to CNS depression and toxic delirium.

In some instances, the combination of TCAs with other medications is beneficial; the antidepressant effect is enhanced. Some examples of this positive result of drug combinations include TCA with lithium carbonate, TCA with thyroid, and TCA with tryptophan. There have also been reports of synergistic effects from the combination of TCAs with other TCAs, with MAOIs, and with antipsychotics.

Lithium Preparations

The therapeutic pharmacological action(s) of lithium in bipolar affective disorder or other disorders remains unknown. Typically, the agent is very well tolerated in nontoxic dosage ranges, though there are patients who experience significant adverse effects, including signs of toxicity, at low serum levels. Thus, clinical response as well as serum level assays should be used to identify and monitor adverse and toxic effects.

Adverse effects are relatively common and involve the following systems: the central nervous and neuromuscular systems (fine hand tremor, drowsiness, muscular weakness, lethargy, confusion, etc.), the genitourinary (oliguria, polyuria, incontinence, impotence/sexual dysfunction, etc.), cardiovascular (arrhythmia, hypotension, bradycardia, etc.), autonomic nervous system (blurred vision, dry mouth, etc.), gastrointestinal (nausea, diarrhea, vomiting, fecal incontinence, anorexia, indigestion, etc.), metabolic and endocrinological (thyroid disease, hypercalcemia, hyperparathyroidism, etc.), dermatological (drying and thinning of the hair, itching, exacerbation of psoriasis, etc.), and others (dehydration, mild thirst, weight changes, edema, etc.) (Table 13–2).

Since lithium is an ion, the pharmacokinetics of this agent are considerably different from most of the other psychotropic medications. Lithium is neither protein bound nor metabolized by the liver. The fate of lithium in the body is determined primarily by the kidney, which is its main avenue of excretion. For this reason, the most common cause of significant drug–drug interactions in patients taking lithium are medications that affect the rate of renal excretion of lithium. The end result of changes in the rate of excretion are changes in the serum level of lithium. With increase in serum level comes increased risk of toxicity; with decrease comes increased risk of relapse of affective symptoms.

The effect on central and peripheral receptor sites of combining lithium with other medications is also clinically significant. Some medications work synergistically with lithium to produce an increased therapeutic effect in patients with affective disorder. This synergism has been observed in the treatment of both manic and depressed patients. Other medications increase the risk of neurotoxicity by causing an additive effect.

As with the TCAs, there are populations that are at increased risk for adverse effects from the combination of lithium with other medications. The geriatric population is at risk for several reasons. There is an increase in the number of medications taken per patient with age; renal clearance decreases with age; and elderly patients tend to have diseases that require diuretics. Several diuretics, including the thiazide group, decrease the excretion of lithium; the degree depends on individual sensitivity, pharmacology of the diuretic, dosage of the diuretic, and duration of administration. The older patient is also more sensitive to the neurotoxic effects of lithium.

Obviously, patients with renal disease are also a population at risk, especially those on renal dialysis. Another vulnerable group are

TABLE 13-2 Lithium

Drug	Effect	Mechanism	Clinical Significance
Thiazide diuretics	↑ Plasma lithium levels	↑ Tubular absorption	Yes
Loop diuretics	↑ Plasma lithium levels	↑ Sodium depletion	Yes
Potassium sparing diuretics	↑ Plasma lithium levels	↑ Tubular absorption	Yes
Carbonic anhydrase inhibitors	↓ Plasma lithium levels	↑ Excretion	Yes
Osmotic diuretics	↓ Plasma lithium levels	↑ Excretion	Yes
Xanthines	↓ Plasma lithium levels	↑ Excretion	Yes
Sodium Chloride Sodium Bicarbonate	↓ Plasma lithium levels	↑ Excretion	Yes
Nonsteroidal anti-inflammatories	↑ Plasma lithium levels	↓ Renal clearance	Yes
Methyldopa	Neurotoxicity (in a few cases)	?	?

Phenytoin	Neurotoxicity (in a few cases)	?	?
Neuromuscular blocking agents	Prolongs action NBA	?	Yes
Tetracycline, Metronidazole	↑ Plasma lithium levels (in a few cases)	↓ Renal clearance	?
Digitalis	↑ Risk digitalis toxicity	↓ Intracellular potassium	?
Mazindol	↑ Plasma lithium levels (one case)	?	?
TCAs	? Potentiation antidepressant effect	?	?
Antipsychotics	? Worsen lithium neurotoxicity	?	?
Amiloride	↓ Lithium induced polyuria	Improve renal concentrating capacity	Yes
Carbamazepine	Positive clinical response in some manic patients previously refractory to lithium alone. Combination may ↑ risk neurotoxicity	?	Yes
Verapamil	↓ Plasma lithium levels (in two cases)	?	?

patients with brain damage, especially diffuse disease, as neurotoxicity can occur at lower than usual serum levels of lithium for them. Patients of any age with cardiovascular disease which requires diuretic therapy are also at high risk.

ANTIPSYCHOTIC DRUGS

Chlorpromazine (CPZ) is the historical prototype of the antipsychotic agents. It acts at all levels of the CNS as well as on several organ systems. The principal pharmacological actions are psychotropic but it also has sedative and antiemetic activities. In addition, it has strong antiadrenergic and weaker peripheral anticholinergic activities, slight antihistaminic and antiserotonergic activity. Like other antipsychotic agents, CPZ causes dopamine blockade, the action that may explain its antipsychotic action.

Adverse reactions of CPZ occur in the following systems: CNS [sedation, dizziness, extrapyramidal reactions (EPS), confusion, catatonic states, etc.], hematological (agranulocytosis, leukopenia, etc.), cardiovascular (postural hypotension, tachycardia, etc.), hypersensitivity (jaundice, urticaria, photosensitivity, dermatitis), dermatological (skin pigmentations, etc.), endocrinological (lactation and breast engorgement, amenorrhea, gynecomastia, etc.), ophthalmological (opacities in cornea and lens, pigmentary retinopathy, etc.), autonomic nervous system (dry mouth, nasal congestion, constipation, adynamic ileus, urinary retention, etc.), and others (hyperpyrexia, increased appetite and weight gain, peripheral edema, etc.) (Table 13–3).

All marketed agents have similar efficacy. Thus, agent selection is guided heavily by the desire to retain or to avoid particular adverse effects. In general, the low potency agents (CPZ, thioridazine) have more sedating anticholinergic and antiadrenergic effects, but fewer EPSs. In contrast, the more potent newer neuroleptics (stronger dopaminergic blockade), though having fewer adverse side effects overall, do present a greater risk of extrapyramidal reactions.

The pharmacokinetics of CPZ are similar to those of the TCAs in that distribution and metabolism are the stages primarily affected by drug combinations. Pharmacological action (at the receptor site) of CPZ can also be the site of interactional effects.

Antipsychotic Drugs

Neuroleptics can usually be used safely in combination with lithium, MAOIs, and TCAs. Although there have been isolated reports of serious neurotoxicity with fever, confusion, tremors, ataxia, and coma, with the combination of lithium and antipsychotics, it is now felt that these agents can be safely combined in most patients if doses are moderate and patients are closely monitored. Any sign of toxicity should lead to discontinuation of medication. Severely manic patients may be treated with antipsychotics alone, initially. After symptoms are reduced, lithium can be added. The combination of neuroleptics with antidepressants (TCAs and MAOIs) is generally safe, though it requires some caution as there may be increased sedation and antimuscarinic effects. Theoretically, greater risk of "hypertensive" crises with the MAOIs may follow this increased antimuscarinic activity.

There are numerous drug interactions of proven clinical significance. Patients receiving CNS depressants may experience potentiation of the depressant effect when antipsychotics are added. An additive effect is also evident with antimuscarinic agents; an increased atropine-like effect results. Chlorpromazine also increases the serum level of a given dose of oral anticoagulant. And lastly, CPZ blocks the antihypertensive effects of guanethidine and related antihypertensives.

Patients at special risk when receiving antipsychotics in combination with other drugs include the elderly or demented with cardiovascular, hepatic, or chronic respiratory disorders. Those exposed to extreme heat and those taking atropine or related drugs are also at high risk.

Monoamine Oxidase Inhibitors (MAOIs)

The MAOIs are a series of agents with differing pharmacological profiles but a common action—monoamine oxidase inhibition. This enzyme inhibition results in reduced destruction of serotonin and norepinephrine. These agents are used primarily for the treatment of depression and panic disorders though they may also be effective in the treatment of hypertension. (Pargyline is marketed for the latter indication.) Historically, the MAOI–"cheese" interaction, which causes dramatic and potentially fatal hypertensive crises, forced attention to the drug and food interactions of the MAOIs.

TABLE 13-3 Antipsychotics

Drug	Effect	Mechanism	Clinical Significance
Anticholinergics	↑ Anticholinergic adverse effects/toxicity when used with AP with anticholinergic properties	Additive anticholinergic effect at receptor site	Yes
CNS depressants	↑ Sedation when used with sedative AP	Additive sedating effect at a receptor site	Yes
Antacids (Aluminum Hydroxide)	↓ Plasma AP levels (Chlorpromazine)	↓ Rate of oral absorption	?
Phenytoin	↑ Risk of phenytoin toxicity	↓ Metabolism	Yes
Guanethidine-like antihypertensives	↓ Antihypertensive effect	↑ Antagonism at receptor site	Yes
Barbiturates	↓ Plasma AP levels	↑ Metabolism	Yes
Narcotics (Meperidine)	↑ Narcotic analgesic effects ↑ Hypotension ↑ Respiratory depression	? ↓ Metabolism	Yes
L-Dopa	↓ L-Dopa antiparkinsonian effect	Antagonism at receptor site	Yes
Methyldopa	↑ Risk neurotoxicity with Haloperidol	?	?
Propranolol	↓ Plasma propranolol levels ↑ Plasma AP levels	↓ Metabolism ↓ Metabolism	? ?

Oral anticoagulants	↓ Bleeding	↓ Metabolism	?
Sympathomimetic amine	↑ Hypotension	Alpha-adrenergic blocking effects of AP at receptor site	Yes
Succinylcholine	↑ Duration apnea	↓ Serum cholinesterase levels	?
Valproic acid	↑ Plasma levels valproic acid (Chlorpromazine)	↓ Metabolism	?
Disulfiram	↓ Plasma levels AP (Perphenazine)	↑ Metabolism (Perphenazine)	?
Lithium	Potentiate neurotoxicity of lithium	Additive effect at CNS receptor site	Yes
	↓ Plasma lithium (Chlorpromazine) levels	?↑ Renal excretion	?
	↑ Plasma lithium (Haloperidol) levels	?↓ Renal excretion	?
TCAs	↑ Clinical efficacy (psychotic depression)	? Synergism at CNS receptor sites	Yes
	↑ Plasma antidepressants levels	?↓ Metabolism	?
	↑ Plasma AP levels	?↓ Metabolism	?
Carbamazepine	↓ Plasma Haloperidol levels	↑ Metabolism	?
Anesthetics (Enflurane, Isoflurane)	↑ Hypotension	?	Yes
Attapulgite	↓ Plasma AP levels	↓ Absorption AP	?
Estrogens	↑ Plasma AP levels	↓ Metabolism AP	?

Adverse effects of the MAOIs are common and involve the following systems: cardiovascular (orthostatic hypotension, etc.), hepatic (jaundice, etc.), CNS (dizziness, sedation, stimulation, weakness, fatigue, tremor, confusion, etc.), genitourinary (urinary retention), GI (constipation, dry mouth, etc.), ophthalmological (blurred vision, nystagmus, etc.), and others (edema, sexual disturbances, etc.) (Table 13-4).

The most severe interactions of the MAOIs are with the sympathomimetic drugs and foods high in tyramine. The combination of these agents with an MAOI can lead to a hypertensive crisis, a potentially life-threatening event associated with seizures, fever, sweating, excitation, delirium, tremor, strokes, coma, and circulatory collapse.

The co-administration of MAOIs with CNS depressants requires caution as marked sedation may occur. With narcotic analgesics, especially meperidine, not only can CNS depression be potentiated but severe hypertension and hyperpyrexia can occur. MAOIs reverse the antihypertensive effects of guanethidine, methyldopa, reserpine, and other rauwolfia derivatives. In contrast, they increase the hypotensive effects of other antihypertensive agents, including diuretics. Co-administration with a TCA is controversial and possibly produces a hypertensive crisis and typically a 2- to 3-week "washout" period between agents is recommended. However, when indicated, they can be given together, usually begun simultaneously and slowly increased.

All patients on MAOIs require due caution and even closer monitoring. They must be warned of potential adverse effects with other drugs and substances and be instructed to report promptly any headaches or other unusual symptoms. Perhaps only the trusted and reliable patients should be treated with MAOIs.

Several patient populations are at great risk for adverse interactions. These include the elderly, the demented, and the physically ill. Suicidal patients may overdose or deliberately take potentially toxic combinations.

Benzodiazepines

The benzodiazepines rank with the antidepressants as the most commonly prescribed medications by psychiatrists, primary care practitioners, and other specialists. This is in large part because sleep disturbance and anxiety, the symptoms these agents are primarily

TABLE 13-4 Monoamine Oxidase Inhibitors

Drug	Effect	Mechanism	Clinical Significance
Sympathomimetic amines	↑ Adrenergic effects (especially BP)	↓ Metabolism sympathomimetic amines ↑ Catecholamines at receptor site	Yes Yes
Opiates	↑ Opiate CNS depressant effects	↓ Metabolism	Yes
Meperidine	Excitation, hyperpyrexia, rigidity, ↑ BP	?	Yes
Levodopa	↑ BP or ↓ BP; facial flushing, headaches	↑ Dopamine, ↑ norepinephrine at receptor site	Yes
Barbiturates	↑ Plasma barbiturate levels	↓ Metabolism	Yes
Succinylcholine	Prolonged apnea	↓ Plasma pseudocholinesterase	Yes
Antiparkinson agents (Anticholinergics)	↑ Plasma antiparkinson agent levels	↓ Metabolism	Yes
Phenothiazines	↑ Extrapyramidal reactions	↓ ? Metabolism	Yes
Thiazide diuretics	↓ BP	?	Yes
Insulin and hypoglycemic agents	↑ Hypoglycemia	? Potentiation at receptor site	Yes
CNS depressants	↑ CNS sedation	Potentiation at receptor site	Yes
Guanethidine methyldopa	Antagonize hypotensive effect	Antagonism at receptor site	?
Tricyclic antidepressants	↑ ? Antidepressant effect ↑ ? Toxicity	? Synergism at receptor site ↓ ? Metabolism of TCAs	? ?

prescribed for, are ubiquitous in all fields of medicine. Fortunately, the benzodiazepines infrequently cause clinically significant drug–drug interactions despite the fact that they are often used in association with other medications. They are relatively safe to administer with other drugs primarily because they lack significant hepatic enzyme-inducing effect. This is in striking contrast to the barbiturates, the sedative hypnotics the benzodiazepines replaced (Table 13–5).

The most common clinical problems resulting from the interaction of benzodiazepines with other drugs is excessive CNS sedation; it occurs when they are combined with other CNS depressants. Increased plasma levels are the second major problem encountered. These increases occur when other medications hamper the metabolism of the benzodiazepines. It should be noted that individual compounds within the benzodiazepine family may manifest widely differing abilities to cause adverse effects when combined with other medications. For this reason, generalizations about benzodiazepines do not apply to all drug combinations involving this class of drugs. Attention must be paid to the specific benzodiazepine involved in any case report. Many drug–drug interactions have only been studied using the commonly used diazepam or chlordiazepoxide. Conclusions from these studies cannot necessarily be applied to other benzodiazepines.

ELECTROCONVULSIVE THERAPY-MEDICATION INTERACTIONS

Electroconvulsive therapy (ECT) was first introduced in the late 1930s and became widespread as a major medical intervention for the treatment of major psychiatric disorders, especially the affective disorders. With the advent of psychiatric medications and the increasing reports of complications from ECT, the use of this modality declined in the 1950s and 1960s. Within the past decade, however, ECT seems to have made a comeback. There are several reasons for this return to favor. The use of modern anesthetic techniques has decreased the morbidity of ECT and markedly increased patient comfort. Further, it is now recognized that many patients, especially those with psychotic depression, show a less-than-adequate response to medications. Also, many patients, especially the elderly, cannot tolerate the adverse effects of medications; for them, the potential risks of medi-

TABLE 13-5 Benzodiazepines

Drug	Benzodiazepines	Effect	Mechanism	Clinical Significance
Antacids	Chlorazepate	↓ Plasma active metabolite, desmethyldiazepam levels	↓ Metabolism Chlorazepate desmethyldiazepam	Yes
	Chlordiazepoxide	↓ Diazepam and chlordiazepoxide absorption rate (but not amount)		Yes
Food	Diazepam	↓ Diazepam absorption rate (but not amount)	?	Yes
Digoxin	Diazepam Alprazolam	↑ Plasma digoxin levels	? ↓ Renal clearance of dogoxin	Yes
Oral contraceptives	Alprazolam	↓ Plasma Alprazolam levels	↓ Metabolism	?
	Temazepam	↓ Plasma Temazepam levels	↑ Metabolism	?
	Diazepam	↑ Plasma Diazepam levels	↓ Metabolism	?
Cimetidine	Diazepam	↑ Plasma Diazepam levels	↓ Metabolism	Yes
	Chlordiazepoxide	↑ Plasma Chlordiazepoxide levels	↓ Metabolism	Yes
	Lorazepam	↑ Lorazepam levels	↓ Hepatic blood flow	?
Disulfiram	Diazepam	↑ Plasma Diazepam levels	↓ Metabolism	Yes
	Chlordiazepoxide	↑ Plasma Chlordiazepoxide levels	↓ Metabolism	Yes
Phenytoin	Chlordiazepoxide	↓ Plasma phenytoin levels	↓ Metabolism	?
Valproic acid	Diazepam	↑ Plasma Diazepam levels	↓ Metabolism	?
Propranolol	Diazepam	↑ Plasma Diazepam levels	↓ Metabolism	?
Propoxyphene	Alprazolam	↑ Plasma Alprazolam levels	↓ Metabolism	?
L-Dopa	Diazepam	↓ Antiparkinson effect	?	Yes
Antidepressants	All benzodiazepines	↑ CNS sedation	Additive effect at receptor site	Yes

cations outweigh those of ECT. Lastly, the use of unilateral seizure induction has decreased the incidence of significant memory impairment.

Even with improvement in technique and technology in modern ECT administration, adverse reactions resulting from medication–ECT interactions can occur in two major situations. First, psychiatric medications may interact adversely with the three major agents used in induction of ECT: anesthetics, muscle relaxants, and atropine (19). Second, adverse effects may result from the combination of certain drugs with the convulsion itself. Most reports of adverse reactions in this setting have been with psychotropics and cardiovascular agents.

Psychotropics

There have been recent troublesome reports indicating that patients receiving lithium therapy can experience adverse neurological symptoms after ECT treatment. These have included prolonged confusional states, more severe memory loss, and atypical neurological findings (20,21). Also, therapeutic outcome was less satisfactory in some patients on lithium (21). Currently, most authors recommend that lithium be discontinued before ECT.

The use of antidepressants, both TCA and MAOI, during ECT is controversial. Most textbooks recommend discontinuation of these agents at least 10 days to 2 weeks before beginning ECT, the same as the standard recommendation for elective surgery. Recent scientific controlled studies have challenged this clinical lore. One recent study suggests that patients taking TCA during ECT are at no greater risk for cardiovascular changes than patients in whom these agents were discontinued at least 2 weeks before the procedure (22). Another study, however, showed that patients with high anticholinergic drug levels (all on TCA) were at greater risk for developing post-ECT confusional states compared to those patients with low anticholinergic levels (23). Perhaps it is only the anticholinergic potency of an agent that is significant.

Most anesthesiologists recommend that MAOIs be discontinued 2 weeks prior to any procedure requiring anesthesia to prevent adverse reactions. However, in the only prospective controlled experiment studying this issue in both ECT and elective-surgery patients, no significant cardiovascular complications were observed in the patients receiving MAOIs (24).

Benzodiazepines are commonly used as preoperative medication in patients undergoing surgery. The use of these agents has been questioned in patients receiving ECT because of their anticonvulsant properties. One recent study did demonstrate that the administration of diazepam during the ECT procedure, compared with ECT in the same patients without diazepam, resulted in a significant reduction in mean seizure length (25).

There have been no controlled studies evaluating the hazards of antipsychotic use during ECT. These agents are commonly continued during ECT without apparent risk. However, it would seem prudent to discontinue antipsychotics with significant anticholinergic properties to avoid the post-ECT confusional states described above (23).

Cardiovascular Medications

The other major category of medication that has been identified as the probable cause of adverse effects when combined with ECT is the cardiovascular medication. The following agents have been specifically incriminated: propranolol, reserpine, lidocaine, and clonidine.

Propranolol has been used to attenuate the hypertensive response to ECT as well as to suppress the ectopy seen in some patients with cardiac disease after the experience of a seizure from ECT (26, 27). Two recent case reports suggest this use of propranolol can be associated with cardiac arrest (28,29).

In the 1950s, when reserpine was used in patients receiving ECT, several morbid events were noted. These included prolonged apnea, severe hypotension, cardiac arrhythmias, and even sudden death in some cases (30). For this reason, it is recommended that reserpine be discontinued 2 weeks before ECT is started.

The antiarrhythmic agent lidocaine has been well studied in patients receiving ECT. It has been found that in therapeutic doses this agent can decrease the duration of seizures from ECT (31,32). For this reason, it is contraindicated during the procedure.

Clonidine is currently used as an antihypertensive agent. A recent case report suggested that clonidine may have an anticonvulsant effect in patients during ECT (33). The authors of this report postulated that clonidine may raise the seizure threshold in humans. Although this finding awaits reduplication, it is probably prudent to avoid clonidine in patients undergoing ECT.

REFERENCES

1. Boston Collaborative Drug Surveillance Program. (1972). Adverse drug interactions. *Journal of the American Medical Association* 220:1238-1239.
2. Griffin, J. P., and D'Arcy, P. F., eds. (1984). *Manual of Adverse Drug Interactions*. Bristol: John Wright.
3. Salzman, C., and Hoffman, S. A. (1983). Clinical interaction between psychotropic and other drugs. *Hospital and Community Psychiatry* 34:897-902.
4. Tyrer, P. J., ed. (1982). *Drugs in Psychiatric Practice*. London: Butterworths.
5. Shader, R. I., ed. (1975). *Manual of Psychiatric Therapeutics*. Boston: Little, Brown.
6. Davis, J. M. (1985). Other pharmacological agents. In *Comprehensive Textbook of Psychiatry*, vol. 4, ed. H. I. Kaplan and B. J. Sadock, pp. 1556-1558. Baltimore: Williams and Wilkins.
7. Bussuk, E. I., Schoonover, S. C., and Gelenberg, A. J., ed. (1984). *Practitioner's Guide to Psychoactive Drugs*. New York: Plenum.
8. (1976). *Evaluations of Drug Interactions*, 2nd ed. Washington: American Pharmaceutical Association.
9. (1978). *Evaluations of Drug Interactions*, 2nd ed. suppl. Washington: American Pharmaceutical Association.
10. Hansten, P. D. (1979). *Drug Interactions*, 4th ed. Philadelphia: Lea and Ferbiger.
11. Bernstein, J. G. (1983). *Handbook of Drug Therapy in Psychiatry*. Boston: John Wright/PSG.
12. Jefferson, J. W., Greist, J. H., and Baudhuin, M. (1981). Lithium: Interactions with other drugs. *Journal of Clinical Psychopharmacology* 1:124-134.
13. Plon, L., and Gottschalk, L. A. (1984). Antianxiety agents-drug interactions. In *Drugs in Psychiatry*, ed. G. D. Burrows, T. R. Norman, and B. Davies, pp. 157-175. New York: Elsevier.
14. Breckenridge, A. (1983). Interactions of benzodiazepines with other substances. In *The Benzodiazepines: From Molecular Biology to Clinical Practice*, ed. E. Costa, pp. 237-246. New York: Raven Press.
15. Baldessarini, R. J. (1977). Interactions of the antidepressants with other agents. In *Chemotherapy in Psychiatry*, pp. 109-111. Cambridge, MA: Harvard University Press.
16. Siris, S. G., and Rifkin, A. (1981). The problem of psychopharmacotherapy in the medically ill. *Psychiatric Clinics of North America* 4:379-390.
17. (1981). Alcohol-drug interactions: What we should consider. *Resident and Staff Physician*, pp. 97-103, August. (Reprinted from *FDA Drug Bulletin*, June 1979.)
18. Blackwell, B., and Schmidt, G. L. (1984). Drug interactions in psychopharmacology. *Psychiatric Clinics of North America* 7:625-637.
19. Janowsky, E. C., Risch, S. C., and Janowsky, D. S. (1981). Psychotropic agents. In: *Drug Interactions in Anesthesia*, ed. N. T. Smith, R. D. Miller, A. N. Corbascio. Philadelphia: Lea and Febiger.
20. Weiner, R. D., Whanger, A. D., Erwin, W., and Wilson, W. P. (1980). Pro-

longed confusional state and EEG seizure activity following concurrent ECT and lithium use. *American Journal of Psychiatry* 137:1452–1453.
21. Small, J. G., Kellams, J. J., Milstein, V., and Small, I. F. (1980). Complications with electroconvulsive treatment combined with lithium. *Biological Psychiatry* 15:103–111.
22. Azar, I., and Lear, E. (1984). Cardiovascular effects of electroconvulsive therapy in patients taking tricyclic antidepressants (letter). *Anesthesia and Analgesia* 63:1139–1144.
23. Mondimore, F. M., Damlouji, N., Folstein, M. F., and Tune, L. (1983). Post-ECT confusional states associated with elevated serum anticholinergic levels. *American Journal of Psychiatry* 140:930–931.
24. El-Ganzouri, A. R., Ivankovich, A. D., Braverman, B., McCarthy, R. (1985). Monoamine oxidase inhibitors: Should they be discontinued preoperatively? *Anesthesia and Analgesia* 64:592–596.
25. Standish-Barry, H. M., Deacon, V., and Snaith, R. P. (1985). The relationship of concurrent benzodiazepine administration to seizure duration in ECT. *Acta Psychiatrica Scandinavica* 71:269–271.
26. Weiner, R. D., Henschen, G. M., and Pellasega, M. (1979). Propranolol treatment of ECT related ventricular arrhythmias. *American Journal of Psychiatry* 136:1594–1595.
27. London, S. W., and Glass, D. D. (1985). Prevention of electroconvulsive therapy-induced dysrhythmias with atropine and propranolol. *Anesthesiology* 62:819–822.
28. Decina, P., Malitz, S., Sackeim, H. A., Holzer, J., Yudofsky, S. (1984). Cardiac arrest during ECT modified by beta-adrenergic blockade. *American Journal of Psychiatry* 141:298–300.
29. Wulfson, H. P., Askanazi, J., and Finck, A. D. (1984). Propranolol prior to ECT associated with asystole. *Anesthesiology* 60:255–256.
30. Foster, M. W., and Gayle, R. F. (1955). Dangers in combining reserpine with electroconvulsive therapy. *Journal of the American Medical Association* 154:1520–1522.
31. Hood, D. D., and Mecca, R. S. (1983). Failure to initiate electroconvulsive seizures in a patient pretreated with lidocaine. *Anesthesiology* 58:379–381.
32. Ottosson, J. O. (1960). Experimental studies of the mode of action of electroconvulsive therapy. *Acta Psychiatrica et Neurologica Scandinavica (Suppl.)*: 145.
33. Elliot, R. L. (1983). Case report of potential interaction between clonidine and electroconvulsive therapy. *American Journal of Psychiatry* 140:1237–1238.

14

Psychotherapy and Psychopharmacology

David S. Harnett, M.D.

The title of this chapter is an awesome one and is used with some trepidation. First, I refer to the work of Dr. Eric Kandel (1,2), which has implications, albeit quite speculative, as to how we categorize our "therapies." A few years ago, he wrote an article for the *New England Journal of Medicine* with the admittedly provocative title, "Psychotherapy and the Single Synapse." Kandel has reviewed the literature suggesting that sensory and possibly social deprivation in early childhood can alter the structure and function of the cerebral cortex. He has also studied the nervous system of the marine snail *Aplysia californica*. In this model he found that learning is associated with changes in gene expression and chemical connections between synapses. Learning or experience may then result in the long-term disruption or reactivation of synaptic connections. Thus, for *Aplysia*, learning may have long-term biological consequences. The implication is that psychotherapy joins pharmacotherapy in the ranks of the *biological* therapies.

Moving from the conjectural to the pragmatic, Beitman and colleagues (3) have surveyed psychiatrists in the state of Washington who prescribe psychotropic medication to patients in psychotherapy with nonmedical psychotherapists. They note that such pharmacotherapy–psychotherapy–patient triangles are becoming increasingly frequent and raise a number of issues. These include questions such as, who is responsible for monitoring suicidal ideation, how to handle confidentiality, and when should the patient be present during therapists' communication. Finally, the authors wonder to what extent psychopharmacology consultations represent covert requests for supervision or transfer.

There are indeed many theoretical and practical concerns when one attempts to judiciously combine drugs and psychotherapy. This chapter briefly reviews some issues in the treatment of schizophrenia, where our therapeutic success is modest, affective disorders, and finally panic and agoraphobia, where many treatments work but where confusion still reigns.

SCHIZOPHRENIA

It has been clear for some time now that antipsychotic medication is the most effective treatment for schizophrenia as well as for prophylaxis against future exacerbations (4). Prophylactic failures have often been attributed to medication noncompliance. However, more recent data suggest that despite ensured compliance with depot neuroleptics, a significant number of patients will still relapse (5,6). Some of these patients relapse despite neuroleptic maintenance, then stop their medication secondarily while in the throes of a psychotic episode and have mistakenly then been considered to be primary noncompliers. Can psychosocial treatments, then, aid the medication responders who relapse despite medication maintenance, the medication responders who won't take medication, and the medication nonresponders (including those that do and don't take medication)?

It is also clear that most research does not support the use of psychosocial treatments*, especially individual psychodynamically oriented psychotherapy, in schizophrenia. These various studies have been summarized and critiqued elsewhere (7,8). In fact, a leading

---

*It is my contention that the more encompassing "psychosocial treatments," rather than "psychotherapy," are more pertinent in current discussion of schizophrenia. Psychosocial treatments are roughly defined to include individual psychotherapy, group psychotherapy, milieu therapy, social casework (aftercare and rehabilitation), behavior therapy (including social skills training), family modalities, and psychoeducation.

authority has suggested that there are no effective psychosocial treatments for schizophrenia (9). Nonetheless, there is evidence that social factors, including psychosocial treatments, can influence the course of schizophrenia in positive and negative ways. These influences may, in turn, co-vary with medication status. A consideration of these social factors might be useful in designing relevant psychosocial therapies.

There is a long-standing literature suggesting a more benign outcome for schizophrenia in the Third World or nonindustrial nations as compared with industrial societies (10–12). (The possible relevance of these findings to the British "expressed emotion" data is discussed later on.) These cross-cultural differences have been interpreted a number of ways and have been criticized for diagnostic and other methodological faults. One can, for example, postulate an exclusively biological cause with different gene pools having different vulnerabilities. But since the World Health Organization study and others showed consistently superior outcome in varying "developing" areas (Ibadan, Nigeria; Agra, India; Mauritius; Sri Lanka) as opposed to the "developed" cities (Aarhus, Denmark; London; Washington; Moscow), sociocultural factors have been considered. Urbanized and industrial environments were associated with the worst outcome. A study in Sri Lanka (11) indicated that good outcome was not simply an artifact of family willingness to tolerate and underestimate psychopathology. One explanation is folk or supernatural explanations of psychosis. Neither patient nor family is blamed, and stigma, alienation, and isolation are reduced. Moreover, such societies are often characterized by community involvement and responsibility for the mentally ill. Another possibility is a more flexible use of labor in such societies where disability is not absolute and psychotic individuals can find tasks to match their varying abilities (12).

The cross-cultural data are not inconsistent with the stress-diathesis (13) model of schizophrenia that has been receiving increasing attention. This model suggests that affected patients suffer from organically based cognitive and perceptual deficits. These are manifest by difficulties filtering stimuli and the inability to smoothly shift sets or focused alertness. A consequence is vulnerability to extremes of arousal including affective stimulation. This in turn might lead to an intensification of the so-called positive symptoms ("positive" because they are notable for their presence, such as hallucinations and delusions) of schizophrenia. There is also recent data suggesting that high-dose neuroleptics and tardive dyskinesia may worsen these patients' attentional and information-processing abilities (14). This lends further support to the low-dose strategies discussed later on.

Regardless of the correctness of this model, there is an impressive British literature linking stress to psychotic relapse in schizophrenia. If the withdrawal secondary to hyperarousal is prevented, then manifest psychosis may be precipitated (15,16). The existence of an increased number of independent life stresses in the 3 weeks prior to schizophrenic relapse as compared to a control population was also found (17). In addition, medication status seemed to influence the role of stress. Those patients receiving neuroleptics relapsed only after significant stress, whereas the nonmedicated group's relapses were preceded by routine events as well as stresses (18,19). This suggested that neuroleptics might be protective against the routine demands of daily living but not against major stresses.

Further work has led to the development of the concept of expressed emotion (EE). Two separate British groups (16,20) found that for patients returning to live with relatives, a significant predictor of psychotic relapse (reappearance or exacerbation of positive symptoms in the 9 months after discharge) were certain emotions expressed by relatives toward the patient (in the patient's absence) during a standardized interview. Expressed emotion is a calculation of the number of critical comments, hostility, and emotional overinvolvement as determined by standardized rating scales. The notion is not that EE is a cause of schizophrenia, but that the course of established schizophrenia may be influenced by the emotional atmosphere of the family. The 9-month relapse rates for 128 schizophrenic patients (combined from the above two groups) varies with EE, medication status, and face-to-face contact hours with relatives (see Figure 14-1).

These results suggest that for the brief period of 9 months, neuroleptic maintenance confers no additional benefit for the low EE group. In addition, the relapsing effect of high EE may be mitigated by either neuroleptics or decreased family contact hours. Moreover, the combination of medication and less contact hours is more effective than either alone.

A 2-year follow-up (21) suggested the continued association between high EE and relapse. However, antipsychotic medication was now shown to be helpful in forestalling relapse in the low EE group. This might be explained by earlier work suggesting the protec-

Schizophrenia

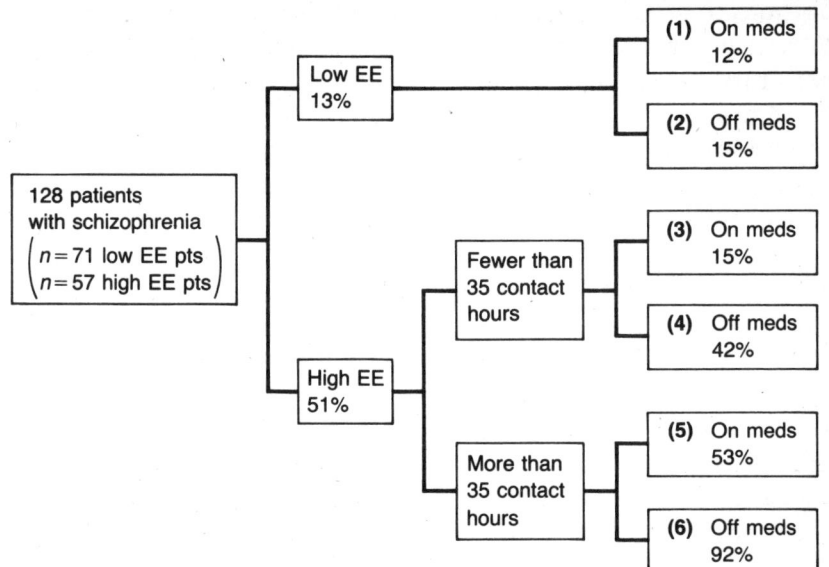

FIGURE 14-1. Nine-month relapse rates.

tive effect of drugs against routine demands but not major stresses. It may be that major stresses don't appear so frequently for the low EE patients.

This relationship between EE and relapse was recently replicated in a southern California population (22). Again, high EE predicted increased relapse 9 months after discharge. However, there were differences in the interrelating factors. In the California group, only the combined effects of antipsychotic medication and decreased family contact hours lessened the relapsing effect of high EE. Neither drug nor decreased contact hours, alone, helped diminish relapse in the high EE group. This may have been related to a higher number of chronic, unmarried, drug-abusing men in the California group who are known to be a vulnerable group. The study has some notable methodological strengths. Relapse was defined as symptomatic worsening of psychosis. Readmission for depression, social disturbance, or relief of family burden is not considered a relapse. A criticism of such research has been that EE may only be an artifact of chronicity. Those who do poorly will tend to elicit negative reactions, according to that argument. However, in this last study, EE was not associated with severity as evaluated upon admission. In addition, equal proportions of patients with high and low EE failed to take their medications. Finally, the relationship between family EE and relapse has been further replicated in an inner-city Chicago population (23).

Carol Howe, a leader of the National Alliance for the Mentally Ill (NAMI), a consumer group, has suggested that EE is one more passing fad in the long tradition in which families of schizophrenic patients are unfairly blamed (24). Perhaps families might be more accepting of the importance of this concept if they were told they are not the sole potential bearers of high EE or, put more generally, of stress. One need look no further than psychiatric inpatient services, the living placements for patients, and outpatient psychosocial treatments for evidence. Examples of each will follow. Thus, high EE can exist outside of the home and, as will be discussed, may have some benefits. Again, the effects of EE sometimes vary with medication status. Surveys of discharged schizophrenic patients living in single-room occupancy hotels in New York City suggest that life satisfaction and favorable social functioning were associated with casual rather than intense relationships with other residents. The suggestion was that a quiet, undemanding, somewhat isolated social atmosphere might be beneficial (13). A Veterans Administration (VA) study suggested that foster care resulted in better social adjustment for schizophrenic patients than continued hospitalization (26). Best results were associated with foster homes that had children, smaller numbers of patients, and smaller numbers of total occupants. Foster homes that provided schizophrenic patients with more stimulation (sponsor-initiated leisure activities), more supervision by sponsors, and more intensive social worker follow-up had poorer outcome. Another VA study suggested that day treatment centers that provide schizophrenic patients with more occupational therapy, recreational activities, and longer duration of treatment had better results (27). Poorer outcome was associated with day treatment that had more professional counseling, more group therapy, and higher patient turnover.

The possible long-term harm of withholding antipsychotic medication in the acute phase, even if medication is later supplied, has been suggested (4). A three-year study at the Massachusetts Mental Health Center (28) compared high (intensive) and low (minimal) social therapy with further subdivision into medication and no-medication groups. The high social therapy/no medication for the initial 6-month group never caught up to the high social therapy/

medication group at 3-year follow-up. Similar results were found in an influential California study (29) that compared individual psychotherapy (by state hospital psychiatry residents) with no psychotherapy again with subdivision into medication and no medication groups. These were first-admission schizophrenic patients who received whatever treatment they and their physician decided on after the initial phase. The 3- to 5-year follow-up again suggested that despite the extensive uncontrolled follow-up period, withholding medications for the relatively brief initial period may have long-standing negative consequences. Another group has found that those receiving major role therapy (a combination of social casework and vocational rehabilitation) without the protection of neuroleptics may do worse than those receiving placebo alone (30). The highly symptomatic schizophrenic patients were most vulnerable to the relapsing effect of this sociotherapy while the asymptomatic patients benefited (31).

In summary, increased demands may enhance performance, but at the risk of increasing positive symptoms and relapse. On the other hand, decreasing demands may diminish positive symptoms and prevent relapse, but with the price of poor performance and possibly more "negative" symptoms (32) (notable for their absence, such as apathy, withdrawal, and blunted affect). One can argue that it may be worth a few extra relapses if overall performance and adjustment can be improved by elevated expectations. From this vantage point, high EE may be beneficial. Similarly, one might wonder if the price of "better outcome" for schizophrenia in the developing countries may be more negative symptoms related to lower cultural expectations.

While there may be an initial, transient improvement of negative symptoms with antipsychotics (33), negative symptoms are generally regarded as nonresponsive to medication. A recent study suggested that nursing homes compared unfavorably to continued hospital care (34) and may represent one of the new negative-symptom-inducing, sterile institutions for the mentally ill. Finally, a recent comparison of schizophrenic outcome in Vancouver and Portland, Oregon, suggested that comprehensive community aftercare was associated with less negative symptoms (35).

What is the implication, then, for psychosocial treatments in schizophrenia? Do all these data spell the death knell for individual psychodynamically oriented psychotherapy in schizophrenia? The data clearly do not support the psychotherapeutic role of the unmedicated regression [though it still has a few remaining adherents (36)] with the preference for issues not being submerged by medication. Rather, the evidence suggests changes in the "timing, intensity and structure" (37) of these psychosocial treatments not previously considered. The earlier mentioned study (30) evaluating major role therapy revealed an important benefit for those that had not relapsed at 18 months. Social therapy plus medication resulted in improved mood and social adjustment as compared to the medication alone (30,38). Various new family therapy approaches, in conjunction with medication, have been shown in controlled trials to reduce relapse in schizophrenic patients (39–44). Such family approaches begin with a supportive, concrete style and attempt to avoid the ambiguity that might otherwise be useful in a traditional, dynamically oriented psychotherapy. Education about schizophrenia, family sessions, and multiple family groups are employed. Coping strategies are suggested and tasks are assigned. Exploratory family approaches may be utilized at a late stage (43). These family modalities have been supplemented by individual social skills training (44,45) which attempts to improve social competence through various behavioral modules that are sensitive to the patient's cognitive and attentional deficiencies.

It is our belief that the stress-reducing psychoeducational approaches must be complemented by a psychotherapeutic approach that empathizes with and helps a patient deal with the subjective experience of his or her psychosis. Strauss and Carpenter (46) have suggested that such an approach can help decrease the patient's sense of isolation. For patients to have some coherent sense of what they are going through and to identify prodromal symptoms and subsequent stages may give them some control over these symptoms. In one study, patients' mechanisms of self-control varied and included self-instruction and both reduced and increased involvement in activity (47).

Low-dose neuroleptic strategies have increasingly been suggested (48-51). High doses may be associated with an increased incidence of tardive dyskinesia. In addition, Kane (52) has suggested that patients receiving lower dosages show various improvements in psychosocial adjustment and family satisfaction despite increased rates of psychotic relapse. Difficulties with high doses may be related directly to side effects, to medication noncompliance secondary to side effects, or to lack of drug efficacy because the dosage is above a presumed therapeutic window (see Chapter 1, "Psychosis"). Intermittent or targeted medication approaches have also been advocated (53,54). Patients would not take continuous medication but would promptly receive it once prodromal symptoms appeared. Hopefully, psychosocial treatments might not only increase medication compliance but, through stress reduction and increase in self-control of symptoms, may themselves permit dosage reduction. In fact, a recent study has given initial support to this notion (42). Family management was not only found superior to individual therapy in reducing psychotic relapse, but was associated with reduced neuroleptic dosage and lower deficit symptoms. Moreover, family approaches appear crucial to help identify prodromal symptoms and to rapidly treat those who are to receive intermittent medication.

Finally, while this review does not find supporting evidence, it also does not militate against intensive dynamic psychotherapies for certain well-compensated, "good prognosis," schizophrenic patients. Perhaps this is not really psychotherapy of schizophrenia, but psychotherapy of character attempting to adapt to the illness schizophrenia. Though not without weaknesses, a 5-year study in Sweden (55–57) suggested that intensive, dynamically oriented psychotherapy plus depot neuroleptics provided benefits as compared to drugs alone. It should also be noted that there still remain a few therapists who claim that neuroleptics interfere with the benefits of psychotherapy (58).

AFFECTIVE DISORDERS

The use of psychotherapy and/or pharmacotherapy in depression is another enormous area that is touched on only briefly here. If psychotherapy for an episode of major depression (DSM-III) is being considered, then by definition one is talking about short-term treatment since the episode itself is unlikely to last more than a year. While hundreds of types of psychotherapy have been described, the field was narrowed to four in a recent critical review of treatments for acute depression (59): cognitive, behavior, interpersonal, and psychodynamic. Group (60) and marital (61) approaches might also be included.

Cognitive, behavioral, and interpersonal approaches are first briefly described. Cognitive therapy (62) is a blend of psychoanalytical and behavioral methods that emphasizes self-understanding and insight but rejects the notion that the behavior is determined by an unconscious over which the individual has little control. Aaron Beck (63), originally trained as a psychoanalyst, considered neurotic depression to be caused by a set of negative thinking patterns by which a person learns about himself, the future, and the world, and which he maintains despite evidence to the contrary. Treatment is then focused on unlearning or correcting these cognitive distortions. Therapy is short-term, collaborative, and present-oriented. It is highly structured, didactic, and involves specific behavioral tasks and homework assignments with specific goals. Rational-emotive therapy (64,65), also developed by a psychoanalyst, could be regarded as a type of cognitive therapy.

Classical behavior therapy has emphasized overt behavior and its modification through external reinforcement. Some behaviorists say that cognitions are acquired and maintained through the same principles that determine behavior (59). In this way, cognitive therapy may be regarded as a type of behavior therapy. The behavioral work of Lewinsohn, McLean, and Rehm, which includes social skills training, is described elsewhere (66). Interpersonal psychotherapy (67) is another short-term treatment that focuses on current depressive symptoms and current depression-related interpersonal difficulties. Klerman (68, 69) has written extensively about the methodological and ideological issues in combining drugs and psychotherapy, especially in regard to affective illness. He has considered a number of potential interactions which are illustrated:

1. *No Interaction.* Cognitive therapy (59) alone, appears to be an effective treatment for many ambulatory nonbipolar depressives without melancholia. Rush (70) has suggested that antidepressants, while effective, do not result in any enhanced improvement of acute depressive symptoms when combined with cognitive therapy.

2. *Negative Effect.* There is little evidence that psychotherapy or medications diminish each other's beneficial effects in depressed patients.

3. *Additive Effect.* Interpersonal psychotherapy has also been found, by itself, to be an effective modality for outpatient nonbipolar, nonendogenous depressives. Yet, Weissman and

Klerman (71) have found that not only are tricyclics helpful, but that the combination yields benefits greater than either treatment alone. This additive effect continues into the maintenance period after resolution of the acute episode.

As noted above, Rush has not been impressed with the additive effect of cognitive and pharmacotherapy for acute depressive symptoms. However, some patients with prolonged vegetative depressions successfully ameliorated with antidepressants may be left with residual negative thinking patterns (cognitive symptoms of depression). Such patients may attain additional benefits from cognitive therapy (70).

4. *Complex Facilitative Effect.* This means that one treatment is ineffective unless accompanied by other treatment and that the combination is most effective. Melancholic and psychotic depression might fit this category, as would bipolar disorder.

The dichotomy between mild and severe depression received further support from a study (72) which looked at patients prematurely terminating treatment. Pharmacotherapy (with and without psychotherapy) was associated with greater dropout in mild depressives. On the other hand, psychotherapy without medication led to more treatment stoppage in the endogenous patients.

Systematic studies of combined treatment in bipolar illness are fewer than unipolar depression. A stimulus-reducing, limit-setting, highly structured psychotherapeutic approach to acute mania is often employed. Whether and which psychotherapy to add to lithium in the maintenance period is less clear. Clinical reports of useful group therapy interventions (73) have included marital groups and educational approaches. Jamison (73) has speculated that cognitive-behavioral techniques might be helpful for lithium compliance, psychodynamic approaches for the interpersonal sequelae of the illness, and group therapy for denial of illness and self-esteem issues. Yet those questions remain to be studied. In one of her studies, Jamison (73) found that the patients receiving lithium considered psychotherapy to be more useful than did the psychotherapists.

Finally, an additional use of psychotherapy for bipolars might be for mild depressions persisting despite the use of lithium. Tricyclic maintenance, even in the presence of lithium, is increasingly being discouraged (74) since it has been implicated in leading to rapid cycling.

In providing longer-term psychotherapy in the maintenance phase, the question might arise whether one is still treating the affective illness or really dealing with the personality of a patient who additionally has recurrent affective episodes. One can argue that before the advent of lithium, it was difficult to get a clear look at the character style of many bipolar patients.

A number of questions may then arise in attempting to sort out personality from affective illness and what treatment to employ. The long-standing notion that personality predisposes one to affective illness has come under scrutiny (75). The converse hypothesis, that personality may often represent a complication (short and long term) of affective episodes, has also been considered. Furthermore, premorbid character may influence the manifestation of an acute affective illness (76). For example, hysterics may appear quite different from obsessives when they become depressed. Finally, what is called personality may actually represent an attenuated or (atypical) version of affective illness. Thus, what is borderline personality to some may be cyclothymia, dysthymia, or atypical bipolar disorder to others. Akiskal (77) has coined the term "subaffective" which emphasizes the presentation as mild, or forme fruste, but still fundamentally affective illness.

The plethora of terms employed to describe the overlapping symptom constellations generally referred to as atypical depression has made this area even more difficult to understand. (Atypical depression is reviewed in Chapter 11.) That atypical depression is characterized by mood that is reactive to social/environmental change further clouds the distinction between affective illness and patients with personality disorders who are chronically unhappy. It certainly remains possible that such controversial conditions as borderline personality disorders may sometimes represent the combination (and interaction) of a personality disorder as classically defined plus an affective illness.

PANIC AND AGORAPHOBIA

The use of drugs versus psychotherapy remains especially controversial in the area of panic disorder and agoraphobia. Eminent proponents of pharmacological and behavioral approaches have cited controlled studies that seem to contradict each other (78,79). In addition, psychoanalytic approaches to anxiety have had a long and influential tradition (80).

Klein and others have emphasized the importance of panic attacks themselves as the chief cause of patient distress and dysfunction (81,82). The emphasis on pharmacological treatment of panic has become increasingly popular. Moreover, panic is seen as leading to the secondary manifestations of anticipatory anxiety (of further panic attacks) and agoraphobia (avoidance of conditions where attacks might be predicted to occur or that might make attacks particularly uncomfortable) (81). Freud (83) actually anticipated this sequence during his earlier formulation of anxiety. The discovery in the early 1960s that imipramine can block panic attacks without affecting anticipatory anxiety, while benzodiazepines seem to have the opposite effect lends credence to the notion that panic anxiety and anticipatory anxiety might be two qualitatively distinct entities (81).

The eminent British researcher Marks (84) has emphasized that phobic avoidance, not panic attacks, is the major cause of disability in these patients. The argument is that the key to rendering agoraphobic patients functional is to treat their phobic avoidance with behavior therapy. The number and intensity of panic attacks will also be reduced, but by no means entirely. The patients are then presumably able to tolerate the residual number of panic attacks without any further development of phobic behavior. In addition, behavioral theory teaches that the difference between panic anxiety and less severe forms is merely quantitative.

A point of dispute is whether antidepressants such as imipramine and phenelzine are effective for agoraphobics with panic attacks in the absence of depression. In a review of the literture, Marks (85) has suggested that antidepressants are helpful only in phobic patients in the presence of dysphoria or anxious-depressed mood. He suggests that in these patients, medication has a broad-spectrum effect alleviating not only dysphoria, but also panic, hostility, and anger. This is in marked contrast to impressive data suggesting that pretreatment depression is not correlated with outcome (86) or possibly even associated with negative outcome (87).

As further indictment to the overly widespread use of antidepressants in nondysphoric agoraphobics, Marks (88) has pointed to the notable dropout rate in patients taking pills or placebo, the significant incidence of side effects, and perhaps most important, the high rate of relapse when medication is stopped, even after a 6- to 8-month course. He contrasts the broad-spectrum use of antidepressants with the specific use of the behavioral technique "exposure in vivo" which he claims yields much more lasting gains.

Marks has also cautioned against the concurrent use of high-dose benzodiazepines or alcohol during behavior therapy. Included in his caution is the novel benzodiazepine alprazolam which has recently been shown by others (89) to block panic attacks. Although acknowledging he has no controlled data, he suggests (90) that greater than 1.5 ounces of pure alcohol, 7.5 mg diazepam, 1.0 mg alprazolam, or the equivalent, daily, may interfere with habituation (decreased behavioral response after repeated stimulation) in behavior treatment. This would occur, he says, through the principle of state-dependent learning. These substances, then, may be responsible for a number of behavior therapy failures.

Another point of controversy is what type of behavior treatment should be given either in conjunction with medication or without. There are a number of possibilities whether one believes in first blocking the panic attacks with medication and then treating the residual avoidance patterns or focusing on the phobic avoidance immediately. One possibility is to use no behavioral therapy at all. If the phobias are secondary to panic attacks that have been pharmacologically blocked, then perhaps the phobias might dissipate on their own. This might be more likely with early intervention before phobic behavior has become too entrenched.

If one is to use behavior therapy, there are a variety of approaches from which to choose (91). These include gradual (systematic desensitization) or rapid (flooding) exposure to feared stimuli. Exposure may occur in imagination or in real life (in vivo); therapy may be individual or group oriented, and may or may not include relaxation techniques. There may be variable amounts of therapist-assisted versus self-directed exposure, structure, such as homework, and cognitive therapy additions, such as paradoxical intention. Recently, there has appeared a consensus that the key ingredient is prolonged and repeated real-life exposure to phobic stimuli (91). The exposure must be of sufficient duration so that anxiety begins to abate. The gradation of phobic cues, relaxation techniques, and the imaginal phase can often be dispensed with and would therefore be regarded as only occasionally needed preliminaries. The importance of exposure was also anticipated by Freud who said (92),

> One can hardly ever master a phobia if one waits until the patient lets the analysis influence him to give it up . . . one succeeds only when one can induce them through the influence of the analysis to . . . go into the street and to struggle with their anxiety while they make the attempt [pp. 165-166].

Yet the question remains as to whether some sort of formal behavior program is needed as opposed to any nonspecific psychotherapy that through the power of the therapeutic relationship leads to prolonged in vivo exposure. One major study (93) found that supportive psychotherapy (dynamically oriented) plus imipramine achieved the equally good results that behavior therapy (systematic desensitization and assertiveness training) plus imipramine did in a group of agoraphobics and mixed phobics (circumscribed phobia plus panic attacks).

What then is the role of psychodynamic approaches in panic disorder and agoraphobia? Do they offer anything more specific than a vehicle for in vivo exposure? Psychoanalytic theory based on Freud's later formulation of anxiety (94) is similar to the behavioral notion that panic and milder anxiety are only quantitatively distinct. Recent data have demonstrated the efficacy of high doses of the highly potent alprazolam (89) and possibly other benzodiazepines (95,96) in panic disorder. In addition, in a multicenter study, imipramine was found to be more effective than chlordiazepoxide in a group of neurotic outpatients with a predominance of non-panic attack anxious symptoms (97,98). These data do not support the notion of two distinct types of anxiety (panic and anticipatory) described by Klein in his historic paper (81).

Psychoanalytic approaches have traditionally emphasized the usefulness of unmedicated anxiety as a guide to help elucidate underlying intrapsychic conflict. [Self-psychology has modified the conflict origin of agoraphobia instead suggesting the etiological role of a structural deficiency of the self (99)]. The major indication for adjunctive and temporary pharmacotherapy is severity of symptoms. The cost of medication might then be a delay in the patient gaining "ego-mastery" (100). The contrasting so-called biological view would be to identify the specific syndrome (or disease). The lack of severity of symptoms would not, in the biological model, preclude pharmacological treatment.

The gain in the psychoanalytic approach would be to uncover and profitably work with buried issues that are responsible for the current symptoms. For example, in the panic-agoraphobia situation, one might reveal dependency conflicts that could be analyzed and worked through. The contrasting disease model would say that the patient might have trouble with dependency secondary to an untreated illness. If the panics are blocked with medication and the phobias ameliorated with behavior therapy, then perhaps "after the dust clears," the dependency problem will also be gone.

Psychoanalytic practitioners have also noted that there appears to be an ever-rising incidence of panic disorder. This observation is not supported by any systematic data and may simply represent the delayed identification of a patient population that has always existed. However, another possibility is that the furor of media and professional attention to a newly discovered "curable disease" has led a diverse group of people with some anxiety to seek treatment for their "panic attacks." Physicians may encourage this process in an effort not to miss any disguised cases. The result may be a subtle alteration of the clinical picture in some patients. The pressure of insurers for an axis I biological illness to justify reimbursement for outpatient psychotherapy might also have a subtle influence upon patient presentation. Refinements in the diagnosis of panic disorder could potentially help ameliorate this danger.

Nemiah has carefully described cases where conflicted aggressive and sexual themes appear in the associations of patients talking about their panic attacks (80). However, while associations are suggestive, they do not prove etiology (101). Panickers are often perplexed by their attacks and, for example, in the cases described by Nemiah, may have been searching for intrapsychic explanations as a means of coping with a terrifying experience.

Yet, it certainly remains possible that a subgroup of patients will panic exclusively as a result of conflict. More likely, some patients with an inherited or developmentally acquired vulnerability to panic will become symptomatic in the presence of stress. In fact, studies have shown that a large number of adult panic disorder patients have childhood histories of severe separation anxiety. In these particular patients, the later onset of panic is often precipitated by a significant loss (102). In a similar vein, it has been noted that agoraphobics will often refuse to face a phobic stimulus unless accompanied by a companion. This other person seems to raise the panic threshold for the patient. All this suggests is that a biopsychosocial model may be relevant to panic disorder.

Shader (103) has proposed an interactional model where there is a relationship between overall anxiety levels and the frequency of panic attacks. He suggests, "The greater the background level of anxiety, whether related to acute or chronic situational anxiety or to life stress or marked anticipatory anxiety, the greater the frequency of panic attacks" (104). This has been supported by others who have suggested that generalized anxiety may precede as well as follow the onset of panic attacks (96).

Shader further suggests an analogy between epileptic seizures and panic attacks. Stress has been noted to increase frequency of seizures in some patients. Perhaps the kindling process postulated to occur in seizure patients that increases paroxysmal firing might also occur in panic patients as background anxiety level builds. Moreover, a study revealed that psychodynamically oriented psychotherapy markedly reduced seizure frequency in children whose disorders were not controlled by medication alone (105).

Thus, one might treat uncomplicated panic disorder (i. e., without agoraphobia) successfully with medication alone (106) as one typically does with epilepsy. Alternatively, according to the above hypothesis, one might add psychotherapy (psychodynamic or behavioral) to decrease background anxiety which, in turn, will decrease panic. The implication for the usefulness of psychotherapy in this presumed subgroup of patients is profound. What is suggested is that sorting out intrapsychic conflict, for example, might render the patient less vulnerable to panic. This might allow medication dosage reduction, perhaps discontinuance, and a lesser incidence of recurrence of panic attacks. Yet this is all quite speculative. The notion of using psychotherapy to reduce relapse after drugs are stopped is interesting and would be very useful but awaits the confirmation of research studies.

Finally, psychodynamic understanding and approaches are necessary for various types of resistance to pharmacological and behavioral treatments (107). Loss of secondary gains from being ill might result in a patient sabotaging a treatment plan that otherwise seems to be going well. Assessment of the family may also be indicated, since the patient's symptom may play a role in maintaining a family's dynamic equilibrium. Family members may even encourage phobic behavior. Moreover, the patient, fearing that he or she may panic if unaccompanied to a therapy session, may cancel if there is no one "available" to escort him or her. Thus family intervention may be needed to allow other more specific modalities to be effective.

REFERENCES

1. Kandel, E. R. (1979). Psychotherapy and the single synapse. *New England Journal of Medicine* 301(19):1028-1037.
2. Kandel, E. R. (1983). From metapsychology to molecular biology: Explorations into the nature of anxiety. *American Journal of Psychiatry* 140(10):1277-1293.
3. Beitman, B. D., Chiles, J., and Carlin, A. (1984). The pharmacotherapy-psychotherapy triangle: Psychiatrist, nonmedical psychotherapist, and patient. *Journal of Clinical Psychiatry* 45(11):458-459.
4. Davis, J. M., Janicak, P., Chang, S., and Klerman, K. (1982). Recent advances in the pharmacologic treatment of schizophrenic disorders. In *Psychiatry 1982 Annual Review*, ed. L. Grinspoon. Washington, DC: American Psychiatric Press.
5. Hogarty, G. E., Schooler, N. R., Ulrich, R., Mussare, F., Ferro, P., and Herron, E. (1979). Fluphenazine and social therapy in the aftercare of schizophrenic patients: Relapse analyses of a two-year controlled study of fluphenazine decanoate and fluphenazine hydrochloride. *Archives of General Psychiatry* 36:1283-1294.
6. Schooler, N. R., Levine, J., Severe, J. B., Brauzer, B., DiMascio, A., Klerman, G. L., and Tuason, V. B. (1980). Prevention of relapse in schizophrenia. An evaluation of fluphenazine decanoate. *Archives of General Psychiatry* 3:16-24.
7. Heinrichs, D. W., and Carpenter, W. T. (1982). The psychotherapy of schizophrenic disorders. In *Psychiatry 1982 Annual Review*, ed. L. Grinspoon. Washington, DC: American Psychiatric Press.
8. Stanton, A. H., Gunderson, J. G., Knapp, P. H., Frank, A. F., Vannicelli, M. L., Schnitzer, R., and Rosenthal, R. (1984). Effects of psychotherapy in schizophrenia: I. Design and implementation of a controlled study. *Schizophrenia Bulletin* 104:520-563.
9. Klein, D. F. (1980). Psychosocial treatment of schizophrenia, or psychosocial help for people with schizophrenia? *Schizophrenia Bulletin* 6(1):122-130.
10. World Health Organization. (1979). *Schizophrenia: An International Follow-up Study*. New York: Wiley.
11. Waxler, N. E. (1979). Is outcome for schizophrenia better in nonindustrial societies? The case of Sri Lanka. *Journal of Nervous and Mental Disease* 167(3):144-158.
12. Warner, R. (1983). Recovery from schizophrenia in the third world. *Psychiatry* 46:197-212.

13. Liberman, R. P. (1982). Social factors in the etiology of the schizophrenic disorders. In *Psychiatry 1982 Annual Review*, ed. L. Grinspoon. Washington, DC: American Psychiatric Press.
14. Spohn, H. E., Coyne, L., Lacoursiere, R., Mazur, D., and Hayes, K. (1985). Relation of neuroleptic dose and tardive dyskinesia to attention, information-processing and psychophysiology in medicated schizophrenics. *Archives of General Psychiatry* 42(9):849–859.
15. Venables, P. H., and Wing, J. F. (1962). Level of arousal and the subclassification of schizophrenia. *Archives of General Psychiatry* 7:114–119.
16. Brown, G. W., Birley, J. L. T., and Wing, J. K. (1972). Influence of family life on the course of schizophrenic disorders: A replication. *British Journal of Psychiatry* 121:241–258.
17. Brown, G. W., and Birley, J. L. T. (1968). Crisis and life changes and the onset of schizophrenia. *Journal of Health and Social Behavior* 9:203–214.
18. Leff, J. P., and Wing, J. K. (1971). Trial of maintenance therapy in schizophrenia. *British Medical Journal* 3:599–604.
19. Leff, J. P., Hirsch, S. R., Gaind, R., Gaind, R., Rolides, P. D., and Stevens, B. S. (1973). Life events and maintenance therapy in schizophrenic relapse. *British Journal of Psychiatry* 123:659–660.
20. Vaughn, C. E., and Leff, J. P. (1976). The influence of family and social factors on the course of psychiatric illness. *British Journal of Psychiatry* 129:125–137.
21. Leff, J. P., and Vaughn, C. E. (1981). The role of maintenance therapy and relative expressed emotion in relapse of schizophrenia: A two-year follow-up. *British Journal of Psychiatry* 139:102–104.
22. Vaughn, C. E., Snyder, K. S., Freeman, W., Jones, S., and Falloon, I. R. H. (1984). Family factors in schizophrenic relapse. Replication in California of British research on expressed emotion. *Archives of General Psychiatry* 41:1169–1177.
23. Moline, R. A., Singh, S., Morris, A., and Meltzer, H. Y. (1985). Family expressed emotion and relapse in schizophrenia in 24 urban American patients. *American Journal of Psychiatry* 142:1078–1081.
24. Howe, C. W. (1985). Role of families: Shaping the system for recovery. Presented at the Annual Meeting of the American Psychiatric Association, Dallas.
25. Kanas, N. (1985). Inpatient and outpatient group therapy for schizophrenic patients. *American Journal of Psychotherapy* 39(3):431–439.
26. Linn, M. W., Klett, C. J., and Caffey, E. M. (1980). Foster home characteristics and psychiatric patient outcome: The wisdom of Gheel confirmed. *Archives of General Psychiatry* 37:129–132.
27. Linn, M. W., Caffey, E. M., Klett, C. J., Hogarty, G. E., and Lamb, H. R. (1979). Day treatment and psychotropic drugs in the aftercare of schizophrenic patients. A Veterans Administration cooperative study. *Archives of General Psychiatry* 36:1055–1066.
28. Greenblatt, M., Solomon, M. H., Evans, A. S., and Brooks, G. W. (1965). *Drug and Social Therapy in Chronic Schizophrenia.* Springfield, IL: Charles C. Thomas.
29. May, R. P. A., Tuma, A. H., and Dixon, W. J. (1981). Schizophrenia: A follow-up study of the results of five forms of treatment. *Archives of General Psychiatry* 38:776–784.

30. Hogarty, G. E., Goldberg, S. C., Schooler, N. R., and Ulrich, R. F. (1974). Drug and sociotherapy in the aftercare of schizophrenic patients. II. Two-year relapse rates. *Archives of General Psychiatry* 31:603-608.
31. Goldberg, S. C., Schooler, N. R., Hogarty, G. E., and Roper, M. (1977). Prediction of relapse in schizophrenic outpatients treated by drug and sociotherapy. *Archives of General Psychiatry* 34:171-184.
32. Wing, J. K., and Brown, G. W. (1970). *Institutionalism and Schizophrenia.* Cambridge, England: Cambridge University Press.
33. Schooler, N. R., and Levine, J. (1983). Strategies for enhancing drug therapy of schizophrenia. *American Journal of Psychotherapy* 37(4):521-532.
34. Linn, M. W., Gurel, L., and Williford, W. O. (1985). Nursing home care as an alternative to psychiatric hospitalization. A Veterans Administration cooperative study. *Archives of General Psychiatry* 42:544-551.
35. Beiser, M., Shore, J. H., Peters, R., and Tatum, E. (1985). Does community care for the mentally ill make a difference? A tale of two cities. *American Journal of Psychiatry* 142:1047-1052.
36. Feinsilver, D. B., and Yates, B. T. (1984). Combined use of psychotherapy and drugs in chronic, treatment-resistant schizophrenic patients: A retrospective study. *Journal of Nervous and Mental Disease* 172(3):133-139.
37. Hogarty, G. E. (1984). Depot neuroleptics: The relevance of psychosocial factors—a United States perspective. *Journal of Clinical Psychiatry* 45(5, Sect. 2):36-42.
38. Hogarty, G. E., Goldberg, S. C., and Schooler, N. R. (1974). Drug and sociotherapy in the aftercare of schizophrenic patients. III. Adjustment of nonrelapsed patients. *Archives of General Psychiatry* 31:609-618.
39. Goldstein, M. J., Rodnich, E. H., Evans, J. R., May, P. R. A., and Steinberg, M. R. (1978). Drug and family therapy in the aftercare of acute schizophrenics. *Archives of General Psychiatry* 35:1169-1177.
40. Leff, J., Kuipers, L., Berkowitz, R., Eberlein-Vries, R., and Sturgeon, D. (1982). A controlled trial of social intervention in the families of schizophrenic patients. *British Journal of Psychiatry* 141:121-134.
41. Falloon, I. R. H., Boyd, J. L., McGill, C. W., Razani, J., Moss, H. B., and Gilderman, A. M. (1982). Family management in the prevention of exacerbations of schizophrenia: A controlled study. *New England Journal of Medicine* 306(24):1437-1440.
42. Falloon, I. R. H., Boyd, J. L., McGill, C. W., Williamson, M., Razani, J., Moss, H. B., and Gilderman, A. M. (1985). Family management in the prevention of morbidity of schizophrenia. Clinical outcome of a two-year longitudinal study. *Archives of General Psychiatry* 42:887-896.
43. Anderson, C. M., Hogarty, G. E., and Reiss, D. J. (1980). Family treatment of adult schizophrenic patients: A psycho-educational approach. *Schizophrenia Bulletin* 6(3):490-505.
44. Hogarty, G. E., Anderson, C. M., Reiss, D. J., Kornblith, S. J., Greenwald, D. P., Javna, C. D., and Madonia, M. J. (1986). Family psycho-education, social skills training, and maintenance chemotherapy in the aftercare treatment of schizophrenia: One year effects of a controlled study on relapse and expressed emotion. *Archives of General Psychiatry* 43:633-642.

References

45. Liberman, R. P., and Evans, C. C. (1985). Behavioral rehabilitation for chronic mental patients. *Journal of Clinical Psychopharmacology* 5(3):15S-21S.
46. Strauss, J. S., and Carpenter, W. T., Jr. (1981). *Schizophrenia.* New York: Plenum.
47. Breier, A., and Strauss, J. S. (1983). Self-control in psychotic disorders. *Archives of General Psychiatry* 40:1141-1145.
48. Kane, J. M., Rifkin, A., Woerner, M., Reardon, G., Sarantakos, S., Schiebel, D., and Ramos-Lorenzi, J. (1983). Low-dose neuroleptic treatment of outpatient schizophrenics. *Archives of General Psychiatry* 40(8):893-896.
49. Kane, J. (1985). Compliance issues in outpatient treatment. *Journal of Clinical Psychopharmacology* 5(3):22S-27S.
50. Marder, S. R., VanPutten, T., Mintz, J., McKenzie, J., Lebell, M., Faltico, G., and May, P. R. A. (1984). Costs and benefits of two doses of fluphenazine. *Archives of General Psychiatry* 41:1025-1029.
51. Teicher, M. H., and Baldessarini, R. J. (1985). Selection of neuroleptic dosage (letter). *Archives of General Psychiatry* 42:636-637.
52. Kane, J. M. (1986). Dosing strategies with long-acting injectable neuroleptics, including haloperidol decanoate. *Journal of Clinical Pharmacology* 6(Suppl.): 20S-23S.
53. Carpenter, W. T., Stephens, J. H., Rey, A. C., Hanlon, T. E., Heinrichs, D. W. (1982). Early intervention versus continuous pharmacotherapy of schizophrenia. *Psychopharmacology Bulletin* 18(21):21-23.
54. Herz, M. I., Szymanski, H. V., and Simon, J. C. (1982). Intermittent medication for stable schizophrenic outpatients: An alternative to maintenance medication. *American Journal of Psychiatry* 139:918-925.
55. Lindberg, D. (1981). Management of schizophrenia. Long-term clinical studies with special references to the combination of psychotherapy with depot neuroleptics. *Acta Psychiatrica Scandinavica (Suppl.)* 289:1-26.
56. Lindberg, D. (1981). Personality changes in chronic schizophrenic patients during five years' treatment with intensive psychotherapy in combination with depot neuroleptics I. Analysis of changes as measured by the Holtzman Inkblot Technique. *Acta Psychiatrica Scandinavica (Suppl.)* 289:27-55.
57. Lindberg, D. (1981). A controlled study of five years' treatment with psychotherapy in combination with depot neuroleptics in schizophrenia II. Personality changes measured by 10 selected Rorschach variables. *Acta Psychiatrica Scandinavica (Suppl.)* 289:56-66.
58. Karon, B. P., and Vanderbos, G. R. (1981). *Psychotherapy of Schizophrenia. The Treatment of Choice.* New York: Jason Aronson.
59. Kovacs, M. (1983). Psychotherapies for depression. In *Psychiatry Update*, ed. L. Grinspoon. Washington, DC: American Psychiatric Press.
60. Covi, L., Lipman, R., Derogatis, L., Smith, V., and Pattison, J. (1974). Drugs and group psychotherapy in neurotic depression. *American Journal of Psychiatry* 131:191-198.
61. Friedman, A. S. (1975). Interaction of drug therapy with marital therapy in depressed patients. *Archives of General Psychiatry* 32:619-637.
62. Rush, A. J. (1984). Cognitive therapy. In *Psychiatry Update*, ed. L. Grinspoon. Washington, DC: American Psychiatric Press.

63. Beck, A. T., Rush, A. J., Shaw, B. F., and Emery, G. (1979). *Cognitive Therapy of Depression.* New York: Guilford Press.
64. Ellis, A., and Grieger, R., eds. (1977). *Handbook of Rational Emotive Therapy and Practice.* New York: Springer.
65. Strupp, H. H., and Blackwood, G. L. (1980). Recent methods of psychotherapy. In *Comprehensive Textbook of Psychiatry/III*, vol. 2, ed. H. I. Kaplan, A. M. Freedman and B. J. Sadock. Baltimore, MD: Williams and Wilkins.
66. Kovacs, M. (1980). The efficacy of cognitive and behavior therapies for depression. *American Journal of Psychiatry* 137:1495–1501.
67. Klerman, G. L., Weissman, M. M., Rounsaville, B., and Chevron, E. S. (1984). Interpersonal psychotherapy for depression. In *Psychiatry Update*, vol. 3, ed. L. Grinspoon. Washington, DC: American Psychiatric Press.
68. Klerman, G. L. (1983). Psychotherapies and somatic therapies in affective disorders. *Psychiatric Clinics of North America* 6(1):85–103.
69. Klerman, G. L. (1984). Research considerations in evaluating combined treatments. In *Combining Psychotherapy and Drug Therapy in Clinical Practice*, ed. B. D. Beitman and G. L. Klerman, pp. 105–119. New York: Spectrum Press.
70. Rush, A. H. (1984). Cognitive therapy in combination with antidepressant medication. In *Combining Psychotherapy and Drug Therapy in Clinical Practice*, ed. B. D. Beitman and G. L. Klerman, pp. 121–147. New York: Spectrum Press.
71. Weissman, M. M., and Klerman, G. L. (1984). Depression: Interpersonal psychotherapy and tricyclics. In *Combining Psychotherapy and Drug Therapy in Clinical Practice*, ed. B. D. Beitman and G. L. Klerman, pp. 149–165. New York: Spectrum Press.
72. Last, C. G., Thase, M. E., Hersen, M., Bellack, A. S., and Himmelhoch, J. M. (1985). Patterns of attrition for psychosocial treatments of depression. *Journal of Clinical Psychiatry* 46(9):361–366.
73. Jamison, K. R., and Goodwin, F. K. (1983). Psychotherapeutic issues in bipolar illness. In *Psychiatry Update*, vol. 2, ed. L. Grinspoon. Washington, DC: American Psychiatric Press.
74. Prien, R. F., Kupfer, D. J., Mansky, P. A., Small, J. G., Tuason, V. B., Voss, C. B., and Johnson, W. E. (1984). Drug therapy in the prevention of recurrences in unipolar and bipolar affective disorders. *Archives of General Psychiatry* 41(11):1096–1104.
75. Akiskal, H. S., Hirschfeld, R. M. A., and Yerevanian, B. I. (1982). The relationship of personality to affective disorders. *Archives of General Psychiatry* 40(7):801–810.
76. Lazare, A., and Klerman, G. (1968). Hysteria and depression: The frequency and significance of hysterical personality features in hospitalized depressed women. *American Journal of Psychiatry* 124:48–56.
77. Akiskal, H. S. (1981). Subaffective disorders: Dysthymic, cyclothymic, and bipolar II disorders in the "borderline" realm. *Psychiatric Clinics of North America* 4:25–46.
78. Zitrin, C. M., Klein, D. F., Woerner, M. G., and Ross, D. C. (1983). Treatment of phobias: Comparison of imipramine hydrochloride and placebo. *Archives of General Psychiatry* 40:125–138.

79. Marks, I. M., Gray, S., and Cohen, D. (1983). Imipramine and brief therapist-aided exposure in agoraphobics having self-exposure homework. *Archives of General Psychiatry* 49(2):153-162.
80. Nemiah, J. C. (1984). The psychodynamic view of anxiety. In *Diagnosis and Treatment of Anxiety Disorders*, ed. R. O. Pasnau. Washington, DC: American Psychiatric Press.
81. Klein, D. F. (1981). Anxiety reconceptualized. In *Anxiety: New Research and Changing Concepts*, ed. D. F. Klein and J. G. Rabkin. New York: Raven Press.
82. Klein, D. F. (1983). Panic attacks in phobia treatment studies (letter, in reply). *Archives of General Psychiatry* 49(10):1151-1152.
83. Freud, S. (1962). Obsessions and phobias (1895a). In *Complete Psychological Works, Standard Edition*, vol. 3. London: Hogarth.
84. Marks, I. M. (1983). Panic attacks in phobia treatment studies (letter, in reply). *Archives of General Psychiatry* 40:1151.
85. Marks, I. M. (1983). Are there anticompulsive or antiphobic drugs? Review of the evidence. *British Journal of Psychiatry* 143:338-347.
86. Sheehan, D. V., Ballenger, J., and Jacobsen, G. (1980). Treatment of endogenous anxiety with phobic, hysterical and hypochondriacal symptoms. *Archives of General Psychiatry* 37:51-59.
87. Zitrin, C. M., Klein, D. F., Woerner, M. G. (1980). Treatment of agoraphobia with group exposure in vivo and imipramine. *Archives of General Psychiatry* 37:63-72.
88. Marks, I. M. (1982). Anxiety disorders. In *Treatment of Mental Disorders*, ed. J. H. Greist, J. W. Jefferson, and R. L. Spitzer. New York: Oxford University Press.
89. Sheehan, D. V., Coleman, J. H., Greenblatt, D. V., Jones, K. J., Levine, P. H., Orsulak, P. J., and Peterson, M. (1984). Some biochemical correlates of panic attacks with agoraphobia and their response to a new treatment. *Journal of Clinical Psychopharmacology* 4:66-75.
90. Marks, I. M. (1985). Behavioral psychotherapy for anxiety disorders. *Psychiatric Clinics of North America* 8(1):25-35.
91. Mavissakalian, M. (1984). Exposure treatment of agoraphobia. In *Psychiatry Update*, vol. 3, ed. L. Grinspoon. Washington, DC: American Psychiatric Press.
92. Freud, S. (1955). Lines of advance in psychoanalytic therapy. In *The Standard Edition of the Psychological Works of Sigmund Freud*, vol. 17, ed. J. Strachey, pp.165-166. London: Hogarth.
93. Klein, D. F., Zitrin, C. M., Woerner, M. G., and Ross, D. C. (1983). Treatment of phobias: Behavior therapy and supportive therapy; are there any specific ingredients. *Archives of General Psychiatry* 40:139-145.
94. Freud, S. (1959). Inhibitions, symptoms and anxiety (1926). In *Complete Psychological Works, Standard Edition*, vol. 20. London: Hogarth.
95. Fontaine, R., and Chouinard, G. (1984). Antipanic effects of clonazepam (letter). *American Journal of Psychiatry* 141(1):149.
96. Beaudry, P., Fontaine, R., and Chouinard, G. (1984). Bromazepam, another high-potency benzodiazepine, for panic attacks (letter). *American Journal of Psychiatry* 141(3):464-465.

97. Kahn, R. J., McNair, D. M., Covi, L., Downing, R. W., Fisher, S., Lipman, R. S., and Rickels, K. (1981). Effects of psychotropic drugs on high-anxiety subjects. *Psychopharmacology Bulletin* 17(3):97–100.
98. Kahn, R. J., McNair, D. M., Lipman, R. S., Covi, L., Rickels, K., Downing, R., and Fisher, S. (1986). Imipramine and chlordiazepoxide in depressive and anxiety disorders II. Efficacy in anxious outpatients. *Archives of General Psychiatry* 43:79–85.
99. Kohut, H. (1984). *How Does Analysis Cure?* Chicago: University of Chicago Press.
100. Sarwer-Foner, G. J. (1982). Psychotherapeutic management of the severely anxious patient. *American Journal of Psychotherapy* 36(3):318–331.
101. Klein, D. F. (1981). Discussion of "the psychoanalytic view of anxiety." In *Anxiety: New Research and Changing Concepts*, ed. D. F. Klein and J. G. Rabkin. New York: Raven Press.
102. Gittleman, R., and Klein, D. F. (1984). Relationship between separation anxiety and panic and agoraphobic disorders. *Psychopathology* 17 (Suppl. 1):56–65.
103. Shader, R. I. (1985). Some observations on the problem of anxiety. In *Anxiety and Anxiety Disorders*, ed. A. H. Tuma and J. Maser, pp. 591–594. Hillsdale, NJ: Erlbaum.
104. Ibid: 592–593.
105. Gottschalk, L. (1953). Effects of intensive psychotherapy on epileptic children. *Archives of Neurology and Psychiatry* 70:361–384.
106. Garakani, M. D., Zitrin, C. M., and Klein, D. F. (1984). Treatment of panic disorder with imipramine alone. *American Journal of Psychiatry* 141:446–448.
107. Hanrahan, M., Gitlin, B., Martin, J., Leavy, A., and Frances, A. (1984). Behavior therapy of anxiety disorders: Motivating the resistant patient. *American Journal of Psychotherapy* 38(4):533–540.

15

Rational Use of Serum Drug Concentration Monitoring

H. Friedman, M.D.
D. J. Greenblatt, M.D.

How often in the daily practice of medicine do clinicians order a serum drug level determination on a patient thought to be doing well, only to find that the serum concentration is in a potentially toxic range? Or conversely, the drug is not detectable in serum. Such discrepancies between measured serum drug concentrations and observed clinical drug effect may occur for numerous reasons. This chapter reviews some aspects of therapeutic drug monitoring that should help clinicians maximize the likelihood of obtaining useful information from serum concentrations of drugs.

RATIONALE FOR MONITORING SERUM DRUG LEVELS

For monitoring of a drug's serum or plasma concentration to be useful for purposes of therapeutic monitoring, at least two requisites must be fulfilled (1,2). First, serum-free drug level must reflect the concentration of the drug at the receptor site; second, the intensity and duration of the pharmacodynamic effect must be temporally correlated with the receptor-site drug concentration. Common reasons for monitoring serum drug levels include: treatment with drugs having a narrow therapeutic margin or range (Figure 15-1); population variations that may alter clinical response (e. g., aging, prematurity, diseases, race, obesity); lack of desired therapeutic effect; toxic effects; to rule out noncompliance; to rule out pharmacokinetic drug interactions; medico-legal reasons (e. g., suicidal or accidental overdose, and employee screening) (3,4). Classes of drugs often monitored include antibiotics, antiarrhythmics, cardiac glycosides, lithium, anticonvulsants, salicylates, theophylline, neuroleptics, and antidepressants.

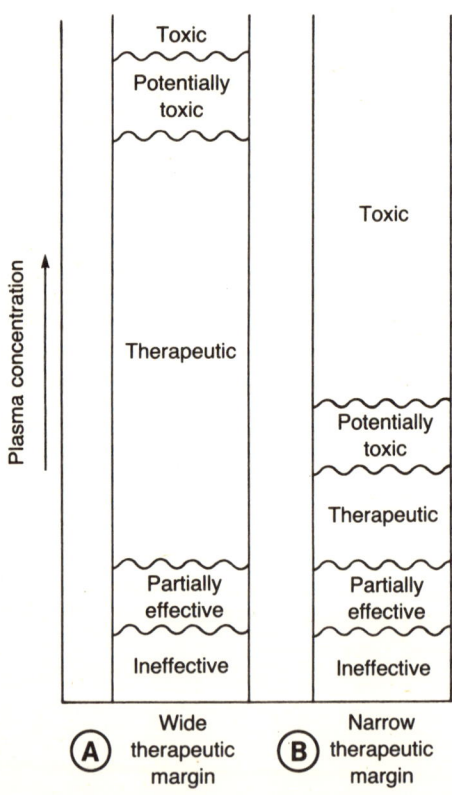

FIGURE 15-1. Schematic relation of serum or plasma drug concentration to clinical efficacy or toxicity for hypothetical drugs having wide (A) or narrow (B) therapeutic ranges. Reprinted from (1), with permission.

DRUG DISTRIBUTION AND ACCESS TO ITS RECEPTOR

When a drug is given by an extravascular route of administration (orally, intramuscular injection, rectally, subcutaneously, etc.), or even by intravenous (I.V.) injection, the entire administered dose does not have immediate and complete access to its receptor site mediating pharmacological activity. After I.V. injection, the entire dose reaches the systemic circulation and, by definition, has 100% bioavailability. However, the drug is distributed not only to the tissue where it is active, but also to a number of other sites (Figure 15-2). Furthermore, once the drug has reached the systemic circulation, it also encounters the plasma proteins. Drugs are bound to plasma proteins to varying degrees (5). The principal binding proteins are albumin and alpha-1 acid glycoprotein. The affinity of a drug for plasma protein limits its freedom to diffuse across cell membranes, hence, further limiting its accessibility to the receptor site.

When a drug is administered by an extravascular route, it reaches the systemic circulation indirectly, often yielding less than 100% bioavailability (6). Oral bioavailability of drugs in tablet and capsule form can be influenced by incomplete absorption due to incomplete dissolution, which in turn depends on packaging and drug particle size. Oral solutions overcome the dissolution problem. Other factors that can influence oral bioavailability include changes in gastrointestinal motility, malabsorption syndromes, and the coad-

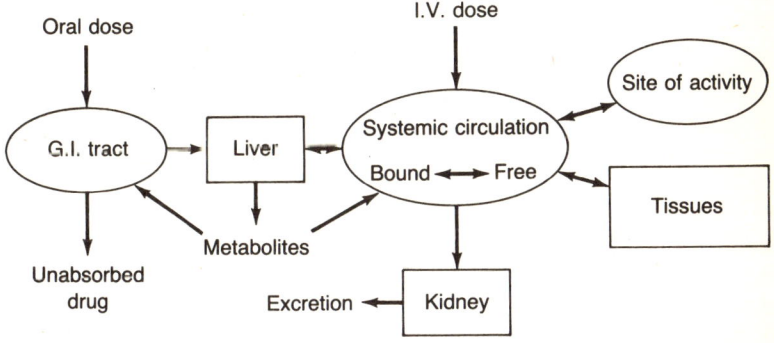

FIGURE 15-2. Schematic representation of pathways of drug distribution and elimination following I.V. or oral administration.

ministration of foods and drugs (especially antacids and chelating agents). In some cases of complete absorption from the gastrointestinal tract, systemic bioavailability is significantly reduced because of extraction from the portal circulation during the first pass through the liver. This is the case with propranolol, lidocaine, tricyclic antidepressants, opiate analgesics, neuroleptics, hydralazine, nitroglycerin, verapamil, and prednisone (7). Reduced bioavailability following intramuscular injection has been attributed to poor drug solubility at physiological pH and/or precipitation at the injection site following administration of chlordiazepoxide, digoxin, phenylbutazone, phenytoin, and quinidine (8).

For all these reasons, drug concentrations in blood, serum or plasma often reflect pharmacological action more closely than administered dosage alone.

FACTORS INFLUENCING INTERPRETATION OF SERUM DRUG CONCENTRATIONS

Total versus Free Serum Concentrations

Although only the unbound or free drug can passively cross cell membranes and leave the circulation to interact with receptors, free drug levels nonetheless are still not routinely monitored. This is partly because their measurement is technically more difficult to perform than that of total levels. Furthermore, for most drugs, the ratio of free to total concentration (free fraction) usually remains constant during a patient's course of therapy. Hence, for most drugs a doubling of the dosing rate will lead to a doubling of both the total and the free serum drug concentrations at steady state. In most clinical situations, interpatient variation in the extent of protein binding of a given drug may be relatively small (9). In some cases, however, protein binding may change substantially, leading to alterations in the therapeutic and toxic ranges for *total* drug concentrations (10,11).

Protein binding of drugs may vary when other drugs present in serum displace them from their binding sites (11). These increased "free" drug concentrations will be transient, however, because the free drug will quickly equilibrate with the tissues, whereas the total concentration will fall. Consequently, a low total serum drug level could be associated with a therapeutic or even a toxic response. In uremia and hypoalbuminemia, drugs may also show reduced binding to albumin. Alternately, alpha-1 acid glycoprotein, an acute-phase reactant, may be transiently elevated in acute inflammatory states (12), causing *increased* binding of some basic drugs and result in increased total serum drug levels without an enhancement of clinical effect. Examples of such drugs include lidocaine, propranolol, imipramine, phenytoin, quinidine, and disopyramide. For drugs with low protein binding, such as cimetidine, digoxin, gentamicin, lithium, procainamide and *N*-acetyl procainamide, changes in protein binding are of far less consequence.

Optimal Sample Timing

Proper choice of sampling time is crucial for the interpretation of serum drug concentrations. In general, it takes four times the drug's half-life at a constant dosing rate for the steady-state condition to be more than 90% attained. Similarly, a reduction in dosage will require the same interval to reach the new steady-state level (Figure 15-3). For example, a drug with a half-life of 3 days will take six times longer to reach steady state than a drug with a half-life of 12 hours (Figure 15-4). Therefore premature sampling, prior to the attainment of the actual steady-state condition, may lead to inappropriate dosage adjustments. Occasionally, the need may arise to

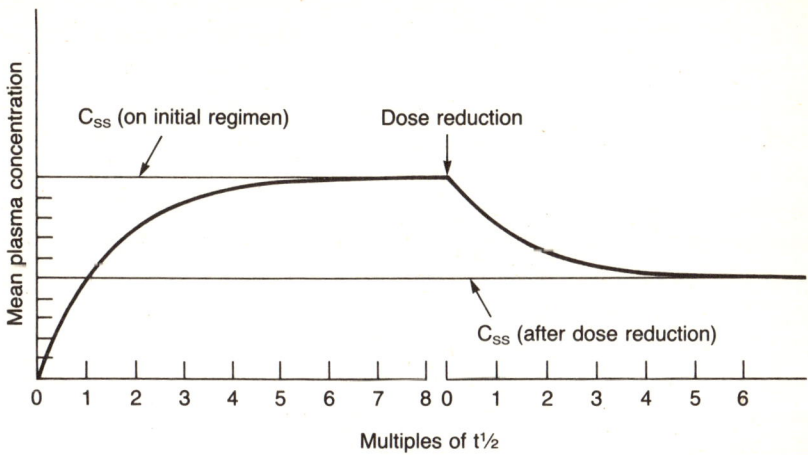

FIGURE 15-3. Time course (in multiples of half-life, $t^{1/2}$) of the mean steady-state serum or plasma drug concentration (Css) during the attainment of steady-state when starting therapy and after reducing the dosage. Reprinted from (1), with permission.

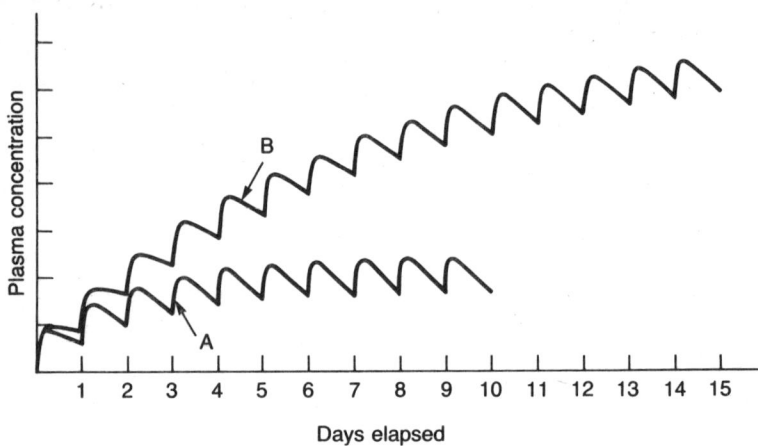

FIGURE 15-4. Time course of the attainment of steady state, assuming drug is given once daily. Case A: drug with short half-life; Case B: drug with a long half-life. Reprinted from (1), with permission.

hasten the attainment of steady state. This can be achieved by giving an initial loading dose (13). However, loading doses also have potential disadvantages, since the rapid attainment of steady state precludes gradual adaptation to drug effects. This is of particular importance for centrally active drugs.

Once steady state has been achieved, the mean serum drug level will be relatively constant. However, the interdose fluctuation depends on the dosage interval and the drug formulation. Sustained release drug formulations are designed to release medication into the systemic circulation at a slow rate. If the rate of drug entry into the systemic circulation precisely mimics a fixed-rate infusion, then the serum drug level will not fluctuate. Although this is an unachievable ideal, some sustained release preparations do in fact allow infrequent dosing with only small fluctuations in serum drug concentrations (14–16).

Usually a drug is absorbed from the intestine during an "absorptive" phase, which is associated with peak serum levels above the mean. The drug then distributes throughout the body and is associated with a fall below the mean into the "trough" phase. The optimal time to sample is just prior to the time of dosing (Figure 15-5). In this way one can ensure that the minimum drug level falls within the therapeutic range. If the trough level is found to be subtherapeutic, the clinician may elect to give smaller doses more frequently while maintaining the same total dose per 24 hours (Figure 15-6). This

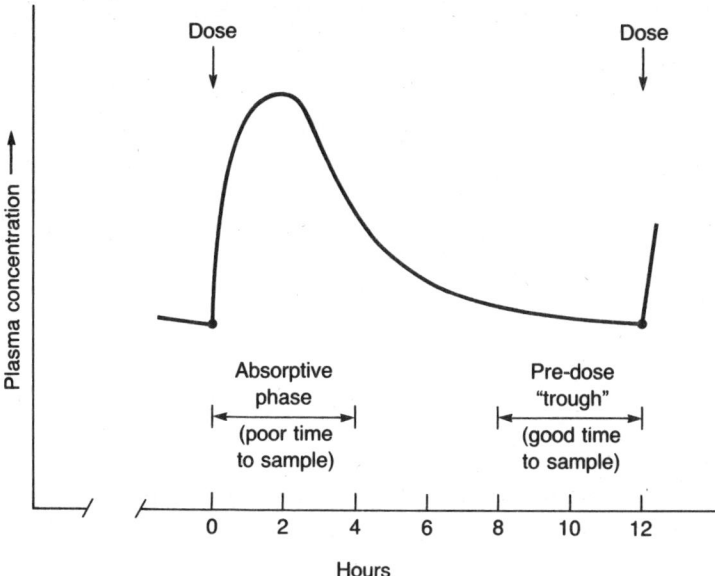

FIGURE 15-5. Time course of plasma drug concentration at steady state during oral dosage every 12 hours, with illustration of optimal sampling time. Reprinted from (1), with permission.

change would reduce the interdose fluctuation and possibly bring the trough level to within the therapeutic range. More frequent dosing is also useful to minimize transient effects due to high peak levels that some people find objectionable, such as sedation and drowsiness from certain psychotropic drugs. On the other hand, dosing schedules that require very frequent dosing are inconvenient, and may be associated with reduced patient compliance.

If the dosage interval is not regular, or if the drug is taken intermittently, then the best time to sample is not necessarily so obvious, since there is no single "trough" concentration (Figure 15-7).

Differences among Collection Tubes

When the blood sample is drawn, it must be into the appropriate type of tube. Vacutainer brand blood collection tubes contain tris (2-butoxyethyl) phosphate (TBEP), a plasticizing agent. Blood samples drawn into these tubes can give spuriously low serum drug levels when the serum is analyzed for imipramine, alprenolol, propranolol, lidocaine, and quinidine (12). The mechanism for the lowering of serum blood levels appears to involve displacement of drugs from alpha-l acid glycoprotein by TBEP (but not from albumin). This in vitro phenomenon results in an increase in unbound drug, which quickly diffuses into and equilibrates with the red blood cells present in the tube. Thus, when the serum is aspirated following centrifugation, the resultant serum drug level is spuriously low. However, the whole blood level is unchanged. Any drug that is extensively bound to alpha-l acid glycoprotein is likely to be influenced by this collection artifact.

Analytical Methodology

Knowledge of the methodology used by a laboratory in analyzing serum for drug levels may be of critical importance for the clinician in interpreting the results. The ideal assay for a particular drug should be able to (a) distinguish among compounds of similar structure, such as the parent drug and its metabolic products or other

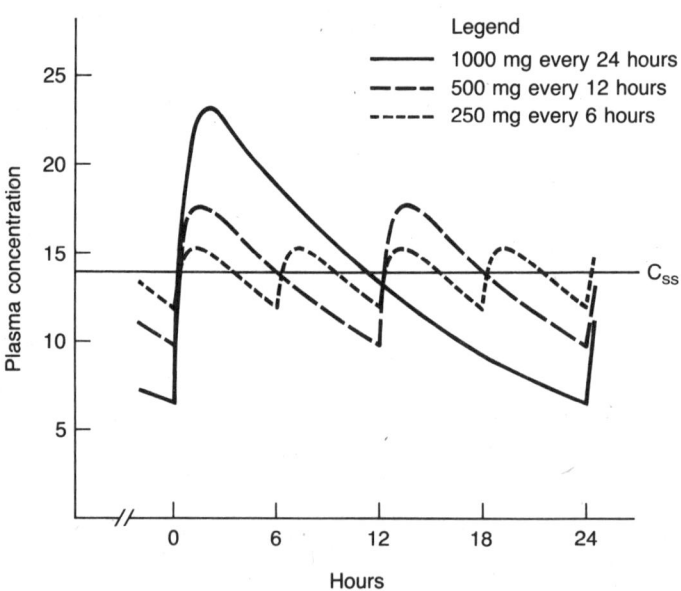

FIGURE 15-6. Interdose fluctuation of plasma drug concentration as function of dosage schedule, assuming that drug is given in overall total dosage of 1.0 g per 24 hours, but with different dosing schedules. Note that Css is the same for each regimen, and that interdose fluctuation is largest for the once-a-day therapy. Reprinted from (1), with permission.

Factors Influencing Interpretation of Serum Drug Concentrations

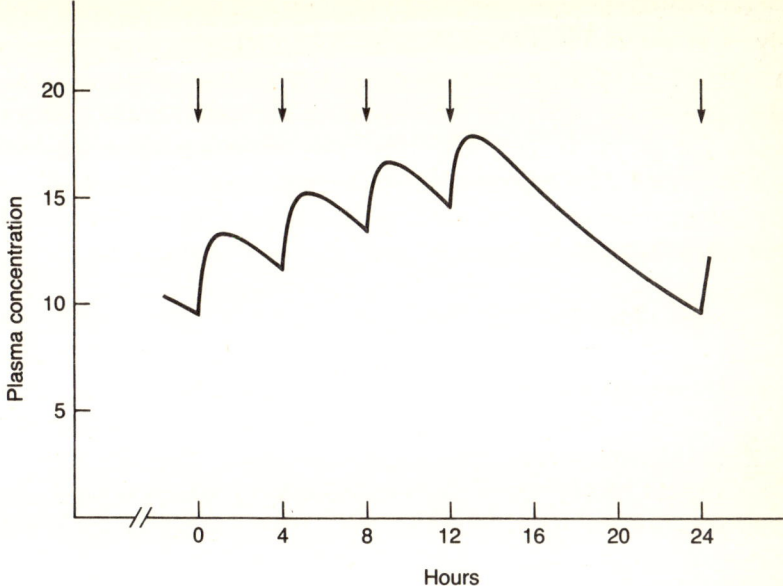

FIGURE 15-7. Plasma concentrations of a drug at steady state with a q.i.d. dosing schedule, with individual doses given at the times shown by the arrows. This complex dosage schedule makes monitoring of plasma drug levels more difficult. Reprinted from (1), with permission.

substances present in the serum (specificity); (b) reliably quantitate blood levels within the therapeutic range (sensitivity and reliability); and (c) be as simple to perform as possible.

Historically, spectrophotometry and colorimetry were the first methods widely used in laboratories for measurement of drug levels. These procedures require multiple solvent extractions, often coupled with chemical reactions, to provide a solution with a hopefully pure drug. The absorption of visible, infrared or ultraviolet light at a specific wavelength by the drug in solution is used to quantitate its presence. The level of sensitivity provided is usually on the order of parts per million to parts per thousand. These methods suffer from poor sensitivity and variable specificity (17).

Immunoassays for drugs have become popular within the last 20 years (18). In principle, they rely on the interaction between a drug acting as an antigen and an antibody to it. Since most drugs are nonimmunogenic, they first must be conjugated by a bridge or linkage group to a substance of high molecular weight such as a protein.

In this conjugated mode, the drug behaves like a hapten and is used to immunize an animal. Antibodies may be generated against the drug if the conjugation bridge or linkage keeps the drug sufficiently far from the larger protein molecule. The necessity for an antibody to seek out a hapten creates the inherent variability in specificity provided by immunoassays. Some antibodies may show cross-reactivity with metabolites and congeners of the drug of interest, thereby rendering the antibodies relatively nonspecific (3,4,19,20). Sensitivity on the order of parts per billion have been claimed for immunoassays.

Chromatography is a method of separating mixtures of diverse or related substances by their physiochemical characteristics so that one or more of those substances may be detected. The main methods used in drug measurement are gas-liquid chromatography (GLC) (21) and high-pressure liquid chromatography (HPLC) (22). The substances to be measured are extracted from serum (e.g., 1.0 ml), concentrated into a small volume (e.g., 0.050 ml) and injected into a column in a mobile phase: gas for GLC and a solution for HPLC. Separation of the components of the mobile phase is affected by interactions with the column's stationary phase. Actual separations are based on lipophilicity, polarity, molecular size, and boiling point (for GLC). High-pressure liquid chromatography separations may be further refined by varying the pH and polarity of the mobile phase.

Often it is possible to detect and quantitate the parent drug and some or all of its important metabolites simultaneously. In some applications, a mass spectrometer is coupled to a chromatograph's effluent and thereby acts as the detector. This combination provides the "gold standard" in specificity and sensitivity in drug analysis. When the drug mixture is well separated by the chromatograph, other less complex detection systems usually suffice. Sensitivity of GLC varies from parts per million to subparts per billion depending on the detection system used. In favorable cases, HPLC can extend sensitivity two orders of magnitude beyond the spectrophotometric range (i. e., subparts per million).

Interpretation of the Serum Drug Level

One should consider what the lab report means. Consider a request for a serum imipramine level on a patient who is on long-term therapy. Assuming the blood was drawn into an appropriate tube at an appropriate time, what does a "good" lab report back?

In the metabolism of imipramine (IMI), it is demethylated to desmethylimipramine (DMI), which itself is pharmacologically active. Therefore, it would be reasonable to measure DMI along with IMI. However, since not all analytical methods are capable of identifying the two distinct compounds, one or the other or a combination thereof may end up being reported. In a few years this problem may become further complicated by the appreciation of other active metabolites of IMI such as hydroxy-IMI and hydroxy-DMI (23).

Finally, using a laboratory with readily available information about its precision and accuracy for drug assays is crucial. After all, what good is a drug level determination if it does not reflect the actual concentration in serum as opposed to the actual plus various nonactive assay-interfering substances (19,20) (Figure 15-8)? Similarly, without knowledge of the minimal detectable level from a lab, a

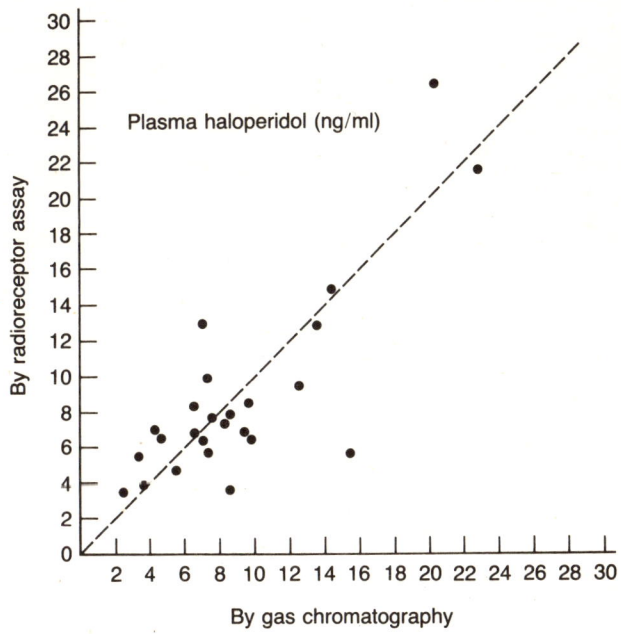

FIGURE 15-8. Comparison of plasma haloperidol concentrations measured by a nonspecific radioreceptor assay (RRA), compared with a specific gas chromatographic technique (24). Dashed line is the line of identity. This indicates that the RRA may be inaccurate and nonspecific.

reported zero may not be the same thing if the laboratory method is not sensitive enough to detect subtherapeutic levels.

The simple act of ordering a serum drug level presupposes its clinical applicability. When one considers such diverse factors as the sample's timing, the patient's clinical state, the drug's pharmacokinetics and metabolism, and the tube type and analytical methodology used, the likelihood of obtaining clinically meaningful and useful results can be maximized (25).

REFERENCES

1. Greenblatt, D. J., and Shader, R. I. (1985). *Pharmacokinetics in Clinical Practice.* Philadelphia: W. B. Saunders.
2. Koch-Weser, J. (1972). Serum drug concentrations as therapeutic guides. *New England Journal of Medicine* 287:227-231.
3. Morgan, J. P. (1984). Problems of mass urine screening for misused drugs. *Journal of Psychoactive Drugs* 16:305-317.
4. Divoll, M. K., and Greenblatt, D. J. (1985). The admissability of positive EMIT results as scientific evidence: Counting facts, not heads. *Journal of Clinical Pharmacology* 5:114-116.
5. Jusko, W. J., and Gretch, M. (1976). Plasma and tissue protein binding of drugs in pharmacokinetics. *Drug Metabolism Reviews* 5:43-140.
6. Greenblatt, D. J., Smith, T. W., and Koch-Weser, J. (1976). Bioavailability of drugs: the digoxin dilemma. *Clinical Pharmacokinetics* 1:36-51.
7. Blaschke, T. F., and Rubin, P. C. (1979). Hepatic first-pass metabolism in liver disease. *Clinical Pharmacokinetics* 4:423-432.
8. Greenblatt, D. J., and Koch-Weser, J. (1976). Intramuscular injection of drugs. *New England Journal of Medicine* 295:542-546.
9. Levy, R. H., and Moreland, T. A. (1984). Rationale for monitoring free drug levels. *Clinical Pharmacokinetics* (Suppl. 1):1-9.
10. Greenblatt, D. J., Sellers, E. M., and Koch-Weser, J. (1982). Importance of protein binding for the interpretation of serum or plasma drug concentration. *Journal of Clinical Pharmacology* 22:259-263.
11. Koch-Weser, J., and Sellers, E. M. (1976). Binding of drugs to serum albumin. *New England Journal of Medicine* 294:311-316, 526-531.
12. Piafsky, K. M. (1980). Disease-induced changes in the plasma binding of basic drugs. *Clinical Pharmacokinetics* 5:246-262.
13. Wilder, B. J., Serrani, E. E., and Ramsay, R. E. (1973). Plasma diphenylhydantoin levels after loading and maintenance doses. *Clinical Pharmacology and Therapeutics* 14:797-801.
14. Kelly, H. W., and Murphy, S. (1980). Efficacy of a 12-hour sustained release

preparation in maintaining therapeutic serum theophylline levels in asthmatic children. *Pediatrics* 66:97–102.
15. Locniskar, A., Greenblatt, D. J., Zinny, M. A., Harmatz, J. S., and Shader, R. I. (1984). Absolute bioavailability and effect of food and antacid on diazepam absorption from a slow release preparation. *Journal of Clinical Pharmacology* 24:255–263.
16. Ochs, H. R., Greenblatt, D. J., Woo, E., Franke, K., Pfeifer, H. J., and Smith, T. W. (1978). Single- and multiple-dose pharmacokinetics of oral quinidine sulfate and gluconate. *American Journal of Cardiology* 41:770–777.
17. Thienes, C. H., and Haley, T. J. (1964). *Clinical Toxicity*, 4th ed. Philadelphia: Lea and Febiger.
18. Marks, V. (1981). Immunoassays for drugs. In *Therapeutic Drug Monitoring*, ed. A. Richens and V. Marks. London: Churchill Livingstone.
19. Blyden, G. T., Franklin, C., Cho, S. I., Kaplan, M. M., Hirsch, C. A., and Greenblatt, D. J. (in press). Cyclosporin-A blood concentrations determined by specific versus nonspecific assay methods. *Journal of Clinical Pharmacology*.
20. Ko, G. N., Korpi, E. R., Linnoila, M. (1985). On the clinical relevance and methods of quantification of plasma concentrations of neuroleptics. *Journal of Clinical Pharmacology* 5:253–262.
21. Sherma, J. (1972). Gas chromatography. In *Handbook of Chromatography*, vol. 2, ed. G. Zweig and J. Sherman. Cleveland, OH: CRC Press.
22. Kabra, P. M., and Morton, L. J., ed. (1981). *Liquid Chromatography in Clinical Analysis*. Clifton, NJ: Humana Press.
23. Potter, W. Z., Calil, H. M., Manian, A. A., Zavadil, A. P., and Goodwin, F. K. (1979). Hydroxylated metabolites of tricyclic antidepressants: Preclinical assessment of activity. *Biological Psychiatry* 14:6–1613.
24. Smith, R. C., Baumgartner, R., Misra, C. H., Mauldin, M., Shvartsburd, A., Ho, B. T., and DeJohn, C. (1984). Haloperidol. *Archives of General Psychiatry* 41:1044–1049.
25. Friedman, H., and Greenblatt, D. J. (1986). Rational therapeutic drug monitoring. *Journal of the American Medical Association* 256:2227–2233.

16

Liability Issues and Malpractice Prevention

Thomas G. Gutheil, M.D.

Few terms strike more terror in the clinician than "malpractice." It is cold comfort that all types of citizens are taking to the courts in unprecedented numbers to settle disputes that formerly called for other means of resolution; rather, the imputations of incompetence, clinical and even personal inadequacy, and outright malfeasance remain intensely traumatizing aspects of the allegation of malpractice.

Psychiatry as a profession can take ambiguous pride in the fact that it remains one of the least-sued medical specialties; we like to think that this has something to do with the centrality of the alliance with the patient in our work. Be this as it may, the numbers of psychiatrists being sued is still increasing, in tardy emulation of the other specialties.

For the psychopharmacologist (by which generic term I shall refer from here on to all psychiatrists who prescribe medications as a part of their practice), the issue is complicated by the fact that medication use appears to offer a conceptual concreteness reassuring to the attorney who is attempting to get a case clearly in mind. No matter how rich the growth of theories of psychotherapy, that field remains amorphous, cloudy, rent by faction and schism, and altogether unsatisfactory for the attorney seeking hard, unambiguous, expensive facts with which to proceed. The consequence is greater vulnerability for the psychopharmacologist to allegation of liability.

This chapter is designed to familiarize the clinician with issues of liability and malpractice peculiar to psychopharmacology and to offer guidelines aimed at reducing liability. While anyone can be sued for anything, and while absolute malpractice prevention is a fantasy, these guidelines may yet stack the deck in favor of suit prevention in the first place, or in favor of a good outcome should litigation ensue. I draw not only on theoretical understanding based on review of case–law and on empirical research in liability assignment, but on practical experience gained from serving as an expert witness in malpractice cases in nine states and as a forensic consultant to clinicians and attorneys concerned about liability.

FUNDAMENTALS OF MALPRACTICE

While this topic is extensively addressed elsewhere (1), a brief review of this central concept may here be in order. Malpractice exists in a given situation when four elements are present and proven; these elements are conveniently recalled through the mnemonic of the "four Ds": Dereliction of a Duty Directly causing Damages. Each of these will be considered in relation to psychopharmacology.

Dereliction refers to negligence in practice, representing dereliction from a particular standard: The standard of care. The standard of care is defined in different ways in different jurisdictions, but it usually falls along three major lines: the community or locality standard (what the average clinician in that community would do under the same circumstances); the "average prudent practitioner" standard (self-explanatory); and the standard of whether a risk–benefit assessment was performed in relation to the procedure, regimen, or medication in question. Note that, because of national publications, meetings (and textbooks like this one!), the community with which the clinician is effectively being compared is a national one. Note also that the "prudence" noted above is retrospectively assessed, inevitably, by hindsight: The damage is already done by the time the case gets to court.

The duty in question is usually quite straightforward—the actual doctor–patient relationship—since the prescriber defines the duty by the act of prescription for that patient. Recall, however, that even the offer of help creates a duty, a point that may be relevant in some various situations. That is, when the clinician is even in the process of evaluating or consulting directly on a patient, sees a patient in an emergency room, gives treatment advice over the phone, or otherwise offers help (regardless of whether a decision has been made to embark on a treatment regimen or longer therapeutic relationship), he or she is viewed as having assumed the "duty" here described.

Direct causation (also known as proximate cause) is the third element that must be proved: The plaintiff-patient must demonstrate that the harm he or she suffered flowed directly from the negligence. A "but-for" test is commonly invoked: "But for" that negligence, the damage would not have occurred.

Finally, actual (in some jurisdictions, physical) damages or harms must be present for malpractice to exist. To grasp this point, consider this hypothetical vignette:

> A physician whose license has expired, while drunk, prescribes over the phone the wrong medication for a patient whom he has never seen and whose condition he misdiagnoses. Is that malpractice? The answer is no, because—though there is negligence aplenty—no statement of damages is given. Appalling as the example may seem, if nothing happens, it is not malpractice.

It should be clear from the foregoing that the questions of dereliction (negligence) and damages will be paramount in psychopharmacology. Direct causation will at times be an issue, while duty will almost always be a given in most clinical situations. The duty of consultants constitutes a special case and will be separately addressed.

IMPORTANT LIABILITY ISSUES IN PSYCHOPHARMACOLOGY

While a listing here cannot presume to be exhaustive, this section addresses the most salient and frequent risk issues in psychopharmacology.

Informed Consent and Special Issues

Elements of Informed Consent. Informed consent consists of three elements: information, voluntariness, and competence, each of which will be separately addressed. The relevance for our present theme is this: Absence of simple consent coupled with an unconsented touching is a battery; absence of informed consent is malpractice, since informed consent is now considered to be a part of the standard of care for medical practitioners.

A major pitfall in informed consent is stated by Blackwell (2): "Too often the prescription signals the end of an interview rather than the start of an alliance" (p. 252). This remark captures the notion held by some clinicians that informed consent is a legalistic ceremony occurring only once when a patient signs a form, and then is over with forever. To be at all meaningful, not only as a clinically important procedure but as a defense against the allegation of malpractice, informed consent must be seen as a dialogue—what I have called elsewhere (3) the "prescribing alliance"—that persists for the duration of the medication regimen.

A pivotal conceptualization related to this is that of the "experiment with an 'n' of one." When a patient tries a medication for the first time, the uncertainty is great and the future, unknown. An important feature of the prescribing alliance that must be formed at the outset is evoking in the patient a sense of facing this uncertainty together with the physician (4). The physician might say something like: "You've never tried this medication before, and it isn't written down anywhere that it is sure to work—I certainly wish it were guaranteed—but we'll be seeing if it helps you and monitoring it together. Your job is to tell me what it feels like and how it is working, and I will be following the effects together with you."

Such a conversation clarifies the uncertainties as inevitable but not unmanageable, and conveys that the clinician will "be there for the patient" during this uncertain time.

The language also serves to disabuse the patient of the ultimately destructive notion that results are guaranteed, an extremely common, often unconscious, fantasy that patients bring to encounters with physicians of all specialties (4). Rather than weakening the authoritative posture of the physician, however, this gentle, alliance-based confrontation with the realities of uncertainty strengthens the patient's collaborative working tie to the physician, thus diminishing the patient's feeling of a betrayed promise of certainty, a promise that not uncommonly leads to litigation as an expression of this frustration.

Information. The element of information always raises the question, how much information is appropriate? Some general guidelines can be given here. First, reading the entire *Physician's Desk Reference* to the patient is not required. The core information that should be conveyed is the risks and benefits of the proposed treatment, the risks and benefits of alternative treatments, and the risks and benefits of no treatment at all.

In discussing risks, the major risks should be described, using the following scale as a guide: The greater the seriousness of the risk or the greater its likelihood of occurrence, the more it should be covered by the clinician's discussion. By this formula, tardive dyskinesia for neuroleptics (discussed more fully later in this chapter) and dry mouth for tricyclics should be highlighted.

The data base in question should be individualized for the particular patient. Somatizing or body-conscious patients require special attention to physical symptoms; patients narcissistically invested in mental functioning require attention to any dulling of clarity of thought.

The single most important point here, however, is not selecting an ideal data base to share with the patient. Rather, it is creating a climate that invites and welcomes the patient's inquiries and active participation on an ongoing basis. The clinician attempts to open a door to the patient's doubts, fears, concerns about whether the new symptom is, indeed, a side effect, and so on. This atmosphere of availability is a potent malpractice preventer in its own right.

Voluntariness. The issue stemming from this element of informed consent is simply that consent is not consent when the response is coerced. To tell patients that if they do not take the medication you will not give them their pants back or fill out their welfare forms is clearly to create a climate low in voluntariness.

There are two common situations where voluntariness does not apply. The first is emergencies, which do not require consent, informed or otherwise; if a patient becomes violent on an inpatient ward, immediate intervention, perhaps including medication given intramuscularly, may be required. Almost without exception, courts recognize the validity of documented emergencies as exceptions to the consent requirement.

The second situation is when the patient is not competent to consent; hence, any consent is not truly voluntary. This topic is addressed in the next section.

Implicit in the above discussion is the question of the right to refuse treatment, an important and highly current medicolegal topic, which would require a chapter in itself. Fortunately, I have written one, and the reader is referred thereto (5).

Competence: A Threshold Issue. When, as earlier noted, the information about risks and benefits relating to proposed treatment are shared with the patient, the patient must be capable of weighing them as an aid to autonomous decision-making. This capacity to weigh the elements of a decision corresponds to competence to make that decision. Only competent consent is valid consent.

An immediate paradox must strike the psychopharmacologist: Many of the medications used in the field are aimed at restoring a competence that has been impaired or abrogated by the very mental illness for which the medicines are the treatment of choice. Despite this point, many patients, though mentally ill, are competent in this area, partly because of their familiarity with the medications from past usage. Those patients who are incompetent require an alternative approach, outlined below.

What makes the assessment of competence difficult is the fact that there is no universally accepted standard or criterion for competence to consent to medications; "the capacity to weigh the relevant risks and benefits" comes closest to serving as a general measure. Some useful references on this complex topic are supplied in the readings at the end of this chapter (see particularly 1, 6, and 7).

If the clinician believes or determines that the patient is incompetent to engage in decision-making because of illness, organic impairment, youth or other reason, a substitute decision-maker must be sought. Note that the clinician's view of the patient's incompetence is only an opinion. The clinician bears the affirmative burden of seeing to it that the matter is brought before the relevant court for judicial ratification; preferably, the patient's family or, alternatively, the hospital's attorney may undertake this task.

What happens next depends somewhat on the jurisdiction. A judge may make decisions for the patient, a guardian may be appointed (family member, attorney, or other person), or other alternatives may be invoked.

The clinician then carries on the informed consent discussion with that substitute decision-maker thus defined. Note that simply asking family members for approval does not replace this formal substitute consent process, although family approval, insofar as it leads them to a greater sense of participation, is often clinically helpful in emergency interventions.

Consent Forms vs. Progress Notes. Attorneys in general and many clinicians have an almost magical view of consent forms. By serving as a written document, such consent forms satisfy the legal system's hunger for signed papers. In reality, however, the complete consent form is too long or incomprehensible to the average patient, and the clear and simple form is often incomplete.

Even worse, forms are not all that helpful in court, since a patient may say, quite truthfully in many cases, "The doctor said I had to sign that before he could treat me, so I did. I don't really recall what it's all about." Use of these forms may also lull the clinician into believing erroneously (a) that incontestable informed consent has been obtained because the patient signed the paper or (b) that the informed consent process is now finished, never again to intrude on the doctor-patient relationship.

As an alternative approach yielding not only more clinically sound consent but some measure of liability protection as well, the author recommends a two-pronged procedure: the "standard discussion" and the progress note.

The "standard discussion" represents a paragraph developed from what the clinician would usually tell the patient about each of the major categories of medications: tricyclics, phenothiazines, benzodiazepines, and so forth. The clinician should routinely review this paragraph (consisting of risks, benefits, side effects to watch for, etc.) with each patient beginning a medication. In addition, the clinician should add material particular to the patient in question, for example, cautions about operating heavy machinery if the patient does that for a living. The clinician then writes a progress note in the patient's record that this discussion has taken place, with the additions specific to that patient as noted above. It is not necessary that the patient sign this note, or anything else.

Even years later on the witness stand, the clinician, asked what he or she told the patient, can reply, "I always give these instructions and information so I assume that I did then; I see by my notes that I also added cautions x, y, and z." This response is fully adequate to document an informed consent; a physician is not expected to recall every word of a conversation, and the burden lies on the plaintiff to prove that the procedure did not occur (8).

Attorneys for some hospitals may insist on written consent forms for all procedures; if this is the case in your hospital, follow that advice, of course. For the private practitioner, the approach outlined above provides ample protection with no great expenditure of time.

Misdiagnosis

Having explored the basic subject of informed consent and its related components, we turn now to common liability issues particular to psychopharmacology. The first on the list is misdiagnosis.

This topic of liability does not mean what it may appear to mean: that, say, manic-depressive illness was mistaken for schizoaffective illness. Such delicate clinical distinctions are not the stuff of lawsuits (1). What is at stake here is the allegation that the clinician "missed" a diagnosis. Examples of such missed diagnoses include the presence of suicidality, the development of a subtle but damaging side effect, or the existence of an unsuspected underlying medical condition that may have caused some of the presenting symptoms. Careful clinical work, close patient monitoring, ready use of general medical consultation, and maintenance of a high index of suspicion are the preventatives here.

Inadequate Treatment

The allegation here is that the clinician failed to treat, insufficiently treated, or inappropriately treated the condition (presumably, correctly diagnosed) for which the patient presented—again, as measured by the standard of care (see above). A miscellany of examples is included under this rubric, including cessation of treatment before the desired result was obtained; treatment at subclinical or ineffective dosages; failure to use a treatment considered definitive; and failure to try new regimens when the original one failed to show signs of working.

Side Effects and Bad Reactions

These phenomena probably represent the most distressing experiences for clinicians and patients alike: for the clinician, because, while attempting to decrease suffering, he or she is the inadvertent author of the patient's distress; for the patient, because of the actual discomfort of the side effect in question and because the hope of help and relief seems so cruelly betrayed.

It is, of course, a truism in all of medicine that there is no medication (including aspirin, oxygen, and water) without side effects; but this fact is often cold comfort in the courtroom. In the author's experience the single factor that most often turns a minor complication of treatment into a lawsuit is surprise, in the context of unavailability: The patient feels unprepared for the unexpected bad effect and feels also that the doctor doesn't want to hear about or discuss it. The latter situation is often compounded by some physicians taking as a narcissistic injury either the appearance of the side effect or the patient's complaint about it.

The self-evident preventatives here are derivatives of the earlier discussion under informed consent. While physicians may minimize side effects in an effort to avoid dissuading the patient from following a beneficial regimen, the cost of such an approach may be higher in the end. The physician's readiness to hear about and discuss any and all effects of the medication is the central preventative here.

Tardive Dyskinesia

As the most serious and least treatable complication, short of death, by psychopharmacological intervention, and as one that has racked up the highest dollar amount to date in malpractice awards, tardive dyskinesia merits a section of its own, even though it is in a sense no different from other undesired results of treatment. Perhaps because of its irreversibility, its concreteness as an effect compared with the more abstract benefits of improved mental status and functioning, or its inherent grotesqueness, tardive dyskinesia appears to bring out the sadism of courts: punitive damages, over and above compensation for harms, are not uncommon.

In general historical terms, the tardive dyskinesia liability tidal wave is just beginning. Special tension surrounds ambiguous indications for use of neuroleptics, such as for behavioral control of retarded patients (the subject of a famous Iowa case). The clinician is challenged more, perhaps, than elsewhere in pharmacological work to maintain a reasonable perspective.

Severely psychotic patients newly admitted to a hospital are often the primary candidates for beginning neuroleptic treatment;

since they are often least competent to give informed consent as well as being most prone because of their illness to distort information given them, the question frequently arises as to what, when, and how much to tell such patients. A useful approach to this problem involves what might be styled a "sliding scale" of informed consent, which relies in part on the fact that tardive dyskinesia tends to develop after considerable time on medications. While acutely disturbed, the patient is told in general terms the risks and benefits of the treatment for the short haul. As the patient's competence improves under the effects of the medications, more information is supplied. At the threshold of outpatienthood, the entire long-term picture is reviewed with the patient, including explicit discussion of tardive dyskinesia in the context of the total risk-benefit picture. Needless to say, documentation of this process and these discussions is essential.

Recall in this connection, the recurring problem of delayed informed consent with chronic patients who spend long periods of time in the hospital. A clinician may inherit a patient who is "on" his seventh physician during a 20-year span of illness. The physician should never assume that informed consent must surely have been obtained earlier in the patient's course; liability protection accrues only from obtaining this consent again when one picks up the patient. It is particularly the warnings about tardive dyskinesia that may fall between the cracks.

Management of Medications and Suicide Risk

While many medications are very low in toxicity (e. g., the phenothiazines) and difficult for patients to use for self-destructive overdosing, it is a paradox of psychopharmacology that the tricyclic antidepressants (among the most toxic) are appropriately employed with depressed patients, those most likely to be in the frame of mind to use them in this manner.

Clinicians confronting this paradox have often resorted to attempting to exert some measure of control over the situation by prescribing in small (say, weekly) installments. The author has elsewhere (1), disparaged the value of this approach, in both clinical and medicolegal terms. Briefly, the weekly approach may, indeed, convey caring and concern for the patient, who may feel more controlled or protected. The approach overlooks, however, the facts that (a) potentially lethal instruments are always present in all circumstances, (b) patients can save up pills or obtain them from other sources, (c) arguably, patients in clinical states so delicate as to be swayed by how the doctor prescribes should perhaps be in protected settings (1).

From the medicolegal side, (a) the approach cuts two ways: in court it can be portrayed as showing non-negligent caution *or* as proof the doctor knew just how dangerous this patient really was (and by implication, did not prevent the death); (b) courts and juries already have documented difficulty in avoiding a magical view (9), which could be summarized by the aphorism, "If the doctor's medicine killed the patient, it is as though the doctor killed the patient," so that the weekly prescription confirms the illusion of a speciously great degree of physician control over the patient's actions, and thus a greater degree of liability. More disturbingly, the weekly approach may lull patient and prescriber into a false sense of security.

The author suggests instead a two-pronged approach based on an expanded form of informed consent usage and sharing of uncertainty (4). The clinician first assesses the patient's competence (as described above) to participate in a risk-benefit examination, explicitly including the risk of temptation to overdose. Questions might include, "What constructive actions would you take if you felt the impulse to overdose?" "What situations increase that risk, so that you could avoid them and minimize the impulse?" "Do you feel able to control these impulses?" If the response to these and similar explorations are reasonable, the patient should be regarded as competent in the manner described.

Joint planning within the alliance can then take place: The patient can be asked if he or she can handle a supply of pills. If patients declare a preference for weekly prescriptions, the clinician should explore (as one would with other decisions of uncertain meaning) the ambiguity of responsibility this may create; does this approach represent wise planning or a pathogenic crutch, is it regressive, and so on.

Of course, these assessments and conversations must be documented, but the reward for this labor may stand the clinician in good stead. When the patient's adult competence is documented, it is harder (not impossible, just harder) for courts to portray the patient as completely under the clinician's control, so that whatever bad happens must be the result of the clinician's lapse of care. Rather, competent adults make their own decisions, which may, regrettably, include overdosing without telling the clinician of their suicidality; but for such autonomous acts the clinician may not be held liable.

These kinds of discussions may have to recur during treatment, but note that the interactions tend to strengthen the alliance, itself a suicide preventative, rather than, as with defensive medicine, undermining it by an adversarial posture.

STRATEGIES OF MALPRACTICE PREVENTION

A large part of this section has already been implicitly covered in the discussions above. This section underscores some of the important steps that clinicians can take to decrease liability risk and elaborates some of the caveats mentioned earlier.

The Pitfall of Defensive Medicine

It may be valuable to reiterate the difference between malpractice prevention, as taught in this chapter, and defensive practice. The latter approach involves excessive testing, extreme conservatism of practice, rigid pursuit of narrow "safety rules," burgeoning of redundant paperwork, multiple cross-referral and consultation, and the like. The flaw in this approach lies not only in its presenting a caricature of normal practice, but in its destructive posture. By definition, defensive practice places the patient in the role of attacker or adversary; the most powerful and important malpractice preventative—the therapeutic alliance—is jettisoned (4). The clinician's efforts are expended in warding off the patient as a threat, to the detriment of the treatment process. An eminently possible result, ironically, is increased liability risk.

Informed Consent as Preventive Strategy

As implied before and described elsewhere (4), the optimal position for the clinician in decreasing risk is that familiar informed consent discussion. When in doubt, when confronted by threatening situations, or risky choices with possible tragic outcomes (e. g., persistent pyschosis vs. tardive dyskinesia), the clinician can draw some real guidance from the structure provided by the informed consent procedure. Doctor and patient, together as co-workers, explore and

Strategies of Malpractice Prevention

confront the facts and risks, the benefits, and expected outcomes of whatever course of pharmacological action is chosen. A routine of periodic competence assessment serves as a vital component of this process.

In addition to improving clinical collaboration and patient satisfaction, this approach fosters—and establishes—patient autonomy, an issue that may become meaningful in litigation that attempts to paint the patient as a childlike victim of the physician's negligence.

Documentation

Clinician resistance to documenting things usually crystallizes around the idea that the recommender is offering cheap advice to "just write more," an exhortation seen as straining already packed time allotments. I suggest instead that the clinician write smarter, not just more, which actually decreases the total time spent writing. Guidance as to what is truly essential and how to record it can be gleamed from above sections and other sources (1,10,11), but the need for documentation is probably inescapable. No doubt, because of early socialization in law school, courts are inclined to a form of concrete thinking, namely, "If you didn't write it, it didn't happen."

Special points for recording include: indications, dosage, refills; competence and informed consent procedures; appearance of desired responses, side effects, drug interactions, toxicities, and responses thereto; and the like.

Consultation

Perhaps surprisingly, consultation with either peer or expert need not even be formal to be a potent malpractice preventative. Casual telephone exchanges of anonymous patient situations, if documented, also suffice: "Joe, I have this 40-year old man with such and such a history, these drug reactions; this is my planned regimen, does that make sense to you?" If Joe agrees and you write it down, you deliver three blows to the allegation of malpractice: (a) a peer in the community agrees with your plan, so it is unlikely you fall below the community standard; (b) another reasonable doctor agrees, so it is unlikely you fall below the "reasonable prudent practitioner" standard; and (c) more subtly (but equally important to the jury), you took the time and made the effort to get the consultation in the first place, so it is unlikely you are a cavalier and negligent narcissist, self-indulgently following your own pharmacological whims.

Note that this particular scenario places the consultant at no increase of risk, since the latter's duty is to you, the consultee, not to the patient. If the consultant sees or examines the patient, some ambiguity enters into this question, but consultation should not be deferred for this reason; the consultant would not have been chosen if his or her work were likely to fall below the standard of care, and the protection for the treating physician still accrues.

Responses to Suit

This topic is too large to address here, so the reader is urged to consult other sources (1). A few cautions about very common pitfalls are in order, however.

First, at any hint of suit, contact your insurer and that agency's lawyer only; discuss nothing with anyone else, except at that lawyer's advice. Second, *never, ever* attempt to go back and alter, insert, or otherwise change a record. Last, avoid panic, sudden impulsive actions, abrupt changes in prescribing, or other practices and the like; if the patient suing you still needs care, offer or arrange responsible referral, even if the patient requests to continue seeing you (litigation, despite how it feels, is not always identical with disapproval, disrespect, disparagement, or ingratitude). From this point, the insurer's attorney will be your guide.

In summary, absolute malpractice prevention is a myth. Nevertheless, the principles outlined here offer the psychopharmacologist some shelter against the rising storms of litigation.

REFERENCES

1. Gutheil, T. G., and Appelbaum, P. S. (1982). *Clinical Handbook of Psychiatry and the Law.* New York: McGraw-Hill.
2. Blackwell, B. (1973). Drug therapy: Patient compliance. *New England Journal of Medicine* 289(5):249–252.
3. Gutheil, T. G. (1978). Drug therapy: Alliance and compliance. *Psychosomatics* 19:219–225.
4. Gutheil, T. G., Bursztajn, H., and Brodsky, A. (1984). Malpractice prevention through the sharing of uncertainty: Informed consent and the therapeutic alliance. *New England Journal of Medicine* 311:49–51.

5. Gutheil, T. G. (1982). The right to refuse treatment. In *Psychiatry 1982: The American Psychiatric Annual Review*, ed. L. Grinspoon. Washington, DC: American Psychiatric Press.
6. Appelbaum, P. S. (1985). Informed consent. In *Law and Mental Health: International Perspectives*, vol. 1, ed. D. Weisstub. New York: Pergamon Press.
7. Appelbaum, P. S., and Roth, L. H. (1981). Clinical issues in the assessment of competency. *American Journal of Psychiatry* 138:1462–1467.
8. Appelbaum, P. S. (1984). Malpractice prevention for clinicians. Presented at the Annual Meeting of the American Psychiatric Association, Los Angeles.
9. Bursztajn, H., Gutheil, T. G., Swagerty, E., and Brodsky, A. Magical thinking in suicide litigation. I: Causality, modality and confusion in reasoning about negligence. *Bulletin of the American Academy of Psychiatry and the Law*.
10. Gutheil, T. G. (1980). Paranoia and progress notes: A guide to forensically informed psychiatric record keeping. *Hospital and Community Psychiatry* 31:479–482.
11. Gutheil, T. G. (1982). Clinical and legal aspects of the psychiatric inpatient record. In *Inpatient Psychiatry: Diagnosis and Treatment*, ed. L. Sederer. Baltimore, MD: Williams and Wilkins.

17

Glossary of Pharmacological Terms

Joseph R. Magliozzi, M.D.
Joe P. Tupin, M.D.

Acceptor: a constituent of living tissue that binds a ligand without necessarily producing an effect (see also Receptor).

Agonist: a ligand that, when bound to a receptor, triggers or enhances the action of the receptor.

Albumin: the major protein of plasma and principal plasma drug-binding protein. Albumin binds to drugs with acidic and basic properties. Its concentrations can be affected by many disease states and conditions, with implications for dosing strategies, especially if total drug concentrations are utilized as guides to dosage adjustment (see also Plasma binding).

Alpha-1 acid glycoprotein (α_1 acid glycoprotein): a plasma protein which binds some cationic drugs such as chlorpromazine and imipramine. Levels of this protein are increased after surgery and trauma and in inflammation, celiac disease, Crohn's disease, malig-

---

*The authors are grateful to the C.V. Mosby Company for permission to reproduce Figure 17-1. The authors also wish to thank Drs. David G. Greenblatt, Theodore Goodman, and Dorothy Gietzen for their suggestions and critical reviews of this chapter. They also wish to acknowledge the excellent manuscript preparation provided by Pamela Baird-Pipkins and Susan White.

nancy, myocardial infarction, renal failure, rheumatoid arthritis, and stress. Levels are decreased in the nephrotic syndrome, in the fetus, and with oral contraceptive use. (1)

Antagonist: a ligand that, when bound to a receptor, inhibits the action of the receptor or prevents subsequent binding.

Beta phase: see Elimination phase.

Binding: the formation of a chemical bond between one compound and another. In pharmacology, this usually denotes a noncovalent attachment of a drug (ligand) to tissue constituents (plasma proteins or tissue binding sites).

Bioavailability (F): the fraction of an orally or parenterally administered drug that reaches the systemic circulation. It is given by the relationship:

$$F = \frac{AUC_{(oral)}}{AUC_{(iv)}}$$

where $AUC_{(oral)}$ and $AUC_{(iv)}$ are the areas under the curves of drug concentration versus time, extrapolated to infinity, following oral and intravenous administration of the same dose (see also Concentration–time curve; Extraction ratio; First pass effect).

Chromatography: a method of separation of compounds based on their differential adherence to particles of an absorbing substance. **Gas chromatography**: a technique used when the compounds to be separated are volatilized to a gaseous state and eluted by a carrier gas. **High pressure liquid chromatography (HPLC)**: a technique carried out in solution with the liquid effluent under pressure.

Clearance (CL): the apparent volume of blood from which a drug is removed in a given unit of time. In more general terms, it can also be conceptualized as the rate of elimination of a drug at a given concentration of that drug.

$$CL = \frac{\text{Rate of elimination}}{C}$$

where C is the concentration in the biological fluid of interest (2). **Renal clearance**: the volume of blood from which unchanged drug is removed by the kidneys in a given unit of time. **Hepatic clearance**: the volume of blood from which the liver removes a drug by metabolic transformation in a given unit of time. **Total clearance**: in the simplest model, assuming no other routes of drug metabolism or elimination, the sum of hepatic and renal clearances. **Intrinsic clearance**: clearance of an organ or organ system under conditions of unrestricted blood flow. In the case of the liver, this term would be related to the metabolic rates of the enzymes involved in the transformation of the drug (3).

Compartment: a hypothetical space, not necessarily corresponding to an organ or organ system, which is assumed to interact with a drug in a uniform way.

Compliance: the ability of a drug recipient to take a drug as prescribed.

Concentration–time curve: a curve of serum or plasma concentration versus time after administration (oral or parenteral) of a single dose of drug (see Figure 17-1).

Curvilinear: a nonlinear mathematical relationship.

Distribution: the processes whereby drugs are disseminated to different body compartments (see Compartment).

Distribution phase (α phase; λ_1 phase): the time period in a complex (multicompartmental) pharmacokinetic model during which the drug concentration–time curve reflects the distribution of drug from one compartment to another.

Distribution, Volume of: the total volume available for drug distribution, assuming instantaneous dispersion of drug. **Apparent volume of distribution**: the volume into which a drug would appear to disperse uniformly given the initial concentration of drug in extracellular fluid and the dose of the drug administered. This volume may exceed the total body volume because the drug may be concentrated in or have a high affinity for certain tissues or organs. For example, lipophilic drugs may have very large apparent volumes of distribution, especially in obese individuals. In a one compartment model or one compartment approximation to a multicompartment model, the apparent volume of distribution is calculated by:

$$V_d = \frac{\text{Total dose administered}}{\text{Plasma concentration of drug at zero time}}$$

or

$$V_d = \frac{F \times \text{dose}}{K_\beta \times \text{AUC}} \quad [1]$$

where F is the bioavailability of a dose, K_β is the rate constant of elimination, and AUC is the area under the curve of drug concentration versus time.

Distribution, Volume of at steady state: the volume into which a drug would appear to uniformly distribute, given its concentration at steady state. This parameter is calculated by:

$$V_{d_{ss}} = \frac{\text{IV dose} \times \text{AUMC}}{(\text{AUC})^2} \quad [2]$$

where the new term, AUMC, is the area under the first moment of the plasma concentration curve C·t vs. t (the mathematical expression of the first moment curve) extrapolated to infinity (2, 3).

While V_{dss} is a very popular conception in current pharmacokinetic theory, it is often poorly understood and suffers from many unrecognized limitations. In many situations the V_d described in equation 1 (often termed VD_{area}) is to be preferred. The reader may consult reference (4) for a thorough discussion of these issues.

Effective dose–50 (ED_{50}): the dose of drug which produces an effect on 50 percent of the test subjects, or the dose which produces 50 percent of a maximal effect.

Efficacy: the effectiveness of a drug.

Elimination: the sum of the processes of excretion and metabolic transformation of drug. **Elimination half-life (half-life, t ½ β)**: in first-order pharmacokinetic models, the time taken for drug concentration to decrease by one-half because of elimination processes. It is related to the rate constant of elimination by

$$\frac{0.693}{K} = t\ \tfrac{1}{2}_\beta$$

Elimination phase (β phase; λ_2- phase): the period after drug administration during which the rate of decrease in drug concentration over time is primarily due to processes of drug elimination.

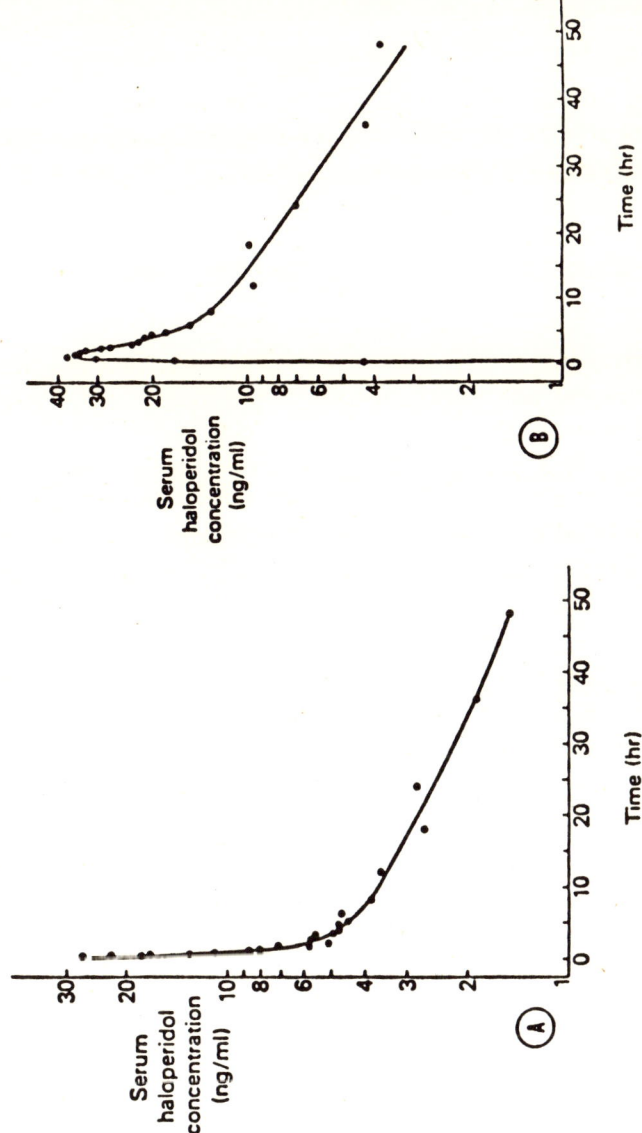

FIGURE 17-1. Concentration–time curves for (A) intravenously and (B) orally administered haloperidol in a single male volunteer subject.

Extraction ratio: the proportion of total blood flow which is cleared of drug in a single pass through an organ of drug elimination or metabolism. It is related to the oral bioavailability of a drug by the relationship

$$E_r = 1 - F_{oral}$$

where F_{oral} is the bioavailability of an orally versus intravenously administered drug. This relationship is based on two assumptions: that a single organ is responsible for drug loss and that drug absorption through the gut is complete.

E_r is also related to clearance by the relationship:

$$E_r = \frac{CL}{Q}$$

where CL is the clearance of an organ and Q is the rate of blood flow to that organ.

In practice, the term extraction ratio is applied primarily to the liver, which is presented with the total amount of an orally administered dose in one "bolus" via the portal vein. It is used to estimate the degree of the first-pass effect, which limits the bioavailability of orally administered drugs such as lidocaine and propranolol (see Bioavailability; First-pass effect) (5).

First-pass effect: the initial extraction of an orally administered drug prior to reaching the systemic circulation (presystemic extraction). The liver and gut wall are the principal agents responsible for this effect which tends to lower the bioavailability of an orally administered drug.

Half-life: in first-order kinetics, the time required for a process to reach 50 percent of completion.

Interaction: the production of alterations in a drug's action by concurrent or recent administration of other drugs. Such alterations may effect attributes such as efficacy, toxicity, untoward drug effects, and may be mediated by influences on drug metabolism, elimination, binding, plasma protein and drug receptors.

Lethal dose–50 (LD_{50}): a dose of drug that is lethal to 50 percent of the test subjects.

Ligand: a substance that binds to an acceptor or receptor.

Linear: a relationship in which the dependent and independent variables are best related by an equation of the form $y = mx + b$ which yields a straight line in which m is the slope and b is the intercept on the y axis.

Lipoproteins: high molecular weight (10^5–10^6 dalton) complexes of lipids, cholesterol, and proteins which circulate in plasma and bind cationic drugs such as propranolol and quinidine. Decreased concentration of lipoproteins have been noted in hyperthyroidism, trauma, and some liver diseases, and increased concentrations in diabetes, hypothyroidism, and the nephrotic syndrome (1).

Log-Linear: a linear relationship between the logarithm of the dependent variable and the independent variable.

Metabolite: a compound formed from metabolic action on another compound.

Multicompartment model: a pharmacokinetic model that takes into account the behavior of a drug in several compartments or spaces (see Compartment).

Pharmacodynamics: the study of the time course of the processes of drug action.

Pharmacokinetics: the mathematical study of the absorption, distribution, and elimination of drugs by living systems.

Plasma binding: the noncovalent interaction of drugs to plasma proteins. This may comprise a sizable fraction of drug in plasma. The bound moiety of a drug is functionally inert and not available for binding to sites of drug action or disposition. Altered levels of plasma-binding proteins lead to changes in total drug levels, without affecting free drug concentrations, which are responsible for therapeutic effects and which interact with dispositional mechanisms. Consequently, misinterpretation of total drug concentrations in cases where binding protein concentrations are changed may lead to major errors in subsequent dose adjustment (6).

Plasma levels: the concentrations, usually at steady state, of a drug in plasma. Plasma is the aqueous component of anticoagulated blood after centrifugation of erythrocytes and leukocytes. Some platelets may remain suspended in plasma if centrifugation does not take place at high centrifugal force. May refer to bound, unbound, or total drug. Expressed in mass or molar units per unit of volume.

Plasma protein binding: see Plasma binding.

Polypharmacy: the practice of using more than one drug concurrently. Although in many situations this is appropriate, care must be taken to avoid deleterious drug interactions or excessive side effects. In psychiatric practice, the term polypharmacy refers to the practice of utilizing several drugs with similar properties to treat a single condition. In most situations, this is rarely justified. An example is the use of several phenothiazine drugs to treat schizophrenia. However, certain combinations, such as the use of lithium plus an antipsychotic or antidepressant, may have legitimate uses.

Radioimmunoassay: an antibody-mediated assay of a given substance. In this type of assay, labeled molecules at a known specific activity and concentration and unlabeled molecules of the same chemical species at an unknown concentration compete for antibody binding sites. At the completion of the reaction, the antibody–antigen complex can be removed and the specific radioactivity of the unbound compound or the antibody–antigen complex determined. From this value the concentration being measured can be determined (see also Receptor binding assay).

Receptor: a tissue constituent that binds a ligand and subsequently produces a physiological effect (see also Acceptor).

Receptor binding assay: a type of assay utilizing receptors to mediate the assay. It is carried out in the same manner as a radioimmunoassay except that in this case receptors are used to form complexes with labeled and unlabeled species instead of specific antibody molecules (see Radioimmunoassay).

Scatchard plot: a linear relationship between applied drug concentrations (expressed in molar units) and the ratio of bound to free drug observed after binding of a drug to its receptor. In such a plot, the x intercept reflects the number or density of binding sites (B_{max}) and the negative inverse of the slope of the line reflects the affinity of drug for receptor (K_D) (see Figure 17–2). This relationship is used typically to display data from in vitro drug-binding studies. Although this relationship was proposed initally to model binding properties of simple proteins by Scatchard in the late 1940s (7), it was not applied to drug- or ligand-binding experiments until Rosenthal did so in 1967 (8) (see Binding; Subsensitivity; Supersensitivity).

Serum levels: the concentration of a drug in serum. Serum is the aqueous phase of whole blood remaining after coagulation has taken

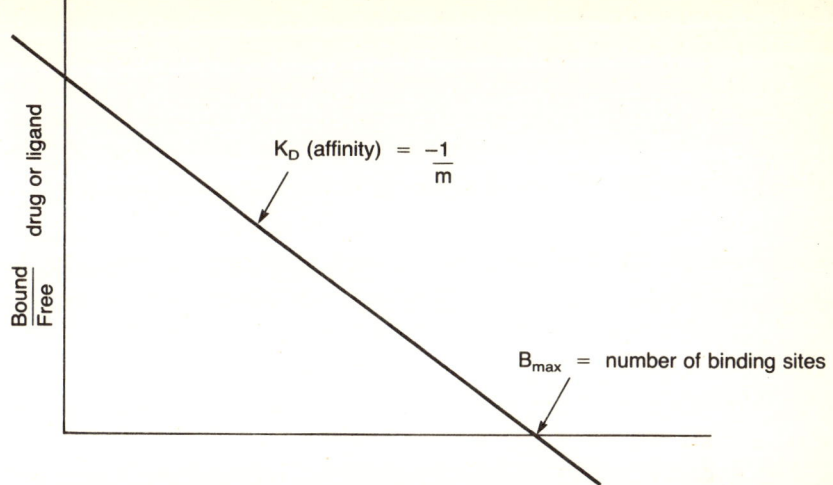

FIGURE 17-2. Scatchard plot representing outcome of in vitro drug binding study. Abscissa: molar concentration of applied drug or ligand. Ordinate: ratio of bound to free drug observed on completion of binding reaction of drug or ligand to receptor. Negative reciprocal of slope: affinity of drug for receptor (K_D). x Intercept: number of binding sites (B_{max}).

place and the clot removed by centrifugation or other separation procedure. May refer to bound, free, or total drug. Expressed as units of mass per unit of volume.

Single compartment model: a model of drug kinetics assuming instantaneous distribution to a single compartment.

Single-dose kinetics: a model describing the time course of absorption, distribution, and elimination of a given drug after a single dose.

Steady state: a state in which the rate of drug elimination is equal to the rate of drug administration so that any resultant plasma levels are constant. The time to attain steady state is approximately four to five elimination half-lives after initiation of therapy at a fixed dosing rate without a loading dose. Steady-state concentrations are given by the equation

$$Css = \frac{D}{\tau \times CL}$$

where Css is the steady-state concentration; D, the fixed dose; τ, the fixed dosing interval; and CL, the systemic clearance (3).

Subsensitivity: a decrease of responsiveness of a tissue or organ to a constant dose of drug (see also Supersensitivity). When mediated by decreases in affinity or number or density of receptors, has been termed down-regulation (see Binding; Scatchard plot).

Supersensitivity: an increase in the physiological or biochemical effect produced by a constant dose or concentration of drug, due to alterations in the properties of the tissue, organ, or cell with which the drug interacts. The increase may be brought about through changes in drug binding or postreceptor effector mechanisms. When these changes are mediated by an increase in drug binding through either increases in affinity of drug to its receptor, or an increase in the number or density of receptor sites, this process has been termed up-regulation (see Binding; Scatchard plot).

Therapeutic range: the range of plasma or serum concentrations, usually at steady state, with which a desirable response has been associated.

Therapeutic window: a rising and falling pattern of response to drug levels in which both high and low levels are associated with suboptimal effect.

Tolerance: a phenomenon of a living system requiring progressively higher doses of a drug to produce a constant effect. This process may be mediated by changes in drug clearance, metabolism, binding, receptor sensitivity, or the initiation by the recipient of compensatory homeostatic mechanisms tending to neutralize the drug's effect.

Toxicity: an unwanted, noxious, or deleterious drug effect.

REFERENCES

1. Tozer, T. N. (1984). Implications of altered plasma protein binding in disease states. In *Pharmacokinetic Basis for Drug Treatment*, ed. L. Z. Benet, N. Massoud, and J. G. Gambertoglio, pp. 173–193. New York: Raven Press.
2. Benet, L. Z., and Massoud, N. (1984). Pharmacokinetics. In *Pharmacokinetic Basis for Drug Treatment*, ed. L. Z. Benet, N. Massoud, and J. G. Gambertoglio, pp. 1–28. New York: Raven Press.
3. Tucker, O. T. (1980). Principles of pharmacokinetics, paper presented at symposium, Drug concentrations in neuropsychiatry, Lasagna, L., Chairman. Ciba Foundation, London, July 4-5, 1979, pp. 13–33. Amsterdam: Excerpta Medica.

4. Greenblatt, D. J., Abernathy, D. R., and Divoll, M. (1983). Is volume of distribution at steady state a meaningful kinetic variable? *Journal of Clinical Pharmacology* 23:391–400.
5. Pond, S. M., and Tozer, T. N. (1984). First pass elimination: Basic concepts and clinical consequences. *Clinical Pharmacokinetics* 9:1–25.
6. Greenblatt, D. J., Sellers, E., and Koch-Weser, J. (1982). Importance of protein binding for the interpretation of serum or plasma drug concentrations. *Journal of Clinical Pharmacology* 22:259–263.
7. Scatchard, G. (1949). The attractions of proteins for small molecules and ions. *Annals of the New York Academy of Sciences* 51:660–672.
8. Rosenthal, H. E. (1967). A graphic method for the determination and presentation of binding parameters in a complex system. *Analytical Biochemistry* 20:525–532.

Index

A type/V type, atypical
    depression, 331–332
Absorption. *See* Drug absorption
Acebutolol, 86
Acetylcholine-rebound syndrome, 59
Acute schizophrenia
  diagnostic factors, 33
  treatment strategies
    fixed standard dose method, 35
    loading dose, 34
    low dose method, 35
    megadose therapy, 34
    rapid tranquilization, 33–34, 35
    research areas in, 36
Adverse effects. *See* Antipsychotics; individual drugs
Affective disorders. *See also* Bipolar disorders; Depressive Disorders; Mania

bipolar disorders, 98
  atypical bipolar disorder, 99
  bipolar affective disorders, 98
  cyclothymic disorders, 99
  depressive only disorders, 99
  and 1970s, 97
  personality factors and, 412
  schizo-affective disorder, 99
Aggression. *See* Violence by individuals
Agoraphobia
  anticipatory anxiety, 413
  panic disorders with, 77–80
  psychotherapy
    and behavior therapy, 414–415
    benefit related to, 416
    psychoanalytic approaches to, 415–417
  stress and panic, 416–417
Akathisia, extrapyramidal reactions, 18, 22–23, 202
Alcohol abuse, dementia and, 172

Alcohol hallucinosis, 129–130
  age of onset, 129
  causes of, 129
  differential diagnosis, 130
Alcohol intoxication,
    antipsychotic agents and, 8
Alcohol withdrawal, 122–129
  anxiety disorders and, 131–132
  depression and, 130–131
  post-detoxification treatment
    antidepressants, 132–133
    benzodiazepines, 133–135
    calcium carbimide, 140
    disulfiram, 137–140
    lithium, 135–136
  symptoms of, 122
  treatment
    alpha-adrenergic agonists, 127
    anticonvulsants, 128–129
    barbiturate, 127
    benzodiazepines, 124–126
    beta blockers, 126
    chloral hydrate, 127
    chlormethiazole, 126–127
    ethanol, 129
    fluid/electrolyte replacement, 123
    general guidelines, 122–123
    lithium, 126
    neuroleptics, 127–128
    nutritional supplements, 123
    paraldehyde, 128
Alpha-adrenergic agonists,
    alcohol withdrawal
    syndrome, 127
Alprazolam, 6, 89, 91, 118, 345
  and children, 238
Aluminum concentrations,
    Alzheimer's disease, 181
Alzheimer's disease, 171, 174–187
  age of onset, 174, 176
  diagnostic criteria, 175–176
  etiology of, 176
  aluminum concentrations, 181
  amyloid accumulation, 180
  cholinergic abnormalities, 180
  diagnostic test results, 179
  genetic disposition, 180
  histological findings, 177
  infections, 180–181
  neurochemical pathology, 178
  phases of
    early, 181, 184
    late, 185
    middle, 184
  secondary psychiatric
      syndromes, 193–194
  sub-groups of patients, 176
  treatment of
    anticoagulants, 185
    anxiety, 197–198
    CNS activation agents, 187
    depression, 194–197
    neuroleptics, 199–203
    neurotransmission promoting
        agents, 185–187
    vasodilators, 185
Amantadine, extrapyramidal
    reactions, 22
Amitriptyline, 95
Amnestic syndrome (amnesia), 170–171
  multiple personality disorder, 171
  psychogenic amnesia, 170–171
  psychogenic fugue, 171
Amoxapine, Alzheimer's
    depression, 196
Amyloid accumulation,
    Alzheimer's disease, 180
Anorexia nervosa, 245–250
  antidepressants, 248–249

cyproheptadine, 247
lithium, 247–248
monoamine oxidase inhibitors
 (MAOIs), 249
zinc therapy, 246–247
Antianxiety drugs, violence by
 individuals, 117–118
Anticholinergic side effects,
 elderly, 202
Anticipatory anxiety
agoraphobia and, 413
antidepressants, 413–414
Anticoagulants, Alzheimer's
 disease, 185
Anticonvulsants
alcohol withdrawal syndrome,
 128–129
children, 241–242
violence by individuals,
 118
Antidepressants
anorexia nervosa, 248–249
anticipatory anxiety, 413–414
combined with antipsychotics,
 13–14
bipolar depression, 279
bulimia, 251–255, 258–261
child psychiatry, 231–235
 disorders treated, 234
 side effects, 235
 tricyclic antidepressants, 231,
  234–235
cocaine abuse, 149
interaction with ECT, 396
post-alcohol detoxification
 treatment, 132–133
postpartum psychosis, 17
violence by individuals, 116
Antihistaminic compounds
advantages/disadvantages of,
 8
child psychiatry, 235, 238
for sedation, 8

Antiparkinson drugs
child psychiatry, 228–229
extrapyramidal reactions, 19
and tardive dyskinesia, 25, 27
Antipsychotics. *See also*
 Neuroleptics; individual
 disorders; individual drugs
adverse effects, 18–32
autonomic effects, 27
cardiovascular effects, 27
dermatological effects, 29–30
drowsiness, 28–29
effect on heart, 28
electrocardiographic (EKG)
 changes, 28
endocrine effects, 31–32
extrapyramidal reactions, 18–
 23
neuroleptic malignant
 syndrome, 23–24
pregnancy/lactation, 30–31
tardive dyskinesia, 24–27
criteria in choice of , 42–44
drug interactions, 388–389,
 390–391
ECT, interaction with, 397
long-acting antipsychotics, 36–
 45
adverse effects, 38–39, 40–41
dosage/treatment period, 40–
 41
effect in schizophrenia, 38
fluphenazine decanoate, 37,
 40
fluphenazine enanthate, 37
haloperidol decanoate, 41–42
indications for, 37–38
injection techniques, 40
polypharmacy, effectiveness of,
 6–7
potencies/affinities for DA-2
 receptor, 5
rise in use of, 1–2

Antipsychotics (*continued*)
  treatment strategies
    fixed standard dose method, 35
    loading dose, 34
    low dose method, 35
    megadose therapy, 34
    rapid tranquilization, 33–34, 35
  violence by individuals, 116
Anxiety
  in Alzheimer's disease, treatment of, 197–198
  definition/scope of, 76–77
Anxiety disorders. *See also* individual topics; individual drugs
  and alcoholism, 131–132
  benzodiazepines (BZDPs), 87–91
  beta blockers, 84–87
  buspirone, 91–93
  childhood, 238
  fear, definition of, 75–76
  generalized anxiety disorder, 77, 78
  monoamine oxidase inhibitors (MAOIs), 93–96
  neurasthenia, 74–75
  panic disorders (PD), 77, 79–80
  phobias, 80–82
  stress, 75, 82–84
Anxiolytics/sedative-hypnotics, in child psychiatry, 235–238
  antihistamines, 235, 238
  benzodiazepines, 235, 238
  disorders treated, 238
Atenolol, 84, 85
Attention-deficit disorder, 116, 117
  clinical guidelines for drug therapy, 366–367
  diagnosis of, 358, 361, 363
    adult criteria, 360
    DSM-III criteria, 358
    rating scales, 361, 371–373
    Utah criteria, 358–360, 368–371
  drug abuse problem, 367–368
  incidence of, 357
  monoamine oxidase inhibitors (MAOIs), 365–366
  psychostimulants, 299, 231, 363–365, 367
    d-amphetamine, 363
    methamphetamine, 364
    methylphenidate, 364
    pemoline, 364–365
  tricyclic antidepressants, 234
Atypical bipolar disorder, 99
Atypical depression, 283, 412
  A type/V type, 331–332
  combination drug therapy, 347
  drug response, problems in study of, 334–335
  electroconvulsive therapy (ECT), 347–348
  historical view, 330–334
  hysteroid dysphoria (HD), 332
  monoamine oxidase inhibitors (MAOIs), 336–347
    irreversible, 341–344
    phenelzine, 336–341
    reversible, 344
  overlapping syndromes, 332–334, 345–346
  practical recommendations, 348–351
  psychotherapy, 350–351
  signs/symptoms of, 330, 331, 332, 334
Autonomic effects, of antipsychotics, 27

Baloperidol, children, 241
Barbiturate detoxification, 141–143
  pentobarbital, 142–143
  steps in, 142–143
  withdrawal symptoms, 141
Barbiturate/opioid intoxication, antipsychotic agents and, 9
Barbiturates
  alcohol withdrawal syndrome, 127
  violence by individuals, 113
Behavior therapy
  depression, 410
  flooding, 414
  key ingredient in effectiveness, 414–415
  medication and, 414
  panic disorders, 414–415
  systematic desensitization, 414
  in vivo exposure, 414, 415
Benign senile forgetfulness, 168–169
Benzodiazepines (BZDPs), 87–91, 113–114, 117
  alcohol withdrawal syndrome, 124–126
  Alzheimer's, anxiety, 198
  children, 235, 238
  dosage and anxiety state, 89
  drug interactions, 392, 394, 395
  evaluating patient for, 88–89
  groups of, 87–88, 90
  interaction with ECT, 397
  post-alcohol detoxification treatment, 133–35
  primary dementias, 8
  side effects, 89
  time factors, 88
  treatment principles, 87
  treatment-resistant schizophrenia, 307
  withdrawal, 89, 91

Beta blockers
  alcohol withdrawal syndrome, 126
  anxiety disorders, 84–87
    contraindications, 86
    effectiveness, case examples, 86–87
    types of BABAs, 84–86
  children, 241
  violence by individuals, 118
Bipolar disorders, 98
  bipolar depression, 279–280
    antidepressants, 279
    electroconvulsive therapy (ECT), 280
    treatment difficulties, 279
  types of
    atypical bipolar disorder, 99
    bipolar affective disorders, 98
    cyclothymic disorders, 99
Blessed Dementia Scale, 167–168, 169, 176
Borderline personality disorder, 281–283
  attention-deficit disorder, adults and, 360
  drug therapy and, 282, 283, 345–346
  episodic dyscontrol, 346
  psychotherapy, 282–283
Brain imaging, 36
Breast changes, antipsychotics, 31
Bromocriptine, 101
  cocaine abuse, 149
  extrapyramidal reactions, 22
  neuroleptic malignant syndrome, 23–24
Bulimia, 250–261
  antidepressants, 251–255, 258–261
  bulimia/depression relationship, 260–261
  bupropion, 257

Bulimia (*continued*)
  carbamazepine, 256
  EEG abnormalities and, 250
  fenfluramine, 255–256
  lithium, 257
  methamphetamine, 255–256
  monoamine oxidase inhibitors (MAOIs), 256–257
  nomifensine, 258
  phenytoin, 250–251
  sodium valproate, 258
  trazodone, 256
Bupropion, 65–66, 346
  Alzheimer's depression, 196
  bulimia, 257
  dosage, 65
  side effects, 65–66
Buspirone, 91–93, 135, 346–347
  advantages to use, 92
  effectiveness, case example, 92–93
Butyrophenones, and pregnancy/lactation, 30

Calcium carbimide, post-detoxification treatment, 140
Carbamazepine, 13, 67
  bulimia, 256
  children, 241
  mania, 102, 106
  treatment-resistant psychoses, 293, 295–296
  treatment-resistant schizophrenia, 308
  violence by individuals, 117
Cardiovascular effects, antipsychotics, 27
Cardiovascular medications, interaction with ECT, 397
Catatonia, 14–15
  characteristics of, 14–15
  classification of, 14

  electroconvulsive therapy (ECT), 15
  monitoring patient, 15
  signs/symptoms of, 15
Characterological depression, 280–284. *See also* individual topics
  atypical depression, 283
  borderline personality disorder, 281–283
  eating disorders, 283–284
  panic disorder, 281
  post-traumatic stress disorder, 284
  symptoms of, 280–281
Characterological pseudodementia, 190–191
Child psychiatry. *See also* Attention-deficit disorder
  anticonvulsants, 241–242
  antidepressants, 231–235
    disorders treated, 234
    side effects, 235
    tricyclic antidepressants, 231, 234–235
  antiparkinsonian agents, 228–229
  anxiolytics/sedative-hypnotics, 235–238
    antihistamines, 235, 238
    benzodiazepines, 235, 238
    disorders treated, 238
  beta blockers, 241
  clonidine, 241
  drug interactions, 222, 224–225
  guidelines for therapy, 212–215
    dosage, 214
    drug holidays, 215
    drug maintenance/monitoring, 218–219
    duration of treatment, 215
    growth/size factors, 213–214
    informed consent, 218

physical exam/lab work-up,
    216–218
  side effects, 214, 219–222
  lithium, 238–241
    disorders treated, 240
    dosage, 240
    monitoring, 241
    side effects, 240
  neuroleptics, 223, 226, 228
    disorders treated, 223, 228
    dosage, 228
    side effects, 228
  psychostimulants, 229–231
    attention-deficit disorder with
      hyperactivity, 229, 231
    drugs used, 229
    side effects, 231
  side effects, 219–222
    avoiding, guidelines for, 222
    common side effects, 220–221
Chloral hydrate, alcohol
    withdrawal syndrome, 127
Chlormethiazole, alcohol withdrawal
    syndrome, 126–127
Chlorpromazine, 388, 389
  autonomic effects, 27
  chronic pain states, 15
  dermatological effects, 29
  drowsiness effect, 28
  electrocardiographic (EKG)
    changes, 28
  and glucose metabolism, 32
  primary dementias, 7
Cholinergic abnormalities,
    Alzheimer's disease, 180
Chromatography, serum drug
    concentration monitoring,
    434
Chronic pain states, 15–16
  headaches, 15–16
    chlorpromazine, 15
    fluphenazine, 15
    phenothiazine, 15, 16

Clonazepam, 13, 89
Clonidine, 102, 117
  children, 241
  opiate withdrawal, 144–148
CNS activation agents,
    Alzheimer's disease, 187
Cocaine abuse. *See*
    Psychostimulant psychosis
Cognitive therapy
  depression, 409–410
  focus of treatment, 410
Colorimetry, serum drug
    concentration monitoring,
    433
Combination drug therapy, 6–7
  atypical depression, 347
  lithium and antipsychotics,
    104–105, 106
  lithium and MAOIs, 62–63
  MAOIs and TCAs, 63–64
  psychotic depression, 13–14
  unipolar depression, delusional,
    66, 278–279
Complex facilitative effort,
    depression, 411
Continuous amnesia, 170
Creutzfeldt-Jakob disease, 180
Cross-cultural differences,
    schizophrenia, 403
Cyclic antidepressants
  Alzheimer's, depression, 195
  unipolar depression,
    nondelusional, 274–275
Cyclothymic disorders, 99
Cyproheptadine, anorexia
    nervosa, 247
Cyproterone acetate, 118

D-amphetamine, attention-deficit
    disorder, 363
Dantrolene, 101
Delirium, 169–170
  drugs related to, 170

Delusional depression, 66–67
  combination drug therapy, 66,
    278–279
  dopamine in, 66–67
Dementia, 171–187. See also
    Alzheimer's disease;
    Primary dementias
  causes of
    alcohol abuse, 172
    Alzheimer's disease, 171,
      174–187
    Huntington's disease, 173
    multi-infarct dementia
      (MID), 167, 172
    normal pressure
      hydrocephalus (NPH), 173
    Parkinson's disease, 173–174
    Pick's disease, 174
  progressive degenerative
    dementia, 171
  treatment of, 191–203
    agitation, 198–199
    anxiety, 197–198
    caretaker education, 192–193
    daily care, 192
    depression, 194–197
    dosage/administration of
      drugs, 199–200, 203
    neuroleptics, 199–203
    paranoia, 198
    propranolol, 203
    side effects of drugs, 200–203
Denervation supersensitivity, 24
Depression/depressive disorders.
    See also Treatment-
    resistant depression;
    individual drugs
  in Alzheimer's disease, 194–197
    amoxapine, 196
    bupropion, 196
    cyclic antidepressants, 195
    electroconvulsive therapy
      (ECT), 197
    maprotiline, 196
    monoamine oxidase
      inhibitors (MAOIs), 197
    trazodone, 196
  bulimia, relationship to, 260–261
  bupropion, 65–66
  children
    lithium, 238–241
    tricyclic antidepressants, 234–
      235
  classification of, 51–53
  delusional depression, 66–67
  medical evaluation, 49–51
  monoamine oxidase inhibitors
    (MAOIs), 62–64
  nomifensine, 59–60
  pharmacological treatment as
    cause, 50–51
  psychotherapy, 409–412
    behavior therapy, 410
    cognitive therapy, 409–410
    complex facilitative effort, 411
    interpersonal psychotherapy,
      410
    and medication, 410–412
  psychotic depression
    combination drug therapy,
      13–14
    electroconvulsive therapy
      (ECT), 13
  serotonin (5-HT) reuptake
    blockers, 64–65
  trazodone, 60–61
  treatment principles, 53–54
  treatment-resistant depression,
    67–68
  tricyclic antidepressants
    (TCAs), 54–59
  typical depression, 330
Depressive pseudodementia, 188–
    190
  diagnostic factors, 190
  signs of, 189–190

Dermatological effects, of antipsychotics
  hyperpigmentation, 29–30
  hypersensitivity reaction, 29
  photosensitivity, 29
Dexamethasone suppression test, 190, 290
Dextroamphetamine, child psychiatry, 229–231
Diazepam, 114, 117
  children, 235, 238
Digitalization, 33–34
Dihydroergotoxine, dementia, 187
Diphenhydramine, extrapyramidal reactions, 22
Disulfiram, 137–140
  adverse metabolic effects, 137–138
  contraindications, 139–140
  disulfiram-ethanol reaction (DER), 137, 138
  pharmacokinetics of, 137
  studies of effectiveness, 138–139
Dopamine agonists
  extrapyramidal reactions, 19, 22
  and neuroleptic malignant syndrome, 24
Doxepin, 95
Droperidol, violence by individuals, 114
Drowsiness, antipsychotics, 28–29
Drug absorption
  absorptive phase, 430
  neuroleptics, 301–302
  trough phase, 430
Drug distribution, and route of administration, 427–428
Drug holidays, children, 215
Drug interactions
  antipsychotics, 388–389, 390–391
    chlorpromazine, 388, 389
  benzodiazepines, 392, 394, 395
  drug-drug interactions
    lithium, 384–388
    tricyclic antidepressants, 379–384
  electroconvulsive therapy (ECT), 394, 396–397
    antidepressants, 396
    antipsychotics, 397
    benzodiazepines, 397
    cardiovascular medications, 397
  monoamine oxidase inhibitors (MAOIs), 389, 392, 393
  pharmacokinetic interactions, 377–378
    absorption, 377
    distribution, 377
    excretion, 378
    metabolism, 377–378
  pharmacological interactions, 376
  reducing, guidelines for, 378–379
Drug-induced behavioral toxicity, treatment-resistant psychoses, 291–292

Eating disorders, 283–284. *See also* individual disorders
  anorexia nervosa, 245–250
  bulimia, 250–261
Elderly akathisia, 202
Electrocardiographic (EKG) changes, due to antipsychotics
  chlorpromazine, 28
  sudden death, 28
  thioridazine, 28
  types of, 28
Electroconvulsive therapy (ECT)
  Alzheimer's depression, 197
  atypical depression, 347–348

Electroconvulsive therapy (ECT) (*continued*)
  bipolar depression, 280
  catatonia, 15
  drug interactions, 394, 396–397
    antidepressants, 396
    antipsychotics, 397
    benzodiazepines, 397
    cardiovascular medications, 397
  mania, 13, 102, 103
  postpartum psychosis, 17
  psychotic depression, 13
  treatment-resistant psychoses, 296–297
Electroencephalogram (EEG) abnormalities, and bulimia, 250
Endocrine effects, of antipsychotics
  breast changes, 31
  glucose metabolism, 32
  menstrual abnormalities, 31–32
  water intoxication, 32
  weight gain, 32
Enuresis, tricyclic antidepressants, 234
Epinephrine, and autonomic effects, 27
Ethanol, alcohol withdrawal syndrome, 129
Expressed emotion (EE), and schizophrenia
  core of behaviors in, 404
  and medication status, 404, 406
  and relapse, 404–406
Extrapyramidal reactions, 18–23
  time for reaction, 18
  types of
    akathisia, 18, 22–23
    drugs used (chart), 20–21
    hypokinesis, 18
    long-acting antipsychotics and, 38–39, 40–41
  neuroleptic malignant syndrome, 19
  rabbit syndrome, 19
  spastic torticollis, 22

Family treatment, schizophrenia, 312–313
Fear, 75–76
Fenfluramine, bulimia, 255–256
Fixed standard dose method, acute schizophrenia, 35
Fluid/electrolyte replacement, alcohol withdrawal syndrome, 123
Fluoxetine, 64–65
  dosage, 65
  side effects, 65
Fluphenazine
  chronic pain states, 15
  schizophrenia, 3
Fluphenazine decanoate, 37, 40
Fluphenazine enanthate, 37
Food reactions, monoamine oxidase inhibitors (MAOIs), 63, 94–95, 96

Generalized amnesia, 170
Generalized anxiety disorder
  DSM-III-R criteria, 77, 78
  symptoms of, 78
Genetic disposition, Alzheimer's disease, 180
Gerovital, dementia, 187
Gilles de la Tourette's syndrome, 16–17
  characteristics of, 16
  haloperidol, 16–17
  neuroleptics, children, 228
  treatment decisions, 17
Glucose metabolism, antipsychotics and, 32

Index

Hachinski ischemia score, 167, 172
Hallucinogenic drugs
  post-LSD syndrome, 10–11, 104
Haloperidol
  Gilles de la Tourette's syndrome, 16–17
  mania, 13
  medical patients with psychotic symptoms, 18
  and pregnancy/lactation, 30
  primary dementias, 7–8
  schizophrenia, 3, 4
Haloperidol decanoate, 41–42
Headaches, 15–16
  chlorpromazine, 15
  fluphenazine, 15
  phenothiazine, 15, 16
Heart, antipsychotics, effect of, 28
Hormonal treatment, sexually associated aggression, 118
Hospitalization, mania, 100, 103
Huntington's disease, 173
Hydergine, dementia, 187
Hyperpigmentation, antipsychotics, 29–30
Hypersensitivity reaction, antipsychotics, 29
Hypokinesis, extrapyramidal reaction, 18
Hypomania, 100, 103
Hysteroid dysphoria (HD), 332

Imipramine, 95
Immunoassays, serum drug concentration monitoring, 433–434
Inadequate treatment, malpractice issues, 446
Infantile autism, neuroleptics, 223
Infections, Alzheimer's disease, 180–181
Informed consent, 441–446
  child psychiatry, 218
  competence of consent in, 444–445
  consent forms vs. progress notes, 445–446
  information to patient and, 442–443
  major pitfall, 442
  as preventive strategy, 450–451
  voluntariness in, 443–444
Injection technique, long-acting antipsychotics, 40
Interpersonal psychotherapy, depression, 410
Isocarboxazid, 62, 94, 341–342

Kuru disease, 180

L-Deprenyl, 343–344, 365
Labetalol, 86
Lithium
  alcohol withdrawal syndrome, 126
  anorexia nervosa, 247–248
  vs. antipsychotics, 12–13
  bulimia, 257
  child psychiatry, 238–241
    disorders treated, 240
    dosage, 240
    monitoring, 241
    side effects, 240
  drug-drug interactions, 384–388
  mania
    combined with antipsychotics, 102, 106
    course of treatment, 101
    maintenance therapy, 104–107
    medical work-up and, 107
    neurotoxicity of, 101
    noncompliance and, 100–101
    side effects, 107

Lithium (*continued*)
  combined with MAOIs, 62–63
  post-alcohol detoxification treatment, 135–136
  postpartum psychosis, 17
  treatment-resistant psychoses, 293
  treatment-resistant schizophrenia, 307–308
  violent behavior, 117
Loading dose, acute schizophrenia, 34
Localized amnesia, 170–171
Long-acting antipsychotics
  adverse effects, 38–39, 40–41
  dosage/treatment period, 40–41
  effect in schizophrenia, 38
  fluphenazine decanoate, 37, 40
  fluphenazine enanthate, 37
  haloperidol decanoate, 41–42
  indications for, 37–38
  injection technique, 40
Lorazepam, 8, 114
Low dose method, acute schizophrenia, 35

Magnesium pemoline, child psychiatry, 229, 231
Malignant neuroleptic syndrome, 101
Malpractice
  basis of, 440–450
    damages, causing, 441
    dereliction of duty, 440–441
  physician responses to suit recommendations, 452
  prevention strategies
    consultation, 451–452
    defensive medicine and, 450
    documentation, 451
    informed consent, 450–451
Malpractice issues
  inadequate treatment, 446
  informed consent, 441–446
    competence of consent in, 444–445
    consent forms vs. progress notes, 445–446
    information to patient and, 442–443
    major pitfall, 442
    voluntariness in, 443–444
  misdiagnosis, 446
  side effects/adverse reactions, 446–447
  tardive dyskinesia liability, 447–448
  suicide risk and medication, 448–450
    recommended approach, 449
    weekly dispensation approach, 448–449
Mania
  antipsychotics vs. lithium, 12–13
  bipolar disorders and, 99
  carbamazepine, 102
    maintenance therapy, 106
  electroconvulsive therapy (ECT), 13, 102, 103
  haloperidol, 13
  hospitalization, 100, 103
  hypomania, 100, 103
  lithium
    combined with antipsychotics, 102, 106
    course of treatment, 101
    maintenance therapy, 104–107
    medical work-up and, 107
    neurotoxicity of, 101
    noncompliance and, 100–101
    side effects, 107
  mood-incongruent/mood-congruent delusions, 99
  new agents, 13

nonlithium therapies, 102
phases of, 102
psychotic mania, 100
rapid cyclers, 106
secondary mania, 103–104
side effects of drugs, 13
tryptophan, 103, 104
Maprotiline, Alzheimer's,
 depression, 196
Meclobemide, 344
Medical patients with psychotic
 symptoms, 18
 haloperidol, 18
Medroxyprogesterone, 118
Megadose therapy, acute
 schizophrenia, 34
Memory loss in elderly. *See also*
 Alzheimer's disease;
 Dementia; individual
 topics
 amnestic syndrome (amnesia),
  170–171
 benign senile forgetfulness,
  168–169
 characterological
  pseudodementia, 190–191
 delirium, 169–170
 dementia, 171–187, 191–203
 depressive pseudodementia,
  188–190
 diagnostic tests
  Blessed Dementia Scale, 167–
   168
  Hachinski ischemia score, 167
  Mini-Mental Status, 168
  physical work-up, 167
 evaluation of, 160, 162
 history taking, 159–160
 mental status examination,
  162–163
 pseudodementia, 187–188
Menstrual abnormalities,
 antipsychotics, 31–32

Mental status examination, 162–
 163
 abstraction, 165–166
 affect/mood, 164
 attention, 162–163
 behavior, 163–164
 calculations, 166
 construction, 165
 general information, 166
 insight, 166–167
 language, 164–165
 memory, short/long term,
  163
 orientation, 162
 personal appearance, 163
 praxis, 165
 sensorium/level of
  consciousness, 162
 thought content, 164
 writing, 165
Mesoridazine
 autonomic effects, 27
 primary dementias, 7
Methadone, 144
 dosage, 144
 maintenance therapy, 146
Methamphetamine
 attention-deficit disorder, 364
 bulimia, 255–256
Methylphenidate
 attention-deficit disorder, 364
 child psychiatry, 229–231
 cocaine abuse, 149
 dementia, 187
Metoprolol, 86
Metropolol, 118
Mianserin, bulimia, 251–252
Mini-Mental Status, 168
Minimal brain dysfunction
 (MBD), 346
Misdiagnosis, malpractice issues,
 446
Molindone, schizophrenia, 3

Monoamine oxidase inhibitors
    (MAOIs), 62-64
  alcoholism depression, 133
  Alzheimer's depression, 197
  anorexia nervosa, 249
  anxiety disorders, 93-96
  bulimia, 256-257
  depression
    dosage, 62, 63, 64
    food reactions, 63, 94-95, 96
    combined with lithium, 62-63
    side effects, 63, 95
    combined with TCAs, 63-64
  drug interactions, 389, 392
  reversibility/irreversibility, 341
    irreversible MAOIs, 341-344
    reversible MAOIs, 344
Multi-infarct dementia (MID),
    167, 172
Multiple personality disorder, 171

Nadolol, 86, 118
Naloxone, 187
Naltrexone, for opiate
    withdrawal, 147-148
Network therapy, schizophrenia, 314
Neurasthenia, 74-75
Neuroleptic malignant syndrome,
    11, 19, 23-24
  causes of, 24
  characteristics of, 23
  dosage, 12
  long-acting antipsychotics, 39
  mania, 12-13
  psychotic phenomena related
    to, 11-12
  receptivity and specific state, 12
  risk factors, 24
  treatment of, 23-24
Neuroleptics. *See also*
    Antipsychotics
  alcohol withdrawal syndrome,
    127-128

Alzheimer's disease, 199-203
  dosage/administration, 199-
    200
  side effects, 200-203
"as needed" antipsychotics,
    304-306
child psychiatry
  dosage, 228
  side effects, 228
extrapyramidal reactions,
    reversing, 19
switching to other drugs, 303-
    304
treatment-resistant psychoses,
    297
treatment-resistant
    schizophrenia, 298-306
Neuroleptization, 33-34
Neurotransmission promoting
    agents, Alzheimer's disease,
    185-187
Night terrors, drugs used, 235,
    238
Nomifensine, 59-60
  advantages of, 60
  bulimia, 258
  dosage, 59
  withdrawal of drug, 59, 60
Normal pressure hydrocephalus
    (NPH), 173
Nutritional supplements, alcohol
    withdrawal syndrome, 123

Opiate withdrawal, 143-148
  clonidine, 144-148
  methadone, 144, 146
  naltrexone, 147-148
  symptoms of, 143-144, 145-
    146
Organic brain syndromes, 7-11
  neuroleptic malignant
    syndrome, 11
  primary dementias, 7-8

Index

substance-induced disorders, 8–11
  alcohol intoxication, 8
  barbiturate/opioid intoxication, 9
  hallucinogen-induced disorders, 10–11
  phencyclidine (PCP) intoxication, 9–10
  stimulant drug intoxication, 9
Organic delusional syndrome, 104

Pain. See Chronic pain states
Panic disorders, 77, 79–80
  with agoraphobia, 77, 80
  DSM-III-R criteria, 79
  psychotherapy, 412–418
    behavior therapy, 414–415
    benefit related to, 416
    psychoanalytic approaches, 415–417
    rise in patients, 416
    seizure frequency and, 417
    stress and panic, 416–417
  seizures and, 417
  symptoms of, 79, 80
Paraldehyde, alcohol withdrawal syndrome, 128
Pargyline, 365–366, 367
Parkinson's disease, 173–174
Pemoline, attention-deficit disorder, 364–365
Penfluridol, Gilles de la Tourette's syndrome, 16
Pentobarbital, barbiturate detoxification, 142–143
Pentylenetretazol, dementia, 187
Phencyclidine (PCP) intoxication
  antipsychotic agents and, 9–10
  phencyclidine psychosis, 115
Phenelzine, 62, 94
  atypical depression, 336–341

Phenothiazines
  chronic pain states, 15, 16
  dermatological effects, 29
  effect on heart, 28
  Gilles de la Tourette's syndrome, 16
  and pregnancy/lactation, 30
Phenytoin, bulimia, 250–251
Phobias, 80–82
  and alcoholism, 131–132
  simple/social phobia, symptoms of, 81
Phobic-anxiety-depersonalization syndrome, 331
Photosensitivity, antipsychotics, 29
Physician's Global Rating scale, 361, 373
Physician's Target Symptoms scale, 361, 373
Pick's disease, 174
Pimozide, 102
  Gilles de la Tourette's syndrome, 16
Pindolol, 86
Post-LSD syndrome, 104
Post-traumatic stress disorder, 284
Postpartum psychosis, 17
  treatment agents, 17
  typical psychosis vs. psychiatric disorders, 17
Postural hypotensive effect, antipsychotics, 27
Pregnancy/lactation, antipsychotics, 30–31
Primary dementias, 7–8
  age factors, 7, 8
  benzodiazepine, 8
  chlorpromazine, 7
  dosage, 8
  haloperidol, 7–8
  high potency/low potency agents and, 7

Primary dementias (*continued*)
  mesoridazine, 7
  thioridazine, 7
  thiothixene, 7
Procaine hydrochloride,
    dementia, 187
Propranolol, 84, 85, 118
  dementia, 203
  treatment-resistant
    schizophrenia, 308–309
Pseudodementia, 187–188
  depressive pseudodementia,
    188–190
  psychiatric illnesses related to,
    188
Psychoanalytic approaches, panic
    disorders, 415–417
Psychogenic amnesia, 170–171
Psychogenic fugue, 171
Psychosis. *See also* Treatment-
    resistant psychoses;
    individual topics
  antipsychotics
    adverse effects, 18–32
    long-acting antipsychotics,
      36–45
  organic brain syndromes, 7–11
  psychotic episodes, 11–18
  schizophrenia, 2–7
  acute schizophrenia, 32–36
Psychosocial treatments
  schizophrenia, 402–408
    best treatment atmospheres,
      406, 407
    and no medication, 406–407
  treatment-resistant
    schizophrenia, 309–315
Psychostimulant psychosis, 148–
    149
  antidepressants, 149
  bromocriptine, 149
  methylphenidate, 149
  symptoms of, 148–149

Psychostimulants
  attention-deficit disorder, 229,
    231
    d-amphetamine, 363
    methamphetamine, 364
    methylphenidate, 364
    pemoline, 364–365
  child psychiatry, 229–231
    drugs used, 229
    side effects, 231
Psychotherapy
  atypical depression, 350–351
  borderline personality disorder,
    282–283
  depression, 409–412
    behavior therapy, 410
    cognitive therapy, 409–410
    complex facilitative effort,
      411
    interpersonal psychotherapy,
      410
    and medication, 410–412
  panic disorders, 412–418
    behavior therapy, 414–415
    benefit related to, 416
    psychoanalytic approaches,
      415–417
    rise in patients, 416
    seizure frequency and, 417
    stress and panic, 416–417
  schizophrenia, 314–315
Psychotic depression, 13–14. *See
    also* Delusional depression
  combination drug therapy, 13–
    14
  electroconvulsive therapy
    (ECT), 13
Psychotic episodes, 11–18. *See
    also* individual disorders
  catatonia, 14–15
  chronic pain states, 15–16
  Gilles de la Tourette's
    syndrome, 16–17

medical patients with psychotic symptoms, 18
postpartum psychosis, 17
psychotic depression, 13–14
Psychotic mania, 100
Psychotolysis, 33–34

Rabbit syndrome, extrapyramidal reactions, 19
Rapid cyclers, 106, 293
Rapid tranquilization, acute schizophrenia, 33–34, 35
Rauwolfia serpentina, 1
Reserpine, and tardive dyskinesia, 26
Reversibility/irreversibility, of monoamine oxidase inhibitors (MAOIs), 341–344

Schizo-affective depression, 287–290
Schizo-affective disorder, 99
Schizophrenia, 2–7. See also Treatment-resistant schizophrenia
  acute schizophrenia, 32–36
    diagnostic factors, 33
    fixed standard dose method, 35
    loading dose, 34
    low dose method, 35
    megadose therapy, 34
    rapid tranquilization, 33–34, 35
    research areas, 36
  combination drug therapy, 6–7
  cross-cultural differences, 403
  dosage/administration, 4
  expressed emotion (EE), 312–313, 404–406
    core of behaviors in, 404
    and medication status, 404, 406
    and relapse, 404–406

high potency agents, 2
  fluphenazine, 3
  haloperidol, 3, 4
  molindone, 3
limitations of chemotherapy, 6
long-acting antipsychotics, 37–38, 41–42
low potency agents, thiothixene, 3
psychosocial treatments, 402–408
psychotherapy, 408–409
response time, 4, 6
schizophrenia-related depression, 285–287
stress and relapse, 404
stress-diathesis model, 403–404
Seasonal energy syndrome, 333
Secondary mania, 103–104
Sedative-hypnotics. See Anxiolytics/sedative-hypnotics
Seizures, panic disorders and, 417
Selective amnesia, 171
Serotonin (5-HT) reuptake blockers, 64–65
  fluoxetine, 64–65
Serum drug concentration monitoring
  analytical methodology, 432–434
    chromatography, 434
    colorimetry, 433
    immunoassays, 433–434
    spectrophotometry, 433
  blood collection tubes, differences in levels, 431–432
  drug distribution/access to receptor, 427–428
  drugs needing monitoring, 426
  interpretation of serum drug level, 434–438

Serum drug concentration monitoring (*continued*)
  reasons for, 425–426
  sample timing, 429–431
  total *vs.* free serum concentrations, 428–429
Side effects/adverse reactions. *See also* Antipsychotics; individual drugs
  malpractice issues, 446–447
  tardive dyskinesia liability, 447–448
Simple phobia, symptoms of, 81
Social phobia, symptoms of, 81
Sodium amytal, violence by individuals, 113
Sodium valproate, 102
  bulimia, 258
Spastic torticollis, extrapyramidal reactions, 22
Spectrophotometry, serum drug concentration monitoring, 433
Stimulant drug intoxication, antipsychotic agents and, 9
Stimulants. *See* Psychostimulants
Stress
  definition of, 75
  and panic, 416–417
  and relapse, schizophrenia, 404
  stress reduction strategies, 82–84
Stress-diathesis model, schizophrenia, 403–404
Substance abuse. *See also* individual topics
  alcohol hallucinosis, 129–130
  alcohol withdrawal syndrome, 122–129
  areas of clinical importance, 121
  barbiturate detoxification, 141–143
  opiate withdrawal, 143–148
  post-detoxification treatment, 130–141
  psychostimulant psychosis, 148–149
Substance-induced disorders, 8–11
  alcohol intoxication, 8
  barbiturate/opioid intoxication, 9
  hallucinogen-induced disorders, 10–11
  phencyclidine (PCP) intoxication, 9–10
  stimulant drug intoxication, 9
Suicide risk and medication, 448–450
  recommended approach, 449
  weekly dispensation approach, 448–449

Tardive dyskinesia, 24–27
  characteristics of, 25
  development of, 24
  interventions, 25–26
  long-acting antipsychotics, 39
  as malpractice liability, 447–448
  prevention of, 26–27
  progression of movements, 25
  risk factors, 25
  withdrawal dyskinesia, 26
Temporal lobe epilepsy, and treatment-resistant depression, 67
Tetrabenazine, and tardive dyskinesia, 26
Thioridazine
  autonomic effects, 27
  drowsiness effect, 28
  electrocardiographic (EKG) changes, 28
  extrapyramidal reactions, 19
  primary dementias, 7

Thiothixene
  primary dementias, 7
  schizophrenia, 3
Timolol, 86
Tranylcypromine, 62, 94, 342–343
Trazodone, 60–61
  Alzheimer's, depression, 196
  bulimia, 256
  dosage, 61
  effects of, 61
Treatment-resistant depression, 67–68
  bipolar depression, 279–280
  characterological depression, 280–284
  evaluation aspects, 67
  schizo-affective depression, 287–290
  schizophrenia-related depression, 285–287
  and temporal lobe epilepsy, 67
  unipolar depression, 271–279
Treatment-resistant psychoses
  carbamazepine, 293, 295–296
  differential diagnosis, 291
  drug-induced behavioral toxicity, 291–292
  electroconvulsive therapy (ECT), 296–297
  lithium, 293
  neuroleptics, 297
Treatment-resistant schizophrenia
  benzodiazepine, 307
  carbamazepine, 308
  lithium, 307–308
  neuroleptic, 298–306
    absorption aspects, 301–302
    "as needed" antipsychotics, 304–306
    dose/response relationship, 300–301
    improvement factors, 298–299
    plasma levels, role of, 302–303
    switching to other drugs, 303–304
  new drugs, 309
  propranolol, 308–309
  psychosocial treatments, 309–315
    family treatment, 312–313
    network therapy, 314
    plan for psychotic/characterological difficulties, 311–312
    psychotherapy, 314–315
TRH stimulation test, 190
Tricyclic antidepressants (TCAs), 54–59
  adverse effects, 55–56, 59
  antidepressants, children, 231, 234–235
  bipolar disorders, 54
  dosage, 56–57, 58
  drug-drug interactions, 379–384
  combined with MAOIs, 63–64
  other options, 58–59
  sedating/activating aspects, 56–57
Tryptophan, mania, 103, 104

Unipolar depression, 271–279
  delusional, 275–279
    combination drug therapy, 278–279
    maintenance treatment, 278–279
  nondelusional, 274–275
    cyclic antidepressants, 274–275
  signs of, 274

Valproic acid, 13, 67
Vasodilators, Alzheimer's disease, 185

Verapamil, 102
Violence by individuals
  drug-related causes, 112
  factors related to, 111, 115–116
  long-term treatment, 115–119
    antianxiety drugs, 117–118
    anticonvulsants, 118
    antidepressants, 116
    antimanic drugs, 117
    antipsychotics, 116
    beta blockers, 118
    goals of, 115–116
  short-term treatment, 112–115
    barbiturates, 113
    benzodiazepines, 113–114
    dosage, 114–115
    droperidol, 114
    goals of, 113
    sodium amytal, 113

Water intoxication, antipsychotics, 32
Weight gain, antipsychotics, 32
Wernike-Korsakoff psychosis, 172

Z track injection technique, 40, 42
Zinc therapy, anorexia nervosa, 246–247